DATE DUE

FEB 2 2 1996			
MAY 1 4 1996			
MAR 1 1 2004			

DEMCO 38-297

Co S D ERS

Ernst Epstein, M.D.

Clinical Professor of Dermatology
University of California, San Francisco
San Mateo, California

Common
SKIN
DISORDERS

W.B. Saunders Company
A Division of Harcourt Brace & Company
Philadelphia London Toronto Montreal Sydney Tokyo

4th
Edition

W.B. SAUNDERS COMPANY
A Division of
Harcourt Brace & Company

The Curtis Center
Independence Square West
Philadelphia, Pennsylvania 19106

Common Skin Disorders, Fourth Edition   ISBN 0–7216–6751–1

Copyright © 1994, 1988, 1983, 1979 by W. B. Saunders Company

Printed in the United States of America.

Last digit is the print number: 9   8   7   6   5   4   3   2   1

To my wife, JAN and our son, STEVE–
for their love, understanding, and patience

Foreword

Dermatology is a deceptive specialty—it appears a simple matter of looking at spots and prescribing ointments. Nothing could be farther from the truth: I've practiced dermatology for two decades and remain amazed at the complexities of diagnosis and treatment.

Ernst Epstein has spent several years refining his clinical practice, including the information and instruction sheets for patients. Here he summarizes his knowledge succinctly in a practical "how-to" text for both physicians and patients.

Some physicians might, at first, consider this approach too impersonal. If, however, you and your staff use the patient instruction sheets systematically, you'll find they actually give you a more personal approach to patient care. By freeing you from the boring repetition of routine information, these instruction sheets will give you more time to discuss your patients' individual needs.

Dermatology is continually changing. You can easily and inexpensively update the instruction sheets to incorporate advances in diagnosis and treatment. The role of this book in patient care should be many times its size.

Howard Maibach, M.D.
Professor of Dermatology
University of California
Medical Center
San Francisco

Preface

Many skin diseases are chronic, requiring years of care. During this time, patients' comfort and appearance depend on following treatment instructions accurately and intelligently. To assure compliance in my own practice, I started writing treatment outlines for my patients from the beginning and was gratified to find that patients not only experienced improved results but also gained reassurance—a definite advantage for a busy physician.

As other doctors have done, I eventually had some of the more common instructions printed in volume. They soon became an essential part of my practice. Colleagues who saw them liked their systematic use and suggested wider dissemination. Thus was born the idea of this book.

A collection of instruction sheets by themselves, however, would have left out someone very important—the physician. Because this book is directed toward nonspecialists in dermatology, I've added practical pointers on therapy—the small but essential details the textbooks omit. The result is a mini-text on the most common skin disorders and methods of treatment.

Unlike traditional dermatology texts, which tend to offer a potpourri of possible therapies for every disease, I've chosen only those I've found the most successful, the easiest for patients, and, when possible, the least expensive. Where there's controversy, I've explained why I prefer one treatment to another.

Proof of the value of this approach is the fact that the book is being published in a fourth edition. It has been enlarged by the addition of new instruction sheets and units for the physician, and by increasing the number of color photographs.

A review of the second edition cautioned readers against photocopying the patient instruction sheets, as they are protected by copyright. Although well-meant, this advice was misguided. The sheets are expressly intended for duplication; you may do so with the publisher's blessing and the full protection of the law.

Throughout the preparation of four editions, I have been greatly indebted to Howard Maibach, M.D., Professor of Dermatology at the University of California, San Francisco, both for providing the stimulus to write and for giving invaluable guidance and advice as the work progressed. Kathy Henne and Adele Seau of my office staff helped with photography, and, through their innovative use of the patient instruction sheets, suggested many practical improvements. The linguistic talents of Polly Miller, a medical economics editor, were instrumental in making the first three editions readable. She kindly consented to clarify my writings for this fourth edition. I am indebted and most grateful to Judith Fletcher, my medical editor at W. B. Saunders Company, for her support, advice, patience, and gentle nudgings.

Ernst Epstein, M.D.

About the Author

Ernst Epstein, M.D., earned his master's degree in biochemistry as well as his doctorate in medicine at Marquette University. After his residency at the University of Pennsylvania Hospital, he became affiliated with the San Mateo, California, Medical Clinic. Since 1971, he has engaged in the private practice of dermatology in San Mateo.

Dr. Epstein is Clinical Professor of Dermatology at the University of California, San Francisco, Medical Center. His professional publications have appeared in the *Journal of the American Medical Association, Archives of Dermatology, British Journal of Dermatology, Cutis, Journal of the American Academy of Dermatology,* and *Journal of Dermatologic Surgery and Oncology.*

Introduction: How to Use This Book

This book is for physicians and assistants who treat diseases. It is not a textbook—absent are the complete disease descriptions that characterize dermatologic texts. Instead, you are provided specific, detailed treatment directions for common skin disorders. I present what appears to be the best single therapy, rather than a bewildering array of possible remedies. The choice of "best" approach reflects my prejudices favoring simplicity, safety, and proven efficacy; some arbitrariness is unavoidable. Where controversies exist, I explain the reason for my position. When there is no satisfactory therapy—as in alopecia areata—this unpleasant fact is stated.

Units covering commonly encountered skin diseases make up the core of this book. For each disease, there is a patient information sheet—sometimes more than one—and a unit for the physician that details therapy. The patient instruction sheet is meant to be copied and given to the patient as an integral part of medical management. These patient information sheets make for more effective therapy, please patients, and save the physician's time.

This introduction describes how the book, particularly the patient information sheets, can be employed for increased effectiveness in treating skin disorders. The following four chapters discuss subjects of particular interest in treating skin diseases: topical corticosteroids, diagnosing dermatitis, treatment of dermatitis, and dermatologic surgical techniques.

Specialist and generalist both will find this book useful. The introductory chapters and the physician portion of each disease unit were written with the nonspecialist in mind. The patient instruction sheets should appeal to all clinicians who treat skin diseases.

THE PATIENT INSTRUCTION SHEET

COMMUNICATING WITH PATIENTS

All clinicians know that successful patient management requires the patient's co-operation. Patients will cooperate fully only if they understand what they have to do, and why. Medical problems may be complex, and patients often fail to understand them. Finally, if the physician relies exclusively on the spoken word to inform and instruct patients, they're all too likely to forget what was said.

How quickly talk is forgotten! We all took copious notes during our professional training. Astute businessmen invariably confirm a verbal discussion or agreement with a written memo. Yet most physicians rely on purely verbal communication to present difficult concepts and unfamiliar instructions. Patients' ability to remember is further impaired by the anxiety most experience in a doctor's office. Little wonder that patients complain they didn't understand what they were told, and remember less of it.

Our knowledge works against us. Without thinking, we use terms that we don't consider technical—*lesion, benign, dermatitis*—with no inkling that they are sailing over the patient's head. We take for granted that patients understand many disorders are idiopathic and chronic. Not so. Patients desire simple explanations as to causes, and they expect cures for their illnesses. Nor do we consider patient's concerns and fears: Who routinely reassures a new patient with psoriasis that it is not contagious and that the lesions are not cancerous? These concepts are of such second nature to us that they don't enter our minds. Yet such worries may lie heavily on a patient's mind.

The inadequacy of talk as the sole means of communicating with patients is obvious. How about writing out the necessary information? Many physicians do write a summary of instructions for patients. Time pressure and the quality of most doctors' handwriting limit the usefulness of this method. It's impossible for even the most conscientious physician to cover all matters relating to every patient complaint—but it isn't impossible to set all this information down clearly once, have it reproduced, and hand it to patients.

PATIENTS LOVE INFORMATION SHEETS

At least once daily, a patient tells me, "These information sheets are great." Then they continue, "Why don't other doctors use them?" Many needless fears are alleviated when an information sheet is reread and digested away from the anxiety-producing doctor's office. Teenagers feel less guilty about their acne after learning it is not the result of poor skin hygiene. Parents stop worrying that their children's eczema results from inadequate care. Patients with psoriasis understand that it is not contagious and feel free to approach their mates sexually.

What might seem a minor misunderstanding to us may lead to major patient concerns. One elderly, retired, skin-cancer patient is deeply grateful, not for my treatment of his skin cancers, but because he again feels free to play golf. His previous—and competent—dermatologist told him that skin cancers resulted from sun damage and he should avoid the sun. Being conscientious, the patient took this literally and gave up his favorite recreation, because he recognized that it was impossible to play golf without sun exposure. Upon reading the information sheets on skin cancer and sun protection, he learned that it is the *cumulative* effect of sunlight over many years that does the damage, and that moderate amounts of sun exposure add little harm. After reading these instructions, he resumed his golf game and made a point of expressing his pleasure. Without the patient information sheets, this problem would never have come to my attention.

WHY YOU WILL LIKE THESE PATIENT INSTRUCTION SHEETS

In addition to pleasing patients, patient instruction sheets will save you time, eliminate most repetitive questions, and decrease telephone calls. They simplify the management of complex as well as routine dermatologic problems.

For example: 17-year-old John comes to have his wart removed; he has his parents' permission but is alone. You explain that the wart is a harmless nuisance easily removed by minor surgery, and remove it. John is given the superficial skin surgery instructions and requested to read them several times, because they tell him how to care for the scab. He is told that warts are caused by a virus and is given the wart information sheet to read at home. You ask John to show both sheets to his parents. Result: John cares for his wound properly, and there is no follow-up telephone call from a parent asking whether the wound can be gotten wet, whether it must be bandaged, whether warts can turn cancerous, and so on.

Another example: 14-year-old Mary, accompanied by her mother, consults you for her acne. When they're taken into the treatment room, they're each given the acne information sheet and asked to read it while waiting for the doctor. After allowing enough time for them to assimilate it, you enter, take the history, and examine Mary. The instruction sheet has answered most questions, and you can concentrate on specific problems (why do you pick?) and therapy. Because the patient information sheet answers routine questions, you are saved the time of repeatedly answering the same questions.

A week later, you see Mary's mother (who is impressed by your patient information sheets) for a troublesome hand dermatitis that has failed to respond to numerous home remedies. You diagnose an irritant hand dermatitis and instruct her in hand protection by going over major points of the hand protection sheet. You ask her to read the sheet once daily at home for 3 days. In this case an instruction sheet is not just a convenient timesaver; it's an essential part of treatment. No patient could remember half this advice if you gave it verbally, even if you had the time.

Next you hand Mary's mother a hand dermatitis treatment sheet and ask her to read it while you're writing a prescription for a topical corticosteroid. You show her how to apply topicals properly, go over the major points (no hand lotions or home remedies), and ask her to reread the instructions at home. Success in treating hand dermatitis often hinges on careful attention to details—far too many to be entrusted to the fragile human memory.

HOW TO USE PATIENT INSTRUCTION SHEETS

The preceding examples illustrate how patient information sheets can be integrated into medical practice. It is not a case of making a diagnosis, handing the patient a prescription and information sheet, and sending him on his way. The patient information sheets supplement and expand verbal explanations. Treatment for many dermatologic conditions is highly individualized; therefore the treatment instructions in many patient sheets are general. Specific instructions for each patient should be written on the information sheet. Some sheets have blank spaces in which you can write the name of the medication you prescribe or recommend. Some parts of information sheets may be irrelevant and should be deleted.

Patient sheets provide a mixture of information and treatment instructions. Some, like the psoriasis sheet, provide mainly background information. Others, such as the various postoperative sheets, consist entirely of specific treatment instructions. Being aware of these two elements will help you make optimal use of patient sheets.

SHEETS CONTAINING PRIMARILY INFORMATION ARE USEFUL—

1. To provide general information before the patient is seen. If the patient has a readily recognized complaint, such as warts or acne, reading the patient sheet will provide information that otherwise would require additional physician time.

2. To inform the patient after he is examined. When examination discloses a condition such as psoriasis, alopecia areata, scabies, or atopic eczema, the patient is told the diagnosis and asked to read the information sheet after getting dressed. I add that I will return to provide treatment instructions and answer any questions. This technique is especially useful if the patient has a disorder that's unfamiliar (e.g., alopecia areata) or widely misunderstood (e.g., scabies). I use this technique when patients return for treatment of a biopsy-proven basal cell carcinoma. They're given the basal cell cancer sheet to read before I see them. My preoperative expla-

nation can then focus on the treatment technique, sutures, scarring, and other problems.

3. As a reasonable way of dealing with "by-the-way" questions. For example, you have just removed a wart from the forefinger of a 28-year-old, fair-skinned woman. As you prepare to dismiss her, she asks if sunlight is bad for her skin and whether she should avoid it. Her reason for asking? Her father has several skin cancers and told her sunlight caused them. Here's an excellent opportunity to practice preventive medicine by spending 10 or 15 minutes discussing solar damage and sun-protective measures. Are you willing to wreck your schedule that way, or do you brush her question off by stating that sunlight *is* bad for the skin and should be avoided? An effective approach is to agree that sunlight damages the skin and then add—while handing her the sheet titled Sunlight and Your Skin—"this sheet explains it and gives you specific advice on how to prevent sun damage to your skin. Please read it carefully at home."

This technique is useful when patients raise questions not related to their own care. Dad wants to know if his teenage son, Billy, has pimples because he is not washing his face enough. It turns out that the few pimples are not bothering Billy, but the face-washing issue has triggered a family war. You reassure Dad that dirt does not cause pimples, give him the acne sheet to read at home, and add, "If Billy's acne does become troublesome, bring him in."

PRIMARILY "OPERATIONAL" SHEETS ARE USEFUL—

1. For routine postoperative care.

2. For performing standard but detailed treatments. Examples are the sheets on hand dermatitis, hand protection, plantar warts, and chemical destruction of warts. Because the treatment varies little from case to case, it can be presented in a standard printed form.

3. As a summary sheet outlining both topical and systemic treatment. An ingenious universal medication summary was devised by Dr. Leonard Katz. It's quickly customized for each patient and has proved a winning patient-pleaser and doctor time-saver in my practice. (The *Universal Medication Summary Sheet* follows *Our Office Information* form.)

MECHANICS: REPRODUCTION AND STORAGE

The patient instruction sheets are meant to be copied and given to the patient. For occasional use, photocopies are fine; when larger numbers are needed, offset printing by a rapid printing shop is inexpensive and fast. Because offset printing uses photocopying techniques, either way of producing copies enables you to alter them by changing the master copy.

Personalize the instruction sheets by adding your name and telephone number. Changes are easy. You can provide additional information by adding a paragraph. Parts of the master can be blocked off with opaque paper; they will appear blank on the copies. An outdated section can be cut out, a new version typed, and the master put together with double-sided, paper-mending tape; the surgery won't show in the copies. There will be a difference in type with this method of change; if that annoys you, use your word processor to produce a new master.

Keep a supply of instruction sheets in each examining room so you can quickly hand your patient the appropriate one. A file cabinet is ideal for storage; if there's no space for one, an expandable compartmented manila file folder works well. Ready availability is important: If the sheets are stored outside the examining room, it will often be too much trouble to get them.

Your master information sheet should be stored in a three-ring binder. With each master sheet, include a blank piece of paper as an ordering record. On this, record the date when the sheet was revised, and also indicate the number ordered and the date, so you can determine how many to order when you run low. In general, order a 1- or 2-year supply of each information sheet, unless you expect to revise it soon.

WRITING YOUR OWN

Every physician should have an information sheet introducing himself and his practice to new patients. Although some offices provide printed booklets, a typed sheet is simple and adequate. Physicians' practices vary so widely that it must be written by you. Check with colleagues in your field and ask to borrow parts of their patient information sheets that you like. The one I use follows this introduction.

Your patient information sheet should briefly describe the nature of your practice and provide specifics as to office hours, appointments, emergency coverage, fees and payments, insurance forms, and anything else your new patients should know. If yours is a group practice, describe your coverage procedure. Keep it short!

Using patient information sheets is habit-forming. They work so well, you'll soon want more. Write your own, using simple words and short sentences. Have it read carefully by a nonmedical person who is not afraid to criticize your writing. It should come back full of suggested changes and half as long. If it does not, either you have a remarkable knack for clear writing or you have chosen the wrong person to criticize your efforts.

A word-processing program greatly simplifies editing and revisions. With some programs you can vary typefaces and sizes. There are even "readability" programs that will tell you when your language is ambiguous or impenetrable.[1] Ecker has summed up the advantages of computers over typewriters.[2] Print out a master copy of the final version, and test it by giving patients photocopies. If the sheet proves worthy and large numbers are needed, have the master reproduced by offset printing.

To sum up the practical points:

1. Keep it short.
2. Use simple language and short sentences.
3. Keep descriptions of therapy sufficiently general so that minor changes won't make your sheet obsolete. When some new, superior fungicides were marketed recently, I had to discard a batch of tinea cruris instructions because they named an older, less effective fungicide in the treatment section.
4. Find a critical editor to proofread your efforts.
5. Leave space at the bottom of the sheet to write specific instructions.
6. Store your sheet on your hard disk for easy revision when updating is needed.

For more information on the mechanics, production, and use of patient instruction sheets as well as interesting articles on the use of audiovisual aids, videotapes, and photographs in the physician's office, consult the June 1991 patient education issue of *Seminars in Dermatology.*

REFERENCES

1. Baker G: Writing easily read patient education handouts. *Sem Dermatol* 10:102, 1991
2. Ecker R: Word processing in the physician's office. *Sem Dermatol* 10:107, 1991

ERNST EPSTEIN, M.D., INC.
Dermatology

100 South Ellsworth Avenue, Suite 707
San Mateo, California 94401
Telephone (415) 348-1242

Our Office Information
Please keep for future reference

1. My specialty

I am a board-certified dermatologist; a specialist trained to diagnose and treat skin diseases such as acne, warts, eczema, psoriasis, poison oak dermatitis, and skin cancer, as well as diseases of the hair and nails. If surgery is required, it will be done in the office. However, I do not treat leg veins or inject collagen.

2. Office hours

Patients are seen *by appointment only*. We answer calls daily, Monday through Friday, 7:45 to 12:00 noon and 1:00 to 5:00 P.M., except Wednesday morning, when the phone hours are 8:30 to 11:30 A.M. We have an answering machine for after-hours calls. It will give you a number to call in case of an after-hours emergency. To change or cancel an appointment, **please call during office hours at least 24 hours before your appointment.**

3. Prescriptions

For accuracy, you are given written prescriptions. For refillable medications, call the prescription number in to the pharmacy that originally filled your prescription. If the medicine is not refillable, an office visit is needed. **By law, we telephone authorization for refills only if you have been seen in the office within the last 12 months.**

4. Fees and billing

After your visit, you will be given a computerized statement giving the diagnosis, procedure, and fee. Payment at this time is requested, by either check or cash. We do not take credit cards.

The fee for office surgery includes a brief, no-charge checkup visit so we can determine that healing has been satisfactory. The surgical fee does NOT include a charge for examination of the tissue, which is sent to a hospital pathology laboratory to determine whether your growth is benign or cancerous. The hospital will bill you for microscopic examination of the tissue.

Should you have questions about the fee, or any problems with payment, please discuss this with me or my aides.

5. Insurance

We do *not* bill private insurance companies—only Medicare. Payment will come to you from Medicare along with the information (EOMB) necessary to bill your secondary insurance company. Please remember that we do not wait for insurance payments—our bill is due and payable when you receive it.

If you have private insurance, submit your claim directly to your insurance company by completing the patient information portion on your insurance form and attaching a copy of our statement. The doctor's signature is *not* needed.

Please remember that your bill is due and payable when you receive it. Most insurance payments are made directly to the patient. If your insurance carrier pays us, we will reimburse you for any overpayment.

If you have any concerns or complaints regarding our services or fees, please tell us. We want to know.

UNIVERSAL MEDICATION SUMMARY SHEET*

In 1991, Dr. Leonard G. Katz in his article *The Use of Printed Instruction Sheets to Enhance Patient Compliance* reproduced the treatment instruction sheet that he gives to most patients. When I first saw this sheet, my reactions were (1) what a clever, useful idea; (2) why hadn't I thought of this? and (3) this will be a great tool in my practice.

Slightly modified, it has proved to be the single most helpful instruction sheet in my office. If you are going to use only one sheet from this book, make it this one—you will appreciate just how much practical information is packed into it. Dr. Katz's sheet lends itself to customizing and clearly distinguishes between topical and systemic medications. It's surprising how often patients get confused in this regard. It provides specific directions for the frequency of topical applications. Like many physicians, I often give patients samples of a medication and a prescription for more, if the samples prove effective ("try before you buy"). However, unless I remember to write out specific directions, the patient must rely on recalling what I told him, and we know how fallible that is.

In treating dermatitis, topical corticosteroids are gradually phased out. Patients often find this a difficult concept, and the information sheet provides specific guidelines. Of course, when treating pyoderma, such tapering is inappropriate. It's simple to cross out those parts of the sheet that do not apply.

Patients are often uncertain about how often to take their oral medications and whether they should be taken on an empty stomach or with meals. This is especially true when samples are provided. It only takes the physician a few seconds to fill in the names and numbers on the sheet and to cross out the inappropriate parts.

It's rare for a patient to be given just one remedy. Often, the assorted samples and prescriptions are confusing. This sheet provides a one-page, easy-to-read summary of treatment and follow up.

A formula for confusion: the patient who has two different disorders that require different treatments. The solution: two separate medication sheets, one for each disorder. Use the same approach when a widespread disorder, such as psoriasis, requires different medications for separate regions. Give this patient a summary sheet for each skin site.

I have deliberately not provided a master copy patient instruction sheet. Please prepare your own to match your practice style, utilizing Dr. Katz's sheet as a model. That is what I did. My current version follows his form. As you use your sheet, you will find modifications to make it more helpful. It's easy to change the format if stored on the hard disc of your word processor.

The medication summary sheet has become an integral part of my practice in the last 4 years. Once you start using it, you will wonder how you got along without it. It's a superb way to prevent misunderstanding and misuse of medications.

---

*Katz LG: The Use of Printed Instruction Sheets to Enhance Patient Compliance. *Sem Dermatol* 10:91–95, 1991 (With permission.)

LEONARD G. KATZ, M.D., INC.

DERMATOLOGY   5 SEVERANCE CIRCLE, SUITE 412
(216) 382-8244   CLEVELAND HEIGHTS, OHIO 44118

NAME _____ DATE _____

EXTERNAL MEDICATIONS (medicines that you put on your skin)

1. Apply _____ to _____ _____ times a day as needed with tapering*
                                                2 days on; 2 or more days off
                                                3 times a week; (ie., Mon., am & pm; Tues., am)

2. Apply _____ to _____ _____ times a day as needed with tapering*
                                                2 days on; 2 or more days off
                                                3 times a week; (ie., Mon., am & pm; Tues., am)

3. Apply _____ to _____ _____ times a day as needed with tapering*
                                                2 days on; 2 or more days off
                                                3 times a week; (ie., Mon., am & pm; Tues., am)

*TAPERING means to gradually decrease your medication from twice a day, to once a day, to three times a week, to two times a week, over a several week period, and then discontinue it. If the rash recurs, restart the medication at twice a day and taper again when improved.

ORAL MEDICATIONS (Medicines that you take by mouth)

1. Take _____ _____ times a day   on an empty stomach
                                                    with food
                                                    does not matter

2. Take _____ _____ times a day   on an empty stomach
                                                    with food
                                                    does not matter

CALL in _____ weeks if NOT improving.

RETURN in _____ WEEKS _____ MONTH _____ YEAR

Figure 1. Oral and topical medication instruction sheet.

ERNST EPSTEIN, M.D., INC.
DERMATOLOGY
100 SOUTH ELLSWORTH AVENUE, SUITE 707
SAN MATEO, CALIFORNIA 94401
—

TELEPHONE (415) 348-1242

Medication Summary For _____ DATE _____

EXTERNAL MEDICATIONS to put on your skin. Apply very thinly.

1. Apply _____ to _____ morning & bedtime
                                                  when better, gradually
                                                  use less often*

2. Apply _____ to _____ morning & bedtime
                                                  when better, gradually
                                                  use less often*

3. Apply _____ to _____ morning & bedtime
                                                  when better, gradually
                                                  use less often*

*For example, if you start at twice a day, when better use once daily, when nearly well use every other night, later on twice a week and when fine, quit.
NOTE: Most external medications are refillable by taking the container to the pharmacy where you purchased it.

ORAL MEDICATIONS to take by mouth.

1. Take _____ _____ times a day   on an empty stomach
                                                    with food
                                                    does not matter

2. Take _____ _____ times a day   on an empty stomach
                                                    with food
                                                    does not matter

RETURN: _____ As scheduled
           _____ If problems arise
           _____ Before supply of oral medicine is used up
           _____ Before last refill of oral medicine is used up

Figure 2. Adaptation of medication summary sheet of Dr. Katz.

Contents

Physician's Section

1 *Rational Use of Topical Corticosteroids*

Patient sheet page P–19*

Topical corticosteroids are the most commonly prescribed agents in dermatologic treatment. They are remarkably effective for numerous—but by no means all—disorders.[1] Many physicians use them on a trial-and-error basis. This is unfortunate, as the effectiveness of topical corticosteroid therapy can usually be predicted if you consider: (1) the disorder that is being treated; (2) the site; (3) the potency of the preparation; and (4) the nonspecific effects of the vehicle.

ROLE OF THE DISORDER IN DETERMINING CORTICOSTEROID THERAPY

Topical corticosteroids are the sovereign remedy for a wide variety of eczematous dermatoses, including atopic dermatitis, asteatotic eczema, nummular eczema, and the many eczematous dermatoses that don't fit conventional classifications. Pruritus vulvae and idiopathic pruritus ani usually respond to topical corticosteroid therapy. Contact dermatitis is responsive to topical corticosteroids in the subacute and chronic stages, when swelling has diminished. In the acute edematous and vesicular stages, most topical corticosteroids are ineffective; the newer, superpotent corticosteroids may be of limited benefit. Stasis dermatitis improves with topical corticosteroids; additional treatment of the venous insufficiency is usually necessary for satisfactory control of this condition. How various dermatoses respond to topical corticosteroids is summarized in Table 1–1.

The response of psoriasis to topical corticosteroids varies with the individual and the skin site. Intertriginous (skin-fold) psoriasis responds well to topical corticosteroids, whereas the response of glabrous (smooth) skin is variable, and scalp psoriasis responds to topical corticosteroids only if the scale is removed before application. The corticosteroid must be carefully matched with the site.

While topical corticosteroids are of benefit in certain infrequent disorders such as discoid lupus erythematosus, most other disorders respond poorly or not at all. In the United States, 1 percent hydrocortisone topical preparations are available without a prescription. These preparations are effective in controlling mild atopic or seborrheic dermatitis. However, many persons use 1 percent hydrocortisone for poison ivy or oak contact dermatitis, where it is of no value, or, in the case of pyodermas, where it is contraindicated.

ROLE OF THE SKIN SITE

Topical corticosteroids are most effective in intertriginous areas, have an intermediate effect on glabrous skin, and are least effective on the palms and soles. In

*Refer to the *Universal Medication Summary Sheet*, page xxi.

Table 1–1. **RESPONSIVENESS OF DERMATOSES TO TOPICAL CORTICOSTEROIDS**

Highly Responsive
Low-potency corticosteroids usually suffice
  Atopic dermatitis
  Seborrheic dermatitis
  Asteatotic dermatitis
  Pruritus ani
  Intertriginous psoriasis
  Stasis dermatitis
Moderately Responsive
Potent corticosteroids, possibly with occlusion, are
    required, but a satisfactory response is usually
    obtained
  Nummular eczema
  Plaque-type psoriasis
  Subacute and chronic contact dermatitis
  Lichen simplex chronicus
Less Responsive
Potent or superpotent (class 1) corticosteroids are needed;
    not all cases respond
  Acute contact dermatitis
  Discoid lupus erythematosus
  Lichen planus
  Palmo-plantar psoriasis
  Lichen sclerosus et atrophicus

general, efficacy parallels the inherent potency and the penetration of the specific preparation. Side effects accompany benefits; skin atrophy and striae from topical corticosteroids occur most rapidly in skin-fold areas.

The differing responses of skin sites are of practical importance. Low-potency corticosteroids, such as 1 or 2 percent hydrocortisone, are preferred for skin-fold areas, because they usually produce an adequate response with minimal risk of skin atrophy. Corticosteroids of intermediate potency will often be necessary on glabrous skin; the face is an exception, as it usually responds well to low-potency corticosteroids. Palms and soles require the most potent corticosteroids, usually with occlusion to increase their effectiveness.

The site influences the choice of vehicle. On the hairy scalp, creams and ointments tend to make the hair greasy. Solutions, gels, and aerosol sprays are best for treating hairy areas. It is possible to apply almost any type of vehicle to other skin areas; however, ointments are often poorly tolerated in skin-fold areas. Dermatitis of skin folds is treated more effectively with a cream or lotion. On glabrous skin, the choice of vehicle will be determined by the acuteness of the dermatitis and by the effect desired—drying or lubricating.

POTENCY OF TOPICAL CORTICOSTEROID PREPARATIONS

There are great differences in the potencies of commercial topical corticosteroid formulations, which range from weak 0.5 percent hydrocortisone cream to highly potent fluorinated compounds. The potency of corticosteroids depends on three variables: (1) the molecular structure; (2) the concentration; and (3) the vehicle.

1. Corticosteroids differ in their anti-inflammatory effects. For example, topical triamcinolone acetonide is many times more potent than hydrocortisone. The relative effectiveness of these drugs can be determined only by careful paired comparison trials in a variety of steroid-responsive dermatoses—a tedious task. We do not yet have such data for many of the newer corticosteroid preparations.

2. The role of concentration in determining potency is recognized by many

manufacturers, who produce preparations of varying concentrations. Hydrocortisone concentrations of less than 1 percent are an obsolete heritage from times when the drug was costly. Triamcinolone acetonide topical preparations are marketed in concentrations of 0.025, 0.1, and 0.5 percent; the 0.025 percent preparation is adequate for most uses.

3. The vehicle plays an important role in determining efficacy. Corticosteroid creams were first prepared by dispersing the drug in a water-washable cream base, while a petrolatum base was used for ointments. The greasy ointment is usually more potent than the cream. Topical corticosteroids are most potent when incorporated in a vehicle that solubilizes the drugs. Specialized corticosteroid vehicles should not be mixed with other topical agents, creams, or ointments, because the unique effect of the vehicle may be destroyed. The technique of solubilizing corticosteroids in their vehicles has led manufacturers to upgrade their older preparations by revising the vehicles, resulting in a bewildering set of new trade preparations. Fluocinolone is sold by Syntex as Synalar when using the old vehicle, old base and as Synemol when incorporated in the new base. Lederle has revised its triamcinolone formulation so there is Aristocort (original preparation) and Aristocort A (new formulation). Because of higher solvent concentrations, some newer cream and gel vehicles are more irritating than older ointment bases, especially when occluded.

The Schering Corporation dramatically increased the potency of betamethasone dipropionate by modifying the vehicle. The more efficacious topicals are marketed under the trade name of Diprolene, while the older preparations are marketed as Diprosone; both contain the identical 0.05 percent concentration of the active agent, betamethasone dipropionate. Clobetasol propionate (Temovate) was the first of a new class of super-potent (ultra-high, class 1) topical corticosteroids. It is somewhat more potent than Diprolene or Psorcon. Halobetasol propionate (Ultravate) is close to the potency of Temovate. However, clinically, these four agents are similar in efficacy, and all are expensive. The super-high-potency corticosteroids must be used with caution, because systemic effects can be demonstrated with 30 g of ointment per week. Atrophy occurs more rapidly with these preparations. The ultra-high-potency drugs should be used only on limited areas, and usually for no more than 7 to 10 days. After that, they should be used intermittently once, twice, or three times per week. Super-high-potency topical corticosteroids should be reserved for special situations, notably for dermatoses not responding to lower-potency agents.

Table 1–2 provides a rough classification of the potencies of some of the topical corticosteroids commonly used in the United States. To avoid a myriad of names, I omitted many topical corticosteroids that, although effective, have no real advantage over older preparations. Detailed listings of the relative potencies of commercial topical corticosteroids are periodically published by *The Medical Letter* and can also be found in review articles. These tables should be used as approximations; potency is measured by a vasoconstrictor assay, which does not always correlate with clinical effectiveness.

The relative potencies of corticosteroids may differ depending on the disease treated. Thus, many of the newer highly potent formulations provide similar excellent results in atopic dermatitis but show significant variation in their effects on psoriasis. Acquaint yourself thoroughly with a few topical corticosteroid formulations. Prescribe only one or two preparations in each category rather than the latest miracle drug described by salesmen or glowingly advertised.

NONSPECIFIC EFFECTS OF THE VEHICLE

The type of vehicle—ointment, cream, lotion, gel, solution, or aerosol—has a significant nonspecific effect on dermatitis. Prior to the advent of corticosteroids, treat-

Table 1–2. **GUIDE TO THE RELATIVE POTENCIES OF COMMONLY USED CORTICOSTEROIDS**

Potency	Generic Name	Trade Name(s)	Strength (%)
Ultra-high	Clobetasol propionate	Temovate	0.05
	Diflorasone diacetate	Psorcon	0.05
	Halobetasol propionate	Ultravate	0.05
	Optimized vehicle formulation of betamethasone dipropionate	Diprolene	0.05
Very high	Desoximetasone	Topicort	0.25
	Diflorasone diacetate	Maxiflor, Florone	0.05
	Fluocinonide	Lidex	0.05
	Halcinonide	Halog	0.1
High	Betamethasone valerate	Valisone	0.1
	Fluocinolone	Synalar, Synemol	0.025
	Triamcinolone acetonide*	Aristocort, Kenalog	0.1
Medium	Desonide	Tridesilon	0.05
	Fluocinolone acetonide	Synalar	0.01
	Flurandrenolide	Cordran	0.025
	Hydrocortisone butyrate	Locoid	0.1
	Hydrocortisone valerate	Westcort	0.2
	Triamcinolone acetonide*	Aristocort, Kenalog	0.025
Low	Hydrocortisone U.S.P.†		1, 2.5

Corticosteroids within each group are roughly equal in activity. The ratings for triamcinolone acetonide and hydrocortisone U.S.P. refer to generic forms in ordinary vehicles; specially formulated vehicles may increase the potency.

*Generic forms are widely available and usually are less expensive. However, not all corticosteroid generics are equally effective.

†Applies only to hydrocortisone itself; certain salts of hydrocortisone are more potent. Thus 0.2 percent hydrocortisone valerate (Westcort) and 0.1 percent hydrocortisone butyrate (Locoid) are medium-potency corticosteroids.

ment of dermatitis depended chiefly on such nonspecific effects. Although the nonspecific effects of a vehicle are less important today, they play a significant and often underappreciated role in treating dermatitis.

The aim of the vehicle is to help normalize dermatitic skin. Solutions and gels generally have a drying effect; greasy ointments have a pronounced lubricating effect. Creams and lotions have a slight lubricating effect. Physicians often err in relying on just one type of preparation—usually a cream—to treat all corticosteroid-responsive dermatoses. Cream preparations are ideal for most acute and subacute rashes but not for dry, fissuring dermatoses, which do best with ointments. Ointments are messier than creams, although if applied thinly, they are usually acceptable. In more acute processes, an ointment's occlusive effect may irritate the skin; creams or lotions are usually better choices. Even an experienced dermatologist may be in doubt as to which vehicle will produce the best response. A simple solution is to have the patient apply a corticosteroid cream to one site and the same drug in ointment form to a matched contralateral site. Any significant difference in effectiveness, and in the patient's subjective preference, will be evident in a few days.

OTHER CONSIDERATIONS IN PRESCRIBING CORTICOSTEROIDS

COST

There are significant cost differences between corticosteroids of approximately equal potency. Many of the newer preparations are much more expensive than the correspondingly potent triamcinolone acetonides. Some brands of 1 percent hydrocortisone are double the cost of others. The difference can be significant to patients who may need several refills. When prescribing topical hydrocortisone, you can save your patients money by prescribing generic brands, and 1 percent hydrocortisone can be purchased without a prescription. Spend a few minutes comparing prices in your pharmacist's book of wholesale costs. As a basic intermediate-strength corticosteroid, 0.025 percent triamcinolone acetonide is usually the best buy.

HOW MUCH TO PRESCRIBE?

How much corticosteroid to prescribe depends on the patient's needs, the price, and the packaging. If the patient applies the corticosteroid sparingly, his or her needs can be estimated accurately. The amount applied by trained individuals is remarkably consistent; what untrained persons apply may vary nearly 20-fold. Most patients tend to apply far too much topical corticosteroid. Show them on a small area of dermatitic or normal skin how to apply a thin film and gently massage it in.

The amounts of topical corticosteroid necessary for two daily applications are shown in Table 1–3. These figures are generous approximations based on precise studies.[2] If the medication is applied only once daily, halve the numbers in Table 1–3. Remember that 30 g (about 1 oz) will suffice for one application to the entire skin of an adult patient.

FREQUENCY OF APPLICATION

How many times should your patient apply the corticosteroid? The usual advice of three or four daily applications is based on custom rather than reason. With the less potent corticosteroids, applications two or three times a day are probably helpful; with the newer, highly potent formulations, one application daily is usually sufficient. On the scalp, one daily application suffices, as the drug usually is not rubbed off. With a highly potent drug, one application daily suffices for optimal corticosteroid effect. If additional emollient action is desired, suggest frequent applications of a plain, nonmedicated lotion or ointment.

There are exceptions to these general rules. When the emollient effect of the corticosteroid vehicle is desired—as in atopic eczema or irritant (housewife's) hand dermatitis—more frequent applications are desirable. Similarly, if the corticosteroid is likely to be washed off, as in hand dermatitis, as many as 10 to 15 applications per day may be beneficial. Increasing the number of applications is an excellent way to get more effect from hydrocortisone. A flare-up of atopic eczema previously controlled with nightly applications of 1 percent hydrocortisone may subside with four or five daily applications of the same steroid, thereby avoiding the need for a more potent preparation.

Table 1–3. **GRAMS OF CREAM OR OINTMENT REQUIRED FOR TWO SPARING APPLICATIONS FOR ONE DAY**

Body Part	Approximate Grams
Face and ears	3
Neck	3
Upper extremity	5
Lower extremity	10
Anterior trunk	8
Posterior trunk	8

Note: 30 g (approximately 1 oz) will suffice for one sparing application to the entire skin of an adult. Because of rounding, the figures above come out to only 26 g per application.

SIDE EFFECTS

SYSTEMIC

Reassure your patients that topical corticosteroids, unlike systemic corticosteroids, are usually well tolerated on a long-term basis and seldom produce undesirable effects. Many patients confuse topical corticosteroids with systemic corticosteroids and are concerned about adverse effects from the ointment you prescribe. The patient instruction sheet Cortisone Ointments will help dispel this misconception, and it also gives tips on treatment techniques and topical side effects. This instruction sheet is important for patients with atopic eczema or other corticosteroid-responsive dermatoses who will be using them on a long-term basis.

Systemic absorption of a topical corticosteroid does occur; with hydrocortisone, approximately 1 percent of the applied dose is absorbed from noninflamed forearm skin. Corticosteroid absorption increases when skin is inflamed and when occlusion is used. Infants and children are more susceptible than adults to systemic effects of topical corticosteroids.

In most patients treated with low- and intermediate-strength topical corticosteroids, it is impossible to demonstrate any systemic effect. In patients with extensive dermatitis treated with topical corticosteroids, especially if the corticosteroid is potent or is used with occlusion, depression of adrenal cortical function may be demonstrable. This adrenal suppression is usually a laboratory finding without clinical significance; normal adrenal function generally returns less than 1 week after the drug has been discontinued. However, patients undergoing long-term topical corticosteroid treatment of extensive dermatitis should be alerted to the possibility that adrenal suppression may pose a health threat in case of surgery or systemic illness.

CAUTION. These reassuring words about the paucity of systemic effects from topical corticosteroids do not apply to ultra-high-potency corticosteroids such as clobetasol propionate (Temovate), halobetasol propionate (Ultravate), diflorasone diacetate (Psorcon), and optimized betamethasone dipropionate (Diprolene). Ultra-high-potency topical corticosteroids should be reserved for special situations and used for brief periods, and patients should be carefully monitored.

Frank adrenal hypercorticism (i.e., Cushing's disease) as a result of topical corticosteroids is rare. It occasionally occurs in children whose severe dermatoses require prolonged topical corticosteroid administration; in these instances, it is an unavoidable complication. In treating children with extensive atopic dermatitis, continuous efforts should be made to decrease the strength of the corticosteroid to the minimum required for reasonable control.

Potent corticosteroids should be prescribed only in limited amounts and then used. Patients are often denied the benefits of topical corticosteroids because of unwarranted fears concerning systemic effects. All too often I encounter children who are miserable with uncontrolled atopic dermatitis because of their parents' unjustified fears of corticosteroid side effects. It is cruel to the child and the family to forgo the topical medication. Augment your discussion of the safety of topical corticosteroids with the Cortisone Ointments patient instruction sheet.

LOCAL SIDE EFFECTS

Atrophy

Cutaneous adverse effects of topical corticosteroids are a more common and more vexing problem than systemic side effects. The ability of potent corticosteroids—

especially the newer, highly potent products—to produce atrophy and acneiform eruptions has not been fully appreciated. In part, this is because such changes are gradual and often attributed to the underlying disease rather than the topical drug. Corticosteroids interfere with cellular replication; this effect is minimal with hydrocortisone, but may be severe with highly potent corticosteroids. Corticosteroid atrophy involves epidermal, dermal, and subcutaneous thinning (Figures C–2, C–3, C–5, and C–6). In skin folds, striae may result; in other areas, the thinning may cause subcutaneous vessels to be visible. Petechiae and ecchymoses may occur. Such thinning of the skin of the hands and feet may cause patients to complain of easy fissuring of their fingertips or toes.

In the perianal and genital area, corticosteroid atrophy and the resulting irritation, burning, and redness may be mistaken for uncontrolled dermatitis. Consequently, ever-stronger corticosteroids are used, and the dermatitis is compounded in a vicious cycle. With hydrocortisone, there is far less chance of atrophy; it is the drug of choice in treating skin-fold areas, especially genital and perianal areas. Clinically, detectable atrophy from 1 percent hydrocortisone practically never occurs. With 2.5 percent hydrocortisone preparations, low-grade atrophy in skin-fold areas may occur. Using the lowest effective concentration of hydrocortisone in skin-fold areas minimizes the risks of atrophy.

Unfortunately, we continue to see patients whose minor genital or perianal dermatitis has been converted into a major therapeutic dilemma by the use of strong topical corticosteroids. The skin thinning from the potent drug may make the area an exquisitely sensitive, continuous source of burning and misery which is irritated by even the blandest topical therapy (Figure C–1). It is a good general rule to not use anything stronger than 1% hydrocortisone in any skin-fold area, especially the genital and perianal area.

Rosaceaform Dermatitis

On the face, potent corticosteroids can cause or aggravate a peculiar acneiform or rosaceaform dermatitis (i.e., corticosteroid rosacea, perioral dermatitis) (Figures C–89, C–90, C–97, and C–98). The picture resembles a combination of dermatitis and acnelike eruption with erythematous scaly patches as well as papules and pustules. When this corticosteroid side effect is superimposed on a preexisting dermatitis, such as seborrheic dermatitis, it frequently escapes recognition and gets steadily worse while being treated with a succession of ever-more-potent corticosteroids. Discontinuing the medication often causes this rosacea to flare up, which further delays the correct diagnosis. Corticosteroid rosacea usually improves with systemic tetracycline; sometimes a short course of systemic corticosteroids is necessary. This rosaceaform corticosteroid complication can be avoided by using only hydrocortisone on the face. The patient instruction sheet on Perioral Dermatitis (Rosaceaform Dermatitis) explains the deleterious effect of strong corticosteroids applied to the face. The Cortisone Ointments patient information sheet stresses the risk of this and other fairly common local complications.

Rebound Dermatitis

Rebound dermatitis may occur when potent corticosteroids are discontinued. This is common in corticosteroid rosacea, where the rosaceaform dermatitis often flares up when the fluorinated corticosteroid is discontinued. It is not uncommon in the genital, inguinal, and perianal areas. Resuming the fluorinated corticosteroid compounds the problem and delays resolution of the underlying disorder. Sometimes a 2- or 3-week course of prednisone is required to suppress rebound dermatitis.

Contact Allergy

Contact dermatitis from topical corticosteroids was formerly thought to be caused by the vehicle or added fragrance. Unfortunately, allergy to the actual corticosteroid molecule does occur, although infrequently. Allergy to corticosteroids is often over-looked, as it is usually low grade and masquerades as a chronic persistent dermatitis rather than an acute, clinically obvious contact reaction. Adding to the difficulty of detecting this complication is that patch tests with commercial corticosteroid formulations are often false-negative. Documenting corticosteroid allergy may require patch tests with the pure compound in an alcoholic vehicle or intradermal tests with aqueous corticosteroid solutions or suspensions.

OCCLUSION

Occlusion greatly potentiates the effect of topical corticosteroids. Occlusion therapy is used mainly for: (1) dermatoses of the palms and soles; (2) psoriasis of glabrous skin; (3) any localized patch of severely lichenified dermatitis; and (4) extensive, severe, steroid-responsive dermatitis as an alternative to systemic corticosteroids. In addition to potentiating corticosteroid action, occlusion by itself has a beneficial effect on endogenous dermatoses, especially psoriasis.

Thin plastic films such as Saran Wrap are useful for occluding small areas. Plastic gloves work well on the hands, and plastic bags can be used on the feet. The trunk can be occluded with a plastic garment bag or plastic trash-can liner with holes cut for the arms and head. The occluding plastic is best held in place with a light garment (e.g., socks on the feet, a sleeve or thin stocking on the extremities) rather than tape, which may irritate the skin. On skin areas where tape must be used, a relatively nonirritating, porous (i.e., paper) product should be employed. For occlusion of extensive areas, a plastic suit is convenient and effective. Light-weight plastic suits designed for occlusive therapy are available from sources such as Dermatologic Lab and Supply (Appendix B).

Occlusion of extensive areas should not be used for more than 8 hours in a 24-hour period, because continuously occluded skin may become macerated and dermatitic. As little normal skin should be occluded as possible. It is traditional to use plastic occlusion overnight; this works well for the hands, feet, and similar limited areas. For those requiring total body occlusion with a plastic suit, a shorter 3- or 4-hour period during waking hours often suffices. The plastic suit is worn next to the skin; the patient may wear ordinary clothing over it. As the patient improves, occlusive therapy should be gradually withdrawn by using it every other day, and later every third day, to minimize the chance of sudden flare-ups.

CAUTION. Patients must not exercise while undergoing complete body occlusion with a plastic suit, because body heat regulation is severely compromised by the inability to evaporate sweat. Patients should be given written warnings to avoid exercise while wearing the plastic suit.

Because occlusion increases corticosteroid absorption, it also increases the risk of side effects. Systemic corticosteroid effects are generally not a problem when less than 10 percent of the body is occluded and low- or medium-potency preparations are used. When large areas of the body are occluded, the possibility of systemic corticosteroid side effects must be kept in mind, especially if the drug is highly potent.

The local side effects of occlusion are related mainly to its potentiation of the tendency of strong corticosteroids to produce atrophy. In hot weather, miliaria can be a problem. Folliculitis occasionally occurs; occlusion should be discontinued when this happens. Occlusion is contraindicated in the presence of pyoderma.

INTRALESIONAL CORTICOSTEROIDS

Intralesional corticosteroid injections occupy an intermediate position between topical and systemic therapy. All of the injected intralesional corticosteroid is absorbed.

Because the corticosteroid is absorbed slowly, it is usually possible to obtain a local therapeutic effect without measurable systemic effects. When large amounts of corticosteroids are injected intralesionally, systemic effects will be evident.

In intralesional therapy, a suspension of slowly soluble corticosteroids is injected into dermatitic skin. Triamcinolone acetonide suspension is the drug of choice; it provides a therapeutic effect lasting 4 to 10 weeks. In the United States, injectable triamcinolone acetonide (Kenalog) is available in concentrations of 10 and 40 mg/ml. Atrophy at the injection site and adverse effects from systemically absorbed corticosteroid increase dramatically with increasing concentration. For most situations, the undiluted 10-mg/ml suspension is the maximum concentration advisable. Often, more dilute suspension will suffice. When using triamcinolone acetonide for treating acne of the face, dilute the suspension to 2 or 3 mg/ml to minimize the chance of atrophy. The 40-mg/ml concentration should be reserved for special situations such as keloids, which fail to respond to the 10-mg/ml concentration.

INDICATIONS FOR INTRALESIONAL CORTICOSTEROIDS

Intralesional corticosteroids are most commonly used for relatively small areas of lichenified, stubborn psoriasis, atopic eczema, lichen simplex chronicus, nummular eczema, and lichen planus. They are also employed in treating alopecia areata. Inflammatory acne lesions are injected with dilute triamcinolone acetonide (Figures C–7 and C–8). Keloids may regress when injected with the undiluted 10-mg/ml suspension, because steroids inhibit fibroblast proliferation. Keloids that do not respond to intralesional triamcinolone acetonide in a 10-mg/ml concentration may be injected with the 40-mg/ml concentration. Start with small amounts injected deeply, or atrophy may occur (Figures C–7 and C–8). Fortunately, this atrophy is usually temporary. Intralesional injections are used for treating a circumscribed, steroid-responsive lesion requiring corticosteroid penetration into the dermis and subcutis. Extensive dermatoses are not suitable for intralesional treatment, because the large amounts of corticosteroids required would produce significant systemic side effects.

TECHNIQUE

Intralesional repository corticosteroids should be injected into the upper subcutis, not intradermally. Intradermal injection (i.e., injection with wheal formation) may cause skin atrophy. The proper depth of injection ranges from 3 to 7 mm; with practice, one learns to insert the needle with a short, quick jab to penetrate the tough dermis.

A tuberculin syringe should be used for intralesional corticoid therapy, because it is difficult to deliver the 0.05- to 0.1-ml optimal amount at each site with a larger-bore syringe. Luer Lok syringes are ideal, as considerable pressure is needed for intralesional injections, and needles attached to an ordinary friction hub tend to become dislodged and result in a spray of the contents. Disposable syringes with Luer Loks are not widely available; they may be obtained form Acuderm or Dermatologic Lab and Supply (Appendix B).

The discomfort of injection is minimized by using tiny needles. The best is the 13-mm (half-inch) 30-gauge needle. The bore of the 30-gauge needle is too small to permit withdrawal of the corticosteroid suspension from the vial; for this, use a 20- or 22-gauge needle.

Intralesional injections are performed best with the syringe held in one hand (Figure 1–1). After thrusting the needle through the dermis with a short wrist

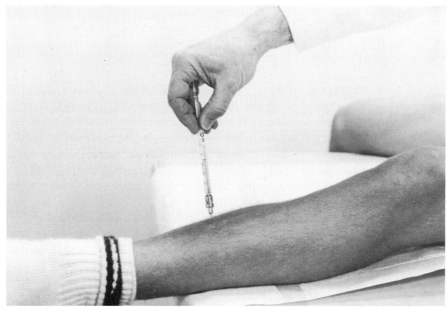

Figure 1–1. Intralesional injection of a corticosteroid into a plaque of psoriasis on a young man's leg. The palm of the hand is squeezed against the plunger to deliver the desired 0.05 to 0.1 ml of suspension to each puncture site. Multiple punctures can be made quickly, because the syringe is gripped in the same way throughout the procedure.

motion, squeeze your palm against the plunger to inject the drug into the subcutis. The following list outlines the procedure:

1. Use a short wrist-motion jab.

2. Insert the needle perpendicular to the skin surface so it will traverse as little tissue as possible.

3. The depth of injection depends on skin thickness and varies from 3 to 7 mm (one fourth to one half the length of a 13-mm needle).

4. Inject 0.05 to 0.1 ml at each puncture. This usually suffices for a 1- to 2-cm² area of dermatitis.

5. For lesions larger than 1 to 2 cm², space the injection sites approximately 2 cm apart.

SIDE EFFECTS

Systemic

The entire amount of corticosteroid deposited intralesionally is absorbed. Not all corticosteroid withdrawn from a vial is deposited in the tissue; a little drips from the needle between injections and a little flows out of each puncture site.

Injections of less than 10 mg of triamcinolone acetonide at intervals of more than 90 days are probably free of detectable systemic side effects. With larger amounts, systemic effects may occur. After receiving 20 to 30 mg of triamcinolone acetonide intralesionally, it's common for patients with eczema or psoriasis to report improvement in lesions that were not injected. Triamcinolone acetonide is slowly absorbed from tissue for 2 to 3 months; injections at more frequent intervals produce a cumulative effect. No firm rules as to the amount and timing of injections can be given; the systemic effects of intralesional corticosteroids must be kept in mind if more than 10 mg of triamcinolone acetonide are injected every 3 months.

In performing intralesional injections, you needn't try to prevent an occasional intravascular injection. Systemic side effects from such occasional intravascular injections have not been reported with triamcinolone acetonide suspensions made in the United States.

Local

Atrophy can be troublesome, although it's nearly always temporary. Whether atrophy occurs depends on the concentration of corticosteroid injected, the depth of injection, the dose per unit area, and the site. On the face, which is highly susceptible to atrophy, only dilute (i.e., 2 to 3 mg/ml) triamcinolone should be used, and it should be injected at least 3 mm deep. In other areas, atrophy can usually be avoided if these guidelines are followed: (1) inject less than 0.1 ml of corticosteroid at each site; (2) inject into the deeper subcutaneous tissue; and (3) use triamcinolone concentrations of 10 mg/ml or less.

Localized infection occasionally follows intralesional corticosteroid injections of the hands or feet, but rarely occurs elsewhere. This factor previously made me reluctant to inject the hands or feet. In the last 6 years, I have prescribed a 2-day course of an oral antibiotic, generally dicloxacillin, erythromycin, or minocycline, whenever I inject the hands or feet. The 2-day course has completely eliminated such hand and foot infections. However, this is anectodal advice; the infrequency of these infections makes documentation by a controlled study difficult.

PUTTING IT TOGETHER

The following examples will illustrate how to employ topical corticosteroids optimally.

1. PATIENT. A 7-year-old girl with dry, scaling patches of low-grade atopic eczema on the face.

TREATMENT. One percent hydrocortisone cream applied thinly three or four times per day. White petrolatum applied after the hydrocortisone at bedtime and during the day as desired if the skin is too dry.

RATIONALE. Highly potent steroids should be avoided in treating the face. As the dermatitis is mild, choose 1 percent hydrocortisone rather than a higher concentration. An ointment is usually more effective for dry dermatitis, but is less cosmetically acceptable than a cream. Compromise by using a cream and have the patient apply petrolatum over the cream at bedtime to provide an ointment effect. The frequent corticosteroid applications are desirable for their emollient as well as their anti-inflammatory effects.

2. PATIENT. A 10-year-old boy with moderately severe, dry, fissured, atopic eczema of the antecubitals, popliteals, and backs of the hands.

TREATMENT. Triamcinolone acetonide 0.025 percent, both cream and ointment. Have the patient use the cream on one side and the ointment on the other, and see which is more beneficial and which is preferred by the patient. One or two daily applications usually suffice. The hands should also receive frequent applications of an emollient. At the 7- to 10-day follow-up visit, instruct the patient in phasing out the triamcinolone acetonide topical, using the base the patient prefers. As he is phasing out the triamcinolone acetonide, he should be phasing in 1 percent hydrocortisone, again in the base of preference, as this should be the topical for long-term maintenance. The goal is to control the eczema with 1 percent hydrocortisone and reserve the triamcinolone acetonide topical for flare-ups not controlled with hydrocortisone.

RATIONALE. An intermediate-strength corticosteroid generally suffices in this situation. While ointments usually are better than creams for chronic atopic eczema, some patients do not tolerate them. The patient has the final word.

3. PATIENT. A 46-year-old man whose chronic seborrheic dermatitis of the glabella, forehead, nasolabial folds, scalp edges, and ears is itchy.

TREATMENT. For the face, 2.5 percent hydrocortisone cream applied thinly at bedtime and massaged in well. Tell the patient that if he isn't better in a week, he should apply it twice daily. If the eyebrows are involved, the cream should be applied with a moist finger to convert it to a liquid for better skin delivery. For the scalp edges and ears, prescribe a medium-potency corticosteroid gel, lotion, or solution applied sparingly at bedtime.

RATIONALE. Using 2.5 percent hydrocortisone, rather than the traditional 1 percent, will result in a faster initial response and require less frequent applications for long-term suppression. A higher concentration of hydrocortisone from 2 to 4 percent could be used; in the United States, hydrocortisone is commercially available in concentrations of 0.5, 1, and 2.5 percent. Hydrocortisone could be used for the scalp edges and ears; however, these sites respond less well to corticosteroids than the face. A medium-potency corticosteroid is preferable and is usually safe in these areas. Once-daily applications to scalp edges and ears generally suffice; bedtime is a convenient and specific treatment time.

4. PATIENT. A 56-year-old woman who has had a patch of chronic, itching, lichenified dermatitis of the occipital scalp and nape of the neck for longer than 10 years. A previous physician prescribed 1 percent hydrocortisone lotion; another gave her 0.1 percent triamcinolone acetonide cream; neither topical controlled her dermatitis. You diagnose lichen simplex chronicus.

TREATMENT. A potent corticosteroid in liquid, gel, or solution form applied once daily. Ask the patient to return in 2 to 3 weeks; if the eruption doesn't improve dramatically, inject 10 mg/ml of triamcinolone acetonide intralesionally. At the follow-up visit, ask the patient to gradually reduce the frequency of applications; for long-term use on the scalp, a potent topical corticosteroid should be applied no more than twice per week.

RATIONALE. Chronic lichenified dermatitis tends to resist corticosteroids; this patient requires a potent drug and a vehicle that delivers it to the scalp. One physician had used the right vehicle but the wrong corticosteroid; the other, the reverse. Always inquire as to previous topical corticosteroid therapy; it may enable you to repeat previous successes and avoid failure. If a lichenified chronic dermatitis fails to respond to a potent corticosteroid, it is either because of inadequate penetration or because the process is not corticosteroid-sensitive. Intralesional injection penetrates the thickened skin.

REFERENCES

1. Robertson DB, Maibach HI: Topical corticosteroids. *Int J Dermatol* 21:59, 1982
2. Schlagel CA, Sanborn EC: The weights of topical preparations required for total and partial body inunction. *J Invest Dermatol* 42:253, 1964

2 *Diagnosing Dermatitis*

Patient sheets pages P–19, P–25

Diagnosing dermatitis is often difficult for the experienced dermatologist. No wonder the generalist may be frustrated when trying to match the patient's rash with such terms as nummular eczema, dyshidrotic eczema, dermatitis venenata, atopic eczema, asteatotic eczema, almost ad infinitum. This chapter describes a simplified way of diagnosing dermatitis that bypasses many traditional diagnostic labels. A simple and therapeutically more useful approach to diagnosing dermatitis recognizes that all dermatoses result from the often complex interaction between exogenous and endogenous factors.

DERMATITIS—A USEFUL CONCEPT

Dermatitis and eczema are interchangeable terms describing skin disorders characterized by superficial scaling, erythema, papules, and vesiculation. Usually these terms are applied to disorders of unknown cause. When the cause of a rash is known, it is given a specific etiologic diagnosis. Thus, dermatitis resulting from poison ivy or oak contact is allergic contact dermatitis. A fungal infection of the feet, although it looks like dermatitis, is diagnosed as tinea pedis. The term dermatitis is used in both a specific way and also in a general sense.

Dermatitis in its more specific sense describes clinical entities with skin eruptions that fit the broad morphologic definition of dermatitis. Atopic dermatitis, seborrheic dermatitis, and psoriasis are all dermatoses. They are well-delineated, endogenous skin dysfunctions. Dermatitis is also used as a general term to describe any eczematous rash of unknown etiology that can't be classified among the major endogenous dermatoses (e.g., atopic dermatitis, psoriasis, seborrheic dermatitis). Unfortunately, most dermatoses encountered by the physician cannot be classified into these three major groupings. Because dermatology began as a morphologic specialty, it was natural for physicians to attempt to classify the mass of dermatoses into morphologic entities. Unfortunately, the resulting welter of terminology has led only to confusion.

Much of the complex terminology attached to dermatitis should be disregarded, because it is largely useless in understanding what is actually occurring. The meaninglessness of much of the terminology becomes clear when presented with patients with chronic dermatitis. These patients have often been given a variety of diagnostic labels by several capable, experienced dermatologists. For example, one of my patients with hand dermatitis had previously been examined by three competent dermatologists and received three different morphologic diagnoses. Initially, the eruption was mild and diagnosed as irritant (housewife's) hand dermatitis. When it got worse and took the form of round, somewhat infiltrated eczematous patches, the next specialist diagnosed nummular eczema. Failing to get relief, the patient consulted a third expert, who diagnosed psoriasis of the hands. When I examined her, she had typical psoriasis of the elbows and scalp; dermatologist number three was correct.

This woman did not have three different skin disorders; she had psoriasis all along. However, in the early stages the condition was not morphologically typical and therefore could not be diagnosed. It would have been simpler to be content with the label of dermatitis until the nature of the process became clear.

No one denies the value of morphologic classifications when they are possible. It is both prognostically and therapeutically useful to distinguish seborrheic dermatitis from scalp psoriasis. The management and prognosis of irritant hand dermatitis differ markedly from those of psoriasis of the hands. Morphology often fails to provide a rational classification; sometimes it is misleading. Rather than struggle with imprecise terminology, we can look in a different way at the many ill-defined dermatoses we encounter.

EXOGENOUS AND ENDOGENOUS FACTORS

Dermatitis results from the interaction of endogenous and exogenous factors. Analyzing a patient's dermatitis from this aspect allows you to understand the processes responsible for the disorder.

Endogenous refers to malfunctioning skin. The mechanism is usually unknown; the dysfunction is genetically determined. Psoriasis, atopic dermatitis, and seborrheic dermatitis are clinically defined disorders that are entirely endogenous in their textbook form. These conditions are prone to spontaneous worsening and remission; these changes frustrate clinicians, because one can never be sure whether the changes are part of the disease process or are caused by external factors.

Exogenous describes the external factors influencing dermatitis. These can be classified as irritants and allergens. Irritants chemically damage skin. Soap, detergents, solvents, and abrasive cleansers are among the many commonly encountered irritants. Persons vary greatly in their response to irritants. Allergens act by an acquired immunologic mechanism. In North America, poison ivy and poison oak are the most common causes of pure allergic contact dermatitis. Sunlight and humidity are other exogenous factors that can affect dermatitis.

DIAGNOSTIC GUIDELINES

Most dermatoses result from a combination of endogenous and exogenous factors. Atopic dermatitis is frequently aggravated by overuse of soap (an irritant) and application of irritating over-the-counter topical remedies. Allergic contact dermatitis caused by a topical medicament may complicate any dermatitis but is especially frequent in stasis dermatitis. It is the clinician's task to sort out the various factors as a preliminary to rational management.

Detecting Endogenous Factors

The directed history is critical. Suspect endogenous factors when there is a long history of dermatitis, especially with intermittent clearing. Did the patient have dermatitis in childhood? Inquire about atopic dermatitis, psoriasis, or any type of chronic skin condition in close blood relatives. If a young woman with patchy hand dermatitis tells you her mother had hand eczema, you can be reasonably certain her dermatitis is basically endogenous.

Examine the entire skin. Dermatitis of the antecubitals and popliteals is evidence of atopic eczema. Don't neglect the perianal skin; a sharply demarcated eruption of the gluteal cleft suggests psoriasis. Pitting of the nails, dermatitis of the glans penis, and chronic scaling of ear canals (Figures C–105 and C–106) all point to psoriasis, mild forms of which are common. Examine the entire skin, even if the patient protests that it is normal. Patients are often embarrassed by, or unaware of, rashes elsewhere. Tell patients reluctant to have their entire skin examined, "I want to examine your normal skin because it will help me treat your rash." Figures C–105 and C–106 illustrate the diagnostic value of examining the patient's entire skin.

Detecting Exogenous Factors

The type of history will depend on the rash's distribution; perform detailed questioning after examining the patient. A patient with hand dermatitis requires completely different questioning from a patient with foot dermatitis. Only a few of the many agents that might cause hand dermatitis could conceivably play a role in foot dermatitis. Taking a suitable exposure history is a challenging art; here are a few guidelines.

Topical applications are some of the most common exogenous causes of dermatitis. Obtain a history of all topical applications the patient has used (e.g., creams, ointments, antibiotics, antiseptics, cosmetics, sun protectives). Details of over-the-counter preparations and prescription items are necessary. Patients' memories are often unreliable; have them bring in everything they have used on their rashes.

Find out if there is any relation to vacation, hobbies, trips, sun exposure, or work. Be cautious and thorough before diagnosing an industrial cause, because such a diagnosis has serious social and medical consequences. In my experience, the diagnosis of industrial dermatitis is often incorrectly applied.

IRRITANTS. Irritants are some of the most common exogenous causes of dermatitis. The diagnosis of irritant factors is circumstantial and unsatisfactory. Everyone is exposed to such irritants as soap and detergents; however, not everyone has dermatitis. On the other hand, any dermatitis will be aggravated by exposure to irritants. There is no test to confirm the diagnosis of irritant dermatitis. A high degree of suspicion leads to elimination of possible causes. Improvement suggests that irritants were responsible, but one cannot be certain, because topical corticosteroids are almost invariably simultaneously employed.

It is universally recognized that soap, solvents, paint, and abrasive cleansers are irritants; however, it is not appreciated that often substances designed for skin application are low-grade irritants. Many cosmetics, skin lubricants, antiseptic creams, and even topical corticosteroids are low-grade irritants. When used repeatedly, they can cause or aggravate dermatitis in a susceptible individual. Irritant dermatitis from preparations designed to improve skin is often overlooked. Irritation from cosmetics is a common cause of facial dermatitis in women. There is enormous individual variation in sensitivity to irritants.

Dry air can irritate by reducing skin moisture. The nonspecific dermatitis labeled asteatotic is common during winter in cold climates, because the low humidity reduces the skin's water content. While most irritants are chemicals, sunlight can produce toxic or irritant dermatitis. Sunlight may also produce allergic dermatitis.

ALLERGENS. Poison ivy and poison oak are common causes of allergic contact dermatitis in North America. Topical medicaments are the next most frequent; often a fragrance or biocide (preservative) is the offender. Allergy to nickel is common in women but infrequent in men. Cosmetics (especially perfumes), rubber, and epoxy glues are at the top of the almost endless list of known sensitizers.

Fortunately, we can test for contact allergy with the patch test. Scratch and immediate-type intradermal tests are useless.* The patch test is simple in theory but tricky in execution, and should be left to experts.

Allergens are a less common cause of dermatitis than endogenous or irritant factors; however, they must be thoroughly searched for. The reward of uncovering a causative allergen is cure. Avoiding further allergen contact cures allergic contact dermatitis. Allergic contact dermatitis is a complex subject; the *Color Text of Contact Dermatitis*,[1] Fisher's clinically oriented book, *Contact Dermatitis*,[2] and the Wilkinson and Rycroft chapters in the *Rook/Wilkinson/Ebling Textbook of Dermatology*[3, 4] provide a wealth of details.

Synthesis

In diagnosing dermatitis, the history, morphology, and distribution of the rash must all be considered in elucidating the role of endogenous and exogenous factors. Sometimes, as in typical psoriasis or atopic eczema, the task is easy. Often it is not. Hand dermatitis presents a formidable diagnostic challenge because it is usually multifactorial, and lesion morphology is often nondescript. A practical, step-by-step approach to diagnosing hand dermatitis is given in Part I, Chapter 15.

UNCERTAINTIES

Diagnosing dermatitis depends on excluding specific causes. As in any other diagnosis based on exclusion (e.g., essential hypertension), there always remains the nagging doubt: Was something overlooked? Even experts occasionally fall into the following traps:

1. A fungal infection mimics another disease. Tinea corporis can perfectly simulate nummular eczema. Dermatophyte infection of the hands often looks just like psoriasis. Do a KOH exam (Appendix A).

2. Scabies can produce eczematous changes and be mistaken for dermatitis—especially on the hands. Suspect scabies with any intensely itching rash; examine the entire skin for burrows.

3. Bowen's disease (intraepidermal squamous-cell carcinoma) often presents as a recalcitrant, localized patch of dermatitis. A biopsy will settle the issue. Biopsying any persistent dermatitis is a good idea. Occasionally, a specific diagnosis, such as lichen planus, will result.

4. Drug eruptions are occasionally eczematous. The localized, fixed drug eruption may mislead the unsuspecting dermatologist.

5. Photosensitivity can mimic an airborne contact dermatitis as well as endogenous dermatitis.

6. The patient may have two disorders. For example, it is not unusual for chronic stasis dermatitis to be complicated by allergy to a topical medicament.

7. The overlooked allergen or irritant is the most common error. There are legions of possible contactants. Allergy to a preservative widely used in ointment bases occasionally maintains a dermatitis while the physician switches from one topical to another. What physician considers the wife's perfume when diagnosing arm dermatitis in a man? Or rubber in eyelash curlers as causing eyelid dermatitis? Persistence, skill, and luck ferreted these diagnoses out. Patch test screening series can help to uncover clinically unsuspected causes.

When a dermatitis fails to improve, question your patient repeatedly about

---

*An exception is contact urticaria, in which erythema and whealing occur 20 to 30 minutes after contact.

what he or she is applying to the skin. Patients may "sneak" cosmetics or consider the use of a hand lotion too inconsequential to mention.

DOCTOR, WHAT'S CAUSING MY RASH?

Physicians dread this question when dealing with dermatitis. People like simple, clear-cut answers. They want to know the cause so they can eliminate it and be cured. They are unhappy when told it is a matter of multiple factors, one of them being endogenous.

An explanation of irritants and allergens is well accepted, but the concept of endogenous factors is troublesome. I tell patients that their skin is "misbehaving" and that this results from a "built-in" skin defect. It helps to point out that other ailments such as arthritis, high blood pressure, and diabetes are results of malfunctioning of the body.

A family history of endogenous dermatitis makes your task easier; point out that defective skin "runs" in their family. Patients with psoriasis will often accept the implications; this is a fringe benefit of advertisements for remedies to heal the "heartbreak" of psoriasis.

Stress the positive. Emphasize that although the underlying cause of the endogenous dermatitis remains unknown, the rash can usually be controlled and often be cleared up. The authority of the written word helps. Be sure the patient receives and reads the appropriate information sheet. Despite your best efforts, some patients will be dissatisfied. They will keep trying to blame their chronic dermatoses on pollution, diet, or nerves. Many will shift from physician to physician in a never-ending search for a cure.

NEURODERMATITIS AND OTHER NONSENSE

It is not only patients who have trouble accepting the concept of endogenous skin dysfunction. Physicians have the same problem. For centuries, toxins and dietary problems were blamed for skin disorders. Bleeding as a method of ridding the body of toxins has long been abandoned, but purging as a treatment for skin diseases was fashionable well into this century. Fortunately, these methods have been discarded. Unfortunately, one delusion persists: That "nerves" cause dermatitis. The erroneous notion of psychogenic dermatitis is maintained in the term neurodermatitis.

The word neurodermatitis was coined by 19th-century physicians who believed that certain dermatoses resulted from dysfunction of cutaneous nerves (i.e., neuritis). The term persisted even after it became clear that cutaneous nerves do not cause dermatitis; however, its meaning was changed. Today, neurodermatitis is applied to the notion that certain chronic dermatoses represent a neurosis (i.e., a psychological disorder); however, there is no evidence that psychogenic disorders cause dermatitis, and a good deal of evidence that they do not. Neurodermatitis is a misleading, archaic label that should be expelled from our vocabulary.

That the nervous system can influence skin disorders is undeniable. Emotional upsets and nervous stress may aggravate psoriasis, atopic dermatitis, and other skin disorders just as they may aggravate hypertension, arthritis, and diabetes; however, no one maintains that the latter conditions are psychogenic in origin. One frequently encounters patients who blame themselves for their psoriasis or eczema because they have been told it is caused by nervousness. Putting the responsibility for such disorders on the patient is not only cruel, it is medically erroneous and therapeutically sterile.

TREATMENT

Basic principles of treatment of dermatitis are outlined in Chapter 3. Fortunately, dermatitis can be managed by treating the appropriate stage of the disorder irrespective of the cause. In other words, an episode of facial contact dermatitis due to a cosmetic can usually be managed identically to an acute flare-up of atopic dermatitis on the face, even though the causes are completely different. By learning the basic principles of treating acute, subacute, and chronic dermatitis, one can manage most patients with dermatitis by simply staging each process.

Well-defined clinical entities involving dermatitis, such as psoriasis, atopic dermatitis, seborrheic dermatitis, and hand dermatitis, have separate instruction sheets and separate physician units to aid in their management. Many patients with dermatitis don't fit the traditional major categories of dermatoses; for these, a catchall instruction sheet, Dermatitis, is included. Its use is described in detail in Chapter 3. Snce most dermatoses are treated with topical corticosteroids, use the Cortisone Ointments information sheet to improve patients' understanding and compliance.

REFERENCES

1. Larsen WG, Adams RM, Maibach HI: *Color Text of Contact Dermatitis.* Philadelphia: WB Saunders, 1992
2. Fisher AA: *Contact Dermatitis,* 3rd ed. Philadelphia: Lea & Febiger, 1986
3. Wilkinson JD, Rycroft RJG: Contact dermatitis. *In* Champion RH, Burton JL, Ebling FJG: *Rook/Wilkinson/Ebling Textbook of Dermatology,* 5th ed. London: Blackwell, 1992
4. Rycroft RJG, Wilkinson JD: Irritants and sensitivities. *In* Champion RH, Burton JL, Ebling FJG: *Rook/Wilkinson/Ebling Textbook of Dermatology,* 5th ed. London: Blackwell, 1992

3 *Treatment of Dermatitis*

Patient sheets pages P–19, P–21, P–25, P–39*

Dermatitis can best be explained to the patient as malfunctioning skin. Dermatitis of varying etiologies is often treated in remarkably similar ways, depending on its stage. This chapter outlines the basic principles of treatment of dermatitis, irrespective of the cause.

Certain endogenous types of dermatitis have been classified into clinical entities: Atopic eczema, psoriasis, and seborrheic dermatitis. Each of these conditions is covered in a separate chapter. Hand dermatitis presents special diagnostic and therapeutic problems and also is considered separately. Poison oak or ivy contact dermatitis is a common, etiologically definable type of dermatitis and is discussed in a separate chapter and has a separate patient instruction sheet.

The separate chapters on these entities augment and extend the general recommendations in this chapter. For example, in seborrheic dermatitis, the general principles of topical corticosteroids, avoiding irritants, and adequate lubrication apply. In addition, seborrheic dermatitis often responds to topical ketoconazole.

Many patients with dermatitis fall outside of these clinical classifications. They have nonspecific dermatitis. Because this diagnosis does not fit neatly into clinical classifications, it does not receive much textbook attention.

Rational treatment of dermatitis is a straightforward process, outlined in Table 3–1. Dermatitis is treated according to its stage—acute, subacute, or chronic—using both specific and nonspecific modalities. Acute poison ivy or poison oak contact dermatitis with blistering and oozing will be managed like acute blistering dermatitis caused by benzocaine in a benzocaine-sensitive patient. Similarly, a low-grade, subacute contact dermatitis of the face from cosmetics will be treated similarly to a low-grade flare-up of atopic eczema of the face. Once the stage of the dermatitis is determined, it is a straightforward matter to initiate the treatment appropriate for that stage.

Nonspecific measures also should not be bewildering. Innumerable substances are recommended to be added to water for soaks and compresses; among them are aluminum acetate (Burow's solution), Epsom salts, oatmeal derivatives, table salt, tea, and copper sulfate. It is easy to lose sight of the fact that water is the active ingredient; the additives are mainly of psychological significance. Because soaks or compresses with plain water may not impress the patient, it is permissible to add some inexpensive, bland agent. My favorite additive is white vinegar, because it is cheap, readily available, and nonsensitizing. The patient is instructed to add 1 or 2 tablespoons (15 to 30 ml) of white vinegar to each liter of water.

*Refer to the *Universal Medication Summary Sheet,* page xxi.

Table 3–1. **TREATMENT OF DERMATITIS**

Acute (Severe) Dermatitis
Systemic treatment
  1. Corticosteroids by mouth, preferably prednisone or prednisolone.
  2. A 10- to 14-day course of systemic corticosteroids usually suffices.
  3. Start with 60 to 100 mg of prednisone the first day.
Topical treatment
  1. Nonspecific soothing compresses or baths with water, aluminum acetate solution (Burow's
     solution), or dilute vinegar (2 tablespoons of white vinegar added to 1 quart of water).*

Subacute (Moderate) Dermatitis
Systemic treatment
  1. Usually none is indicated.
  2. Sometimes a low dose of prednisone (20–40 mg) once daily or every other day is required.
Topical treatment
  Specific
  1. Apply a potent corticosteroid sparingly once or twice daily. Note caution regarding potent
     corticoids.†
  2. Corticosteroid cream or ointment is preferred.
  3. If skin is dry, use greasy corticosteroid ointment at bedtime.
  Nonspecific
  1. At this stage, lubrication is needed; use corticosteroid cream or greasy ointment.
  2. Soaks or compresses are not indicated.
  3. Avoid shake lotions (e.g., calamine lotion); they dry the skin and leave a messy residue.

Chronic Dermatitis
Systemic treatment
  1. None is necessary.
Topical treatment
  Specific
  1. Use a low-, medium-, or high-potency corticosteroid, depending on the degree of lichenification
     (thickening) and severity of the dermatitis.
  2. Corticosteroid cream or ointment (petrolatum) is the best vehicle. Greasy ointments are
     preferable, especially at night.
  3. Use potent corticosteroids only once or twice daily. Note caution regarding potent
     corticosteroids.†
  4. Occlusion overnight with plastic film enhances the corticosteroid effect; use on stubborn,
     severely lichenified dermatoses as well as severe psoriasis.
  Nonspecific
  1. Lubricate the skin with a nonspecific emollient.
  2. Lubricant should be used thinly and frequently.
  3. White petrolatum is the best lubricant. Used sparingly, it is cosmetically acceptable to the
     patient.

---

*This should be called water therapy, because it is the water that is important; additives are mainly of psychological significance. In oozing and crusting dermatoses, water both debrides and soothes. Let the patient choose a comfortable temperature. When the rash is extensive, showers or baths are convenient forms of water therapy.

†CAUTION: Potent topical corticosteroids may cause skin thinning and other significant skin side effects. The face and skin-fold areas are especially vulnerable; avoid medicaments stronger than 1 percent hydrocortisone in these areas. It is often possible to shift to a lower-potency corticosteroid after 1 to 2 weeks of treatment. These cautions apply especially to superpotent corticosteroids, such as clobetasol propionate (Temovate), halobetasol propionate (Ultravate), diflorasone diacetate (Psorcon), and betamethasone dipropionate (Diprolene), which can also cause systemic effects.

PRINCIPLES OF SYSTEMIC TREATMENT

CORTICOSTEROIDS

Corticosteroids are the only systemic anti-inflammatory agents effective in treating dermatitis, and they have revolutionized the treatment of severe dermatitis. The weeks of misery and blistering from severe poison ivy and poison oak contact dermatitis are horrors of the past. Adequate doses of systemic corticosteroids will bring symptomatic improvement of acute dermatitis in 6 to 12 hours. If a patient with acute dermatitis fails to improve within 24 hours after starting systemic corticosteroids, the dose is too low or the diagnosis is in error.

Use enough corticosteroid initially. A useful schedule for moderately severe poison ivy or poison oak contact dermatitis is described in Table 31–1. Severe cases require more corticosteroid, as much as 100 to 200 mg of prednisone daily. The daily dose of prednisone is tapered by 20 to 40 mg/day to a level of 60 mg/day; thereafter, follow the schedule in Table 31–1.

Most acute dermatoses can be controlled within 14 days of initiating systemic corticosteroids. Often, only 3 to 5 days of systemic corticosteroids are required. The aim of systemic corticosteroids is to reduce edema and the acuteness of the process so that topical corticosteroids will be effective. If oral corticosteroid therapy is required for longer than 3 weeks, consider dermatologic consultation and further studies such as patch testing.

Prednisone (or prednisolone*) by mouth is the corticosteroid of choice and can usually be given as a single morning dose. Prednisone is a short-acting corticosteroid; therefore, severe dermatoses may require splitting the daily prednisone ration into morning and evening doses. Other corticosteroids cost more and have the distinct disadvantage of being long-acting. Injectable, repository corticosteroids are not often indicated for systemic therapy because of the difficulty in ascertaining drug release.

Short courses of systemic corticosteroids are remarkably safe. However, caution is required when administering these drugs to patients with peptic ulcers, diabetes, and hypertension. Mild side effects from systemic corticosteroids are common. These usually involve alterations in mood, insomnia, jitteriness, weight gain, and fluid retention. When employing systemic corticosteroids, give patients the instruction sheet (Cortisone Taken Internally) so they understand that these mood changes are not uncommon. If the insomnia and nervousness are annoying, low doses of a tranquilizer such as hydroxyzine (25 to 50 mg) or diazepam (5 to 10 mg) at bedtime are helpful. Avoid barbiturates. Even low doses and short courses of systemic corticosteroids may, on rare occasions, produce severe mood changes, depression, even psychosis. Should this occur, discontinue the drug and consider hospitalizing the patient.

OTHER SYSTEMIC AGENTS

Dermatitis is suppressed only by corticosteroids. Antihistamines, aspirin, and nonsteroidal anti-inflammatory agents do not affect the course of dermatitis. Although the sedating effect of antihistamines may lessen discomfort, it is preferable to make the patient comfortable by suppressing the dermatitis with specific therapy rather than by depressing his or her sensorium. Of course, there are exceptions. When there is much itching, discomfort, and anxiety, mild sedation at bedtime may be helpful. Hydroxyzine or a benzodiazepine is preferable; the barbiturates should be avoided.

PRINCIPLES OF TOPICAL THERAPY

Topical therapy has a dual role: It delivers active agents to the skin, and it has nonspecific debriding, soothing, and lubricating actions. By considering these two effects separately, we remove much of the mystique surrounding topical therapy. In treating dermatitis, topical corticosteroids are the only significant active agent and are discussed in detail in Chapter 1. Corticosteroids have rendered the older anti-

---

*Prednisolone is theoretically preferable, because it is biologically active, whereas prednisone must be converted by the liver to the biologically active compound. In practice, these drugs are used interchangeably; however, prednisone should not be used in patients with liver disease.

dermatitic agents largely obsolete. Avoid potentially sensitizing topical antibiotics (e.g., neomycin) in treating dermatitis. If secondary infection is present or suspected, a systemic antibiotic such as erythromycin is usually superior to a topical antibiotic.

SPECIFIC TOPICAL THERAPY

Specific topical therapy is a matter of choosing the type and concentration of topical corticosteroid. As indicated in Chapter 1, it is simplest to use different concentrations of triamcinolone acetonide when strong corticosteroids are indicated, and various concentrations of hydrocortisone when milder topical corticosteroids are indicated. After evaluating the stage of the dermatitis, choose the appropriate topical corticosteroid from the criteria in Table 1–1.

NONSPECIFIC ASPECTS OF TOPICAL THERAPY

Topical agents may be used for their nonspecific action (e.g., soaks to remove crusts). It is easy to overlook the nonspecific effects of the cream or ointment vehicle. A soothing and lubricating effect is desired. The wrong vehicle may irritate the skin and seriously interfere with the effectiveness of the corticosteroid. The nonspecific effects of topical therapy must be appropriate for the stage of dermatitis (see Table 3–1). Remember the ground rules of topical therapy: Do not irritate, and do not sensitize.

THE APPROPRIATE VEHICLE

In general, acute dermatoses with crusting and vesiculation are best treated with soaks and compresses, whereas chronic, lichenified, scaling dermatoses benefit from the lubricating effect of greasy ointments. Creams and cream lotions are appropriate for acute and subacute dermatoses.

The word lotion applies to both creamy lotions and shake lotions. Shake lotions are a mixture of powder and water; calamine lotion is an example. Cream lotions are oil-and-water emulsions. Shake lotions leave a messy residue on the skin and are obsolete.

AGGRAVATION BY IRRITATING TOPICALS

Avoiding an irritating topical medicament may be difficult. Clinicians understand— but patients often do not—that strong remedies such as undecylenic acid creams and Whitfield's ointment may be suitable for athlete's foot, but will aggravate dermatitis. The patient instruction sheet Dermatitis emphasizes that only water, white petrolatum, and the prescribed medications should be applied to the rash. Because some patients have a compulsion to treat themselves with over-the-counter and home remedies, this point cannot be overemphasized.

Patients often do not consider their over-the-counter skin lubricants, moisturizers, or hand creams to be medications. Many are significantly irritating, and patients must be cautioned not to use these preparations. Petrolatum is the cheapest bland lubricant, but some patients find it messy because they use too much; a microscopically thin layer of white petrolatum is adequate for lubrication and will not render clothes and the environment greasy. Commercial water-washable cream bases similar to hydrophilic ointment (USP) are good alternative nongreasy lubricants, but some are mildly irritating.

It is less well known that many corticosteroid vehicles are irritating. Emulsifying agents or solvents (e.g., propylene glycol) are the usual offenders. Many high-potency topical corticosteroids contain large amounts of propylene glycol to solubilize the drug (see Chapter 1). The irritant effects of propylene glycol are variable and subtle. The newer gel or solution formulations of topical corticosteroids usually contain high concentrations of solvents and should be used with particular caution.

The more acute the dermatitis, the greater the likelihood of irritation from surfactant, emulsifying, or solvent components of the vehicle. Vehicle irritation often manifests itself only in worsening of the dermatitis. When you suspect irritation or sensitivity to the vehicle, the best strategy is to switch to a corticosteroid suspended in petrolatum.

PRACTICAL ADVICE

Treatment of dermatitis is summarized in Table 3–1. Remember that topical therapy boils down to the following elements:

- Application of topical corticosteroids
- Lubricating the skin
- Avoiding irritants
- Eliminating contact allergens

The following guidelines will help you put these principles into practice:

1. Tell the patient not to apply anything to his or her rash except water, white petrolatum, and the medications you have prescribed.

2. Give the patient specific written instructions. These are not a substitute for, but are in addition to, your oral instructions.

3. Limit yourself to prescribing a few topical corticosteroids and one or two lubricants that you have found rarely irritate patients' skin.

4. White petrolatum is the blandest ointment base and rarely irritates the skin. When used sparingly at bedtime, it is acceptable to most patients and can be used on subacute and chronic dermatoses. The two recommended corticosteroids, hydrocortisone and triamcinolone acetonide, are commercially available suspended in white petrolatum. Generic forms of these are usually relatively inexpensive, and 1 percent hydrocortisone is available without a prescription.

5. Skin lubrication is important. When nonspecific dermatitis is extensive, the normal skin should be lubricated to discourage further spread. Techniques for body lubrication are described in the patient sheets for Dermatitis and for Dry Skin (Asteatosis, Xerosis).

6. Avoid producing allergic contact dermatitis to topical medicaments. Do not use topical neomycin, benzocaine, antihistamines, or other well-known offenders; they are of no value and may cause trouble. Use a plain corticosteroid topically.

7. If the dermatitis becomes infected, it is best to use an oral antibiotic such as erythromycin or a synthetic penicillin. If topical antimicrobial therapy is chosen, use mupirocin (Bactroban) ointment, as it is the most effective topical antimicrobial and rarely sensitizes the skin.

8. Be alert. If a dermatitis fails to improve, consider the possibility of irritation by or allergy to a topical agent. A useful maneuver if you are concerned about the safety of the topical regimen is to change to a corticosteroid in a plain, white petrolatum base.

TREATMENT FAILURES

If the dermatitis fails to respond, consider the following explanations:

1. Poor patient compliance. Have the patient describe exactly how he or she

performs treatment. A useful check is to have the patient bring in the unused portion of his medication.

2. Inappropriate treatment. Use of a cream on a dry, fissured dermatitis—which needs an ointment—is a common error. A more potent corticosteroid may be indicated.

3. Irritation or allergy to a home remedy or over-the-counter medicament being used without your knowledge.

4. Irritation or allergy to the prescription medicament. The newer gel vehicles, while elegant, are often irritating. Some corticosteroid lotions, solutions, and creams contain high concentrations of propylene glycol, which may irritate the skin. Allergy to a topical medicament, while always possible, is infrequent, provided the well-known sensitizers are avoided.

5. Incorrect diagnosis. Review the possible diagnoses in Chapter 2.

4 *Dermatologic Surgery*

Patient sheets pages P–103, P–105, P–107, P–109, P–111

Skin lesions that involve only the epidermis can frequently be cured by superficial skin surgery that takes only a few minutes and yields good cosmetic results. These techniques, although simple, are scarcely mentioned in surgical texts. This chapter describes easily mastered techniques for removal of superficial skin lesions. When lesions involve the dermis, conventional full-thickness skin excision is usually best. Full-thickness skin excision is the treatment of choice for most skin cancers, because it gives superior cosmetic results with the advantage of histologic control of the margins of the lesions. The *preoperative* information sheet, Surgery Done in the Office, reassures patients, asks that they avoid aspirin before and after surgery, and alerts us to medications or medical problems that may affect the surgery. Full-thickness skin surgery is well described in several recently published manuals.[1–7] This chapter discusses only some special techniques.

THE TOOLS

CURETTE

The curette is a scraping instrument. Curettes used by bone surgeons and some dermatologists have a spoonlike shape; however, most dermatologists in the United States use the hollow ring curette (Figures 4–1 and 4–2). The ring curette affords superior visibility and control in treating lesions. The opening of the ring curette may be either round or oval; the round is easier to sharpen. Curettes are available in many sizes; I use a 5-mm curette (size indicates diameter of the cutting ring) as a basic tool and a 2-mm curette for small lesions. Ring curettes are available from surgical supply houses specializing in dermatologic instruments (Appendix B).

Curettes must be kept sharp. They will dull rapidly if allowed to rattle against other instruments in a pack or tray; their ends should be covered with tubing (see Figure 4–1). Most rubber and plastic tubing disintegrates during autoclaving. Silastic tubing (Dow), available from laboratory equipment suppliers, does not disintegrate during autoclaving. Surgical firms resharpen curettes; however, you can do it quickly with a special tapering tubular whetstone available from surgical suppliers. Disposable curettes are a useful alternative; these are always very sharp.

CHALAZION CURETTE

The chalazion curette, borrowed from ophthalmologists, is a small, cup-shaped curette with a long, narrow stem. It is sized according to the diameter of the cup

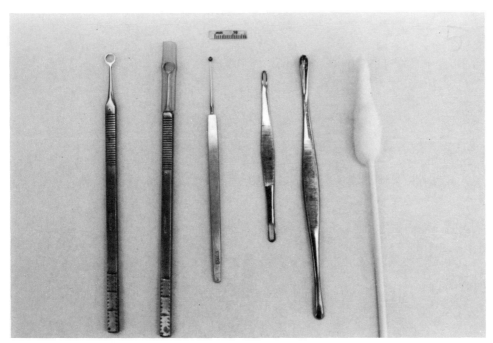

Figure 4-1. From left to right: hollow ring curette, curette protected with Silastic tubing, chalazion curette, Schamberg comedo extractor, Unna comedo extractor, and liquid nitrogen applicator made by shaping a large cotton swab.

(see Figures 4-1 and 4-2). The chalazion curette is a useful instrument for shelling out milia and small cysts; the larger sizes are helpful in scraping the walls of inflamed cysts. You cannot sharpen these curettes, so guard their ends with protective tubing.

SERRATED IRIS SCISSORS

Protuberant benign skin lesions are often treated by snipping them off flush with the surrounding skin. Skin tags, pedunculated nevi (Figure C–61), and protuberant keratoses are among lesions eminently suitable for scissors removal. The ordinary curved iris scissors (see Figure 4–2), no matter how sharp, tends to slip when cutting the tough dermis. Having one blade serrated prevents slippage and vastly improves the usefulness of iris scissors in skin surgery. Scissors with one serrated blade are available from Bernsco, George Tiemann and Co., and Robbins (Appendix B).

GRADLE SCISSORS

The Gradle scissors (see Figure 4–2), a fine, sharp-tipped curved scissors, is an ideal instrument for removing tiny skin tags, dissecting out small cysts, and other delicate surgical procedures.

COMEDO EXTRACTOR

The comedo extractor (see Figures 4–1 and 4–2) puts circumferential pressure on a comedo or milium to "pop" it out. Considerable pressure usually is required and may be painful. There are many types of comedo extractors on the market; all are

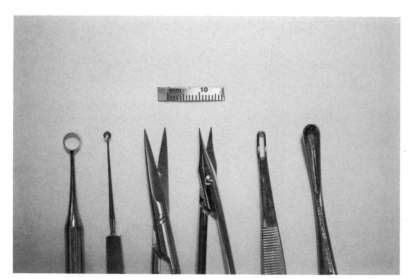

Figure 4–2. Close-up views, from left to right: hollow ring curette, chalazion curette, curved iris scissors with one serrated blade, Gradle scissors, Schamberg comedo extractor, and Unna comedo extractor.

basically of two types. The Unna comedo extractor has a spoonlike end with a central hole, while the Schamberg comedo extractor has wire loops. Both types are useful. For extraction of small comedones, I prefer the Unna type, because it causes less discomfort than the wire loop Schamberg model.

However, when removing large comedones or small cysts, the Schamberg instrument is preferable. Small cysts can often be popped out using the Schamberg extractor after a small nick has been made in the surface with a hypodermic needle or No. 11 blade. The pressure from the wire loop of the Schamberg extractor can be quite painful; when removing milia and small cysts, I inject a small amount of local anesthetic.

PUNCH

The punch, designed for removing the full thickness of the skin, is not an instrument of superficial skin surgery. The smaller sizes are useful for rapid skin biopsies. Various sizes can be used to remove a round lesion precisely.

Punches with small, knurled handles that are rotated by twisting between the fingers are superior to the older, large-handled Keyes punch. Punches are available in 0.5-mm gradations from 1 to 10 mm in diameter. The smallest I use is 1.5 mm in diameter; the largest is 10 mm. The most useful sizes are from 1.5 to 5 mm; it is helpful to have these in 0.5-mm increments. Above the 5-mm size, 1-mm gradations suffice. Punches must be kept sharp. Ends should be covered with tubing to protect their edges during sterilization. They can be sharpened with a tapered, round whetstone. Disposable punches are available in a number of sizes from dermatologic supply houses (Appendix B) and are very sharp and convenient; they are what I now use.

FORCEPS

Jeweler's forceps have tapering, pointed ends with smooth tips and are useful for removing sutures and foreign bodies and gently manipulating tiny bits of tissue. They are inexpensive and available from most surgical suppliers.

Delicate forceps with fine teeth are invaluable for removing tiny cysts, excising small punch biopsy specimens, and other delicate skin surgery. I prefer the Castroviejo model with its comfortable wide handle. Castroviejo forceps are available from Storz (Appendix B) and other surgical suppliers in a variety of sizes; for most dermatologic surgery, the 0.3-mm- or 0.5-mm-tooth size seems ideal. For the tiniest lesions, the 0.12-mm forceps is excellent. Good Castroviejo forceps are expensive but worth the price.

For full-thickness surgery, the standard Adson toothed forceps is the workhorse of the dermatologic surgeon. I strongly urge you to purchase it equipped with a suturing platform. This consists of parallel metal bars that enable you to grasp the needle securely as it emerges from the skin.

HEMOSTATICS

Bleeding after superficial skin surgery may be controlled with: (1) pressure and time; (2) noncaustic packing such as gelatin foam, collagen preparations, or oxidized cellulose; (3) chemical styptics such as ferric chloride, Monsel's solution, aluminum chloride, and trichloroacetic acid; or (4) electrocoagulation of the wound base.

Chemical styptics—Monsel's solution and aluminum chloride are the most popular—are protein precipitants, which cause significant cellular damage and delay healing. I rarely use them. Electrodesiccation thermally destroys protein and cells. Electrodesiccation of the wound base is the most scarring hemostatic technique and should be avoided whenever possible. This stricture against electrodesiccation of entire wounds, however, does not apply to point electrocoagulation of bleeding vessels during excisional surgery.

Simple pressure will stop bleeding; however, bleeding tends to resume when the gauze pressure pad is removed. Using a bland ointment helps to prevent disturbance of the incipient clot when the pressure pad is removed. However, it is easier to use a nondestructive or tissue-neutral hemostatic to control bleeding from superficial wounds. Gelatin foam (Gelfoam), oxidized cellulose (Oxycel), and collagen preparations are commercially available tissue-neutral hemostatics. They are probably equally effective, but differ significantly in cost. I use 7.0-mm-thick Gelfoam packed as 20- by 60-mm strips in individual sterile envelopes. Because only a small part of the package is needed, I tear off a portion with sterile forceps and save the remainder of the envelope. This economy breaches absolute sterility, but this does not matter in skin surgery. These tissue-neutral hemostatics are left in place, because deeper portions are absorbed and superficial fragments can be shed with the crust.

While tissue-neutral hemostatics will adequately control more than 90 percent of superficial wounds, a chemical styptic is preferable in some locations. On lip and scalp wounds, I generally use Monsel's (ferric chloride) solution. When a wound stubbornly continues to ooze blood in spite of the application of Gelfoam and pressure, use of a swab with styptic is indicated.

Chemical styptics should be used with reluctance, and only on superficial intradermal wounds. Full-thickness defects exposing subcutaneous fat are not suitable terrain for ferric iron or other chemical styptics. Hemostasis after full-thickness skin removal can be accomplished by suturing, point electrodesiccation of bleeding vessels, pressure, or packing with an inert hemostatic.

LIQUID NITROGEN

Liquid nitrogen is ideal for removing warts and other lesions such as benign superficial keratoses and hemangiomas, because, when used lightly on superficial lesions, it produces less scarring than other destructive techniques* (Figures C–37 through C–45, C–55 through C–59, and C–116). Liquid nitrogen is either sprayed on the skin, using specially designed equipment, or is applied with a large cotton or rayon swab (see Figure 4–1). The latter method is known as the dipstick technique. The spray technique is faster and does not risk contamination of the liquid nitrogen reservoir. While the dipstick procedure is slower, it allows more precise application of the liquid nitrogen. Each method has its devotees; I prefer the dipstick approach. A number of manufacturers make excellent hand-held liquid nitrogen spray units. Consult colleagues to see which brands they prefer, and then see if the sales representative will permit a trial period before purchase.

If you use the dipstick method, precautions must be taken to prevent contamination of the liquid nitrogen reservoir, because liquid nitrogen is an excellent viral and bacterial preservative. Use a fresh applicator swab for each patient. If more than one application of liquid nitrogen is needed, do not dip the applicator stick in the liquid nitrogen reservoir more than once. Instead, pour some liquid nitrogen into a disposable cup and, after you are finished with the patient, discard the remainder. You can fashion your own dipsticks by adding cotton to an ordinary small cotton swab, but it is more convenient to use the large rayon-wool–tipped applicators used in proctoscopy and other procedures. These blunt-ended applicators are readily shaped to provide a pointed end for liquid nitrogen application. Large, disposable applicators suitable for dipsticks, liquid nitrogen thermos containers, and other liquid nitrogen equipment are available from Dermatologic Lab and Supply Co. (Appendix B).

Liquid nitrogen is available in most larger cities. Liquid nitrogen suppliers provide large steel vacuum drums (Dewar flasks) in sizes holding 20, 30, 40, or more liters. A simple valve permits removal of small quantities, which are conveniently held in small vacuum-walled containers sold for this purpose.

CAUTION. Liquid nitrogen containers must never be tightly stoppered; they will explode. Drill holes in the stoppers. At the end of the day, return unused uncontaminated liquid nitrogen to the large storage flask.

WOUND DRESSINGS

The new wound dressings aim to accelerate skin healing by keeping the wound moist to prevent formation of a crust (scab). Crusts inhibit wound healing by acting as mechanical barriers to re-epithelialization. These dressings have an impermeable or semipermeable membrane to reduce water loss and maintain a moist wound surface.

The simplest type of wound dressing consists of a transparent, water-impermeable plastic film with adhesive on one side to affix it to the skin. It has the disadvantage that exudate collects underneath the dressing.

Other new dressings contain a synthetic colloidal or gel-like mass attached to an impermeable or partially permeable membrane. This plastic mass interacts with the wound surface and absorbs exudate.

All these dressings are expensive and require practice for correct application. Compared with conventional dressings, they accelerate wound healing when large surfaces require re-epithelialization (e.g., after dermabrasion and on donor skin graft sites). However, they probably are not practical for small wounds that follow the removal of warts, keratoses, and similar superficial lesions. Because wound dressing is a rapidly changing field with frequent introduction of new products, I have omitted product recommendations and trade names.

---

*Liquid nitrogen destruction should be limited to clearly benign lesions. If the nature of the lesion is in doubt, use cold-steel surgery to provide a specimen for histology.

The newer, acrylic-based tapes are hypoallergenic and less irritating than cloth tape. Gentlest are the "paper" and other highly permeable tapes. At least one brand, Micropore (3M), is available in a flesh color, which patients prefer to the traditional white. Acrylic tapes made of fabric (Dermicel) are more durable and may adhere better than paper tape. Like paper tapes, fabric tapes are permeable (nonocclusive) and do not macerate the underlying skin. There is no reason to use older kinds of tape for skin wounds.

Using tape to support wounds after excisional surgery permits early suture removal and minimizes wound dehiscence. I use nonsterile, flesh-colored tape. To make the tape stick firmly to the skin, paint spirit gum or Mastisol on the skin before applying the tape. Wound support in hairy areas is a problem because the growing hair quickly loosens the tape. Flexible collodion is an alternative to tape; unfortunately, it usually lasts no more than 1 or 2 days. Flexible collodion will stick longer if spirit gum or Mastisol is applied first.

ADHESIVES

Tincture of benzoin is often painted on patients' skin to make tape stick, but it sometimes causes an allergic reaction with a severe dermatitis. Far better are Mastisol or spirit gum, which are resin-based adhesive solutions. Mastisol (Ferndale Laboratories) is a tape adherent available from the manufacturer, Bernsco, or Dermatologic Lab and Supply (Appendix B). Spirit gum is used by actors to affix wigs and mustaches, and is available from companies that sell theatrical cosmetics. It is cheap, and its high alcohol content assures sterility. If evaporation thickens it excessively, thin it with alcohol or alcohol mixed with acetone. Allergy to either spirit gum or Mastisol is rare. Mastisol and spirit gum have another advantage: They are waterproof. Tape applied over them will stick after getting wet. Patients are pleased that they can shower and bathe, but warn them not to rub or scrub the tape. Remnants of Mastisol or spirit gum can be removed with acetone, nail polish remover, or Detachol (Ferndale).

TECHNIQUES

ALMOST PAINLESS LOCAL ANESTHESIA

With proper infiltration anesthesia, skin surgery is completely painless. If the patient complains of pain during the operation, you either did not inject enough anesthetic, or failed to wait for the anesthetic to diffuse adequately. However, patients are often distressed by pain during injection of the anesthetic. There are two components to injection pain: (1) the pain of the needleprick; and (2) the stinging of the injected anesthetic. The brief discomfort of the needle penetrating the skin can be minimized by using a thin needle; most dermatologists use 30-gauge needles. Thorough chilling of the skin with an ice pack or an ice cube wrapped in a plastic bag largely eliminates needleprick pain. An effective, albeit cumbersome method of eliminating needleprick pain is to use the topical anesthetic, EMLA cream. EMLA cream is a eutectic mixture of lidocaine and prilocaine; unfortunately, to be effective, it requires application under an occlusive dressing for at least 90 minutes.

The brief pain of the needle entering the skin is tolerable for most patients; it is the sharp sting of the anesthetic they object to. The sting of the anesthetic is largely caused by the acid pH required to stabilize the epinephrine. Neutralizing the pH of the anesthetic solution by adding sodium bicarbonate largely eliminates its sting. The procedure is simple: one part of sodium bicarbonate containing 1 mEq/ml is mixed with nine or ten parts of 1 percent lidocaine with epinephrine. Sterile sodium bicarbonate solution containing 1 mEq/ml is available from most hospital pharmacies. This solution is not preservative protected; therefore, a fresh vial should be used each time neutralized lidocaine with epinephrine is prepared. The addition of sodium bicarbonate does not reduce lidocaine's efficacy; however, it does render epinephrine less stable. In the neutralized lidocaine-epinephrine solution, epinephrine loses about 25 percent of its potency in 1 week. The usual commercial 1:100,000 concentration of epinephrine is in excess of what is required; 1:300,000 epinephrine produces adequate vasoconstriction. Consequently, the neutralized lidocaine-epinephrine can be kept for 2 to 3 weeks at room temperature while retaining both its anesthetic and vasoconstrictive effectiveness. Stability can be extended by refrigerating the neutralized lidocaine-epinephrine.

Even neutralized lidocaine produces slight stinging, although most patients do not find it intolerable. Benzyl alcohol is a completely sting-free local anesthetic of brief duration and is ideal for very superficial skin surgery. Multi-dose vials of saline contain a preservative to counteract microbial contamination. Currently, in North America, 0.9 percent benzyl alcohol is the most commonly used preservative. It has mild anesthetic action. Injecting benzyl alcohol–preserved saline is completely sting-free, unlike plain saline, which does sting when injected. Providing the benzyl alcohol containing saline is injected superficially, it produces instantaneous anesthesia of short duration. The anesthetic action is brief, lasting just 2 to 5 minutes, and it is important to completely infiltrate the surgical site so that an edematous area is produced. Then skin tags can be snipped off, seborrheic keratoses curetted off, or lesions shave biopsied completely painlessly. Because the anesthetic action is brief and superficial, benzyl alcohol is not adequate for full-thickness skin excisions or punch biopsies. For this type of surgery, lidocaine, mepivacaine, or similar traditional local anesthetics should be employed. In very tender areas, such as the nose, I sometimes first infiltrate with benzyl alcohol–saline and then painlessly infiltrate lidocaine-epinephrine into the area injected with the benzyl alcohol–saline solution.

Adding epinephrine to benzyl alcohol–saline in a concentration of 1:300,000 extends the period of anesthesia from 2 to 5 minutes to about 15 to 20 minutes. Benzyl alcohol has an excellent safety profile. I am unaware of any reports of immediate allergic reactions or anaphylaxis caused by benzyl alcohol. There have been a few cases of delayed, drug allergy–type reactions from benzyl alcohol used as a preservative in vitamin B_{12} injections.

When using benzyl alcohol–saline as an anesthetic, keep the following points in mind:

1. Benzyl alcohol–saline is only effective for superficial surgery.
2. Inject the benzyl alcohol high in the subcutis so as to balloon-up the tissue.
3. Inject several times as much anesthetic as you would when using lidocaine. It is necessary to render the entire surgical area ballooned-up and edematous.
4. Benzyl alcohol–saline acts instantly, but for only a few minutes; therefore, perform surgery immediately after injecting the anesthetic. This is the direct opposite of the optimal use of lidocaine, in which one should wait a few minutes after injecting the anesthetic before performing surgery.

Supply Hints

Benzyl alcohol–preserved saline is readily available from hospitals and pharmacies in 30-ml multi-use vials. Be sure you use benzyl alcohol–preserved saline, because neither paraben-preserved saline nor plain saline has an anesthetic effect. To prepare 1:300,000 epinephrine in benzyl alcohol–saline, add 0.1 ml of 1:1000 epinephrine solution to a 30-ml vial of benzyl alcohol–saline.

Lidocaine with epinephrine is optimally neutralized by a final concentration of 0.1 mEq/ml of sodium bicarbonate. Mix one part of 1 mEq/ml of sodium bicarbonate solution with nine or ten parts of anesthetic solution. In other words, add 3 ml of sodium bicarbonate 1 mEq/ml to a 30-ml vial of lidocaine; for a 50-ml vial, add 5 ml bicarbonate. A solution of 1 mEq of sodium bicarbonate per ml is equal to 8.4 percent sodium bicarbonate solution, and it is stocked by all hospitals. This solution is only available in single-use vials that are not preservative protected; any leftover bicarbonate solution should be discarded.

ELECTROSURGERY

Electrosurgical† techniques are popular for destroying tissue. The types of currents produced and their actions vary; they all depend on the production of heat. In my opinion, electrosurgical destruction has two applications: (1) point electrocoagulation of bleeding vessels during surgery; and (2) destroying small telangiectases such as vascular spiders. In destroying small blood vessels, bipolar current is superior to monopolar current, and pinpoint epilating needles should be used.

A Brief Diatribe Against Electrodesiccation

Electrodesiccation (electrocoagulation) of skin lesions is fast and simple, yet I believe it should be abandoned for the following reasons:

1. Other techniques cause less scarring. Burn scars are uniquely severe and unsightly (Figures C–116 and C–130 through C–132). Liquid nitrogen, curettage, scissors removal, and scalpel surgery all produce superior cosmetic results with equivalent amounts of tissue destruction.

2. Electrodesiccation is a blind procedure. With curettage, scissors removal, and scalpel surgery, the physician feels and sees the depth of destruction and removal; this is not so with electrodesiccation. Liquid nitrogen destruction has the same handicap as electrodesiccation.

3. Because electrodesiccation thermally "cooks" the tissue, it prevents histologic examination. Curettage, scissors removal, and other cold-steel techniques provide a specimen for histologic confirmation of the diagnosis. The margins of deeper lesions excised with punch or scalpel can be studied for completeness of removal. Again, liquid nitrogen suffers from this same drawback.

Because electrodesiccation suffers from all these handicaps and provides no medical advantage, I have abandoned it except for the two techniques mentioned earlier. Electrodestruction of benign lesions is traditional and popular; unfortunately, it is an inferior technique that should be abandoned by critical physicians seeking the best results.

CURETTAGE

Curettage is best performed using local anesthesia, although some physicians treat multiple superficial keratoses without anesthesia. For keratoses and superficial warts, the curette is held like a pencil in one hand; with short, swift movements, the lesion is scraped from the skin. The fingers of the other hand should stretch the skin tightly during curettage. When warts and deeper lesions are shelled out, it

---

†Electrodesiccation and electrocoagulation are techniques of tissue destruction using high-frequency electric currents. The electrical energy is converted to heat; these methods burn tissue. Electrodesiccation usually refers to superficial destruction with a monopolar current, whereas electrocoagulation refers to the use of a bipolar current to produce a deeper effect.

helps to incise the rim first with a pointed, curved scissors to penetrate the epidermis. Then the curette is used to find the cleavage plane between wart and skin and scoop the lesion out. For optimal healing, stop bleeding by using a tissue-neutral hemostatic (e.g., Gelfoam, Oxycel) and a few minutes of pressure.

Not only does curettage provide tissue for histology, but the feel of lesions during curettage is helpful in diagnosis. Basal-cell carcinomas, for example, have a mushy consistency. Histologic examination of tissue fragments obtained by curettage is simplified when they are allowed to clot together before formalin fixation. Remove bloody fragments from the curette with the point of a scissors or a wooden stick and place them on a piece of smooth paper or on the inside of the specimen bottle, above the formalin. After 5 to 10 minutes, immerse the tissue clot in the fixative. This method will result in a single, easily processed specimen.

USING THE COMEDO EXTRACTOR

When removing comedones (blackheads), use the Unna extractor, centering the opening over the comedo. Then apply firm pressure while wiggling the extractor so as to exert optimal circumferential pressure. If that comedo is not extruded, go on to the next, because comedones often resist removal by reasonable pressure.

The wire-loop Schamberg comedo extractor permits rapid, simple removal of milia (whiteheads) and similar small, superficial cysts. After a tiny nick is made in the overlying skin, firm pressure is applied with the lesion midway in the extractor's loop. Further emptying action is exerted by sliding the extractor's end toward the lesion while maintaining pressure.

CAUTION. Extractors may slip. When working near the eyes, direct pressure on the instrument away from the eyes and shield them with one hand. Pressure with comedo extractors is often painful, especially with the Schamberg model. Before removing small cysts or milia, inject a small amount of local anesthetic into each site.

LIQUID NITROGEN

In using the simple dipstick technique, dip the applicator (see Figure 4–1) in the container of liquid nitrogen and apply its tip to the lesion. As liquid nitrogen runs down the applicator, the skin at the tip turns white; this ice front gradually spreads outward. Stop when the visible freezing extends just beyond the lesion. For a 5- to 10-mm-diameter lesion, 10 to 20 seconds of liquid nitrogen application are generally sufficient. Larger, deeper lesions require longer application. Lesions larger than 15 mm in diameter are best treated by moving the applicator about so as to freeze the entire area without freezing too deeply. Do not dip the applicator back into the reservoir bottle, as viral or bacterial contamination of the liquid nitrogen may occur. Use a fresh applicator or pour a small quantity of liquid nitrogen into a cup and dispose of it when finished (Figures C–55 through C–57).

The duration of freezing also depends on the speed of delivery of liquid nitrogen from your applicator. A large, completely saturated applicator will freeze lesions more rapidly than a small, drier one. Aim to achieve a steady release of small droplets onto the lesion. If large droplets run over the surrounding skin, there is too much liquid nitrogen on the applicator; flick off the excess with a snap of your wrist. The rate of delivery of liquid nitrogen can be adjusted by altering the applicator's angle; the closer to vertical, the more rapid the flow of liquid nitrogen.

Applying liquid nitrogen is an art that can be learned only by experience. If in doubt, err by underfreezing. It is simple to treat residuals a second time; scars from excessive freezing are less correctable. Be suspicious of any lesion that does not respond to liquid nitrogen. If in doubt, biopsy the lesion. Many dermatologists prefer to spray liquid nitrogen using hand-held devices. Manufacturers supply a variety of nozzles and probes. If you are new to liquid nitrogen therapy, try to observe and use both techniques before deciding on which to use in your practice.

Postoperative care after destruction of superficial lesions with liquid nitrogen can be summarized as "ignore." Patients may get the site wet and use makeup, and they need not bandage the site. The necrotic epidermis acts as a protective dressing during skin repair, and infections are very rare. However, healing can be very slow when the feet or lower legs are treated. Garments rubbing on sites treated on the trunk may also delay healing. On the scalp as well as on the dorsa of the hands, blistering and oozing can be an annoying problem. Blisters on the hand often interfere with function. It is perfectly safe and painless for the patient to drain these with a sterile needle. Following liquid nitrogen treatment of eyelid lesions, the loose tissue of the eyelids tends to swell considerably, especially after the patient has been recumbent.

These points are covered in the patient instruction sheet on liquid nitrogen. However, it is wise to alert patients to potential problems when the scalp, eyelids, hands, legs, or feet are treated. Furthermore, the generally uneventful healing and freedom from infection only apply to superficially treated lesions. When liquid nitrogen is used to freeze deeper lesions or is used in skin cancer treatment, deep, draining wounds that require appropriate postoperative care are produced.

PUNCH BIOPSY

When biopsying, mark the area to be biopsied before injecting the local anesthetic. Punch biopsy should always be done with anesthesia. After anesthesia, immobilize the skin with the fingers of one hand while coring out a cylinder of skin by twirling the punch between the fingers of the other. As the punch traverses from the dermis into the fat, resistance lessens. When this lessening of resistance is felt, you are deep enough. When the punch is removed, the core of tissue usually pops up slightly and can be snipped off at the level of the subcutaneous fat with a curved iris scissors without using a forceps. If the tissue cored by the punch does not pop up, you may elevate it with a hypodermic needle or very-fine-toothed forceps (see previous remarks regarding the Castroviejo forceps) and then snip it off. Ordinary forceps may squeeze and distort a small biopsy specimen.

Hemostasis after punch biopsy can be accomplished with Gelfoam packing. Defects from 1.5- and 2.0-mm punches usually do not require suturing and will heal virtually invisibly. Punch defects in the 2-to-3.5-mm range can generally be closed completely with a single suture. Complete closure of larger punch defects frequently leads to dog-earing and should be avoided. Partial closure of a round defect is most practical and is discussed in the next section of this chapter.

With a 1.5-mm punch, you can take biopsy specimens in cosmetically sensitive areas with virtually perfect results. It is better cosmetically to take two or three 1.5-mm samples from a large lesion than one 3- or 4-mm specimen. When several small specimens are taken from a single lesion, they can be combined in one tissue bottle, and the pathologist is informed that they can be mounted on the same slide.

Multiple, small biopsies are an excellent way to delineate the extent of a basal-cell carcinoma with indistinct borders. The location of each biopsy should be sketched out and each specimen submitted in a separate bottle.

The punch is an effective tool for removing small, round lesions. The margins of the lesion should be marked prior to infiltrating the local anesthetic. After the anesthetic has been infiltrated, the diameter of the lesion is measured, the punch chosen, and the lesion removed. This fast method produces excellent results with small lesions.

TANGENTIAL SURGERY FOR REMOVAL OF SUPERFICIAL LESIONS

Superficial lesions can be removed by a slice or shave technique using a sharp blade; the technique is called tangential surgery. Tangential surgery is an excellent way of removing superficial lesions in toto, thereby providing an intact specimen for diagnosis and histologic control of margins. A scalpel blade can be used; however, much more precise control of margins and depths is possible if a straight, rigid blade is employed—much as surgeons use straight, rigid blades for obtaining skin grafts. The single-edge razor blade is an ideal instrument; for lesions smaller than 14 mm wide, cut the single-edge blade in half with tin snips. Tangential surgery is best performed on flat or convex skin surfaces, and should usually be restricted to the trunk and extremities. On the face, other techniques tend to produce better cosmetic results.

You may be reluctant to use a razor blade for surgery. The naked razor blade is not a traditional surgical instrument, and it is easy to be concerned about cutting too deeply. Actually, the usual problem is not cutting deeply enough. Only the central part of the blade is used; the ends remain above the surface of the surrounding skin (Figure C–14), so that on flat surfaces it's almost impossible to cut too deeply. In fact, on flat surfaces, it helps to inject the local anesthetic superficially in order to raise the lesion above the surrounding skin. The procedure is different for convex surfaces, in which the middle of the blade may be cutting quite deeply while the ends are still above the surrounding normal skin. Be careful in performing tangential surgery on strongly convex surfaces such as the fingers.

The following list outlines the procedure for tangential surgery:

1. Using magnification and good illumination, outline the exact margins of the lesion with a pointed, felt-tipped pen.

2. Draw a second line approximately 1.5 mm outside the borders of the lesion. This will be the line of excision (Figure C–13).

3. Just before excision, inject a local anesthetic high in the dermis to elevate the lesion and firm the skin; aim to have the anesthetic spread just beyond the outer line (Figure C–13).

4. Have an assistant stretch the skin by pulling in the line of blade movement. For excisions larger than 14 mm wide, use a single-edge blade. For smaller lesions, use a single-edge blade cut in half (Figure C–14).

5. While excising the lesion with slow, short, sawing movements of the blade, use the fingers of the other hand to elevate and stretch the lesion while depressing the surrounding normal skin (Figure C–14).

6. As a guide to depth, observe the blade edge and the writing on the blade as you cut. If the edge and lettering are discernible through the skin, the depth is less than 0.8 mm.

7. To preserve the specimen in a flat condition, slide it onto cardboard or foam and let the blood clot a few minutes before immersing the specimen and its carrier in formalin.

8. Control bleeding at the excision site with a tissue-neutral hemostatic, such as Gelfoam or a collagen, and pressure. Electrodesiccation, Monsel's solution, and aluminum chloride all increase tissue necrosis, worsen the scar, and are to be avoided.

9. The wound is dressed with antibiotic ointment and a Band-Aid. Tape several layers of gauze over the dressing to absorb any postoperative bleeding. Explain the purpose of this second dressing to the patient; it may be removed in 6 to 12 hours.

10. Tell the patient to change the Band-Aid once or twice daily and apply antibiotic ointment with each dressing change. Provide him or her with wound care instructions such as the patient sheets Care After Superficial Surgery or Wound Care.

11. Healing time depends on the size and location of the lesion. Since most lesions heal by 4 weeks, have the patient return for follow-up in 5 to 6 weeks.

EXCISION WITH PARTIAL CLOSURE

Concern about closing wounds makes some physicians reluctant to excise lesions in locations where the traditional excision and complete closure are not feasible. Complete closure is desirable, but it is by no means necessary. Wounds that are left open often heal with excellent cosmetic results, especially on the face. Simple excision and allowing the wound to granulate are effective in areas such as the nose, where complete closure would require grafting or other plastic surgical procedures. In these situations, my preference is to close the wound partially with sutures, being careful not to distort the tissues. The unclosed portion is allowed to heal secondarily. This technique permits the physician with limited surgical skills to utilize the advantages of excisional surgery in areas where the conventional fusiform excision and complete closure are not possible. A minimum amount of normal tissue is sacrificed, and the tissues are not compromised if additional surgical procedures are needed.

If excision with partial closure is used, it is important that the open portion of the wound not be electrocoagulated or treated with chemical styptics. Bleeding should be controlled with pressure and packing with absorbable material. Sutures can usually be removed 3 to 5 days after the procedure.

BURIED SUTURES FOR WOUND CLOSURE

Buried sutures are useful in closing skin wounds in two ways. Buried sutures remove tension from the wound edges. Subsequent percutaneous sutures can be loosely applied and removed after 3 to 4 days without leaving any marks. Many wounds, especially those on the trunk, can be closed exclusively using buried sutures. The simplest technique—and the one I prefer—is to use interrupted buried subcutaneous sutures placed at a small distance from the wound edge. This requires undermining of the wound edges, which is valuable anyway for optimal cosmetic results. The procedure is illustrated in Figure 4–3.

Wounds on the trunk and proximal extremities tend to stretch, there is little

Figure 4–3. Placement of a buried vertical mattress suture. (A) The suture is started at the base of the skin flap so that the knot will be buried. The skin edge is pivoted over the fingertip using a skin hook (or forceps) to facilitate suture placement. To achieve eversion, it is important to place the suture closest to the epidermis at a point 3 to 4 mm from the skin edge, and deeper in the dermis at the edge. (B) The suture is placed in the opposite skin edge in a mirror-image fashion. (C) Final appearance of the suture, with the knot tied at the base. The edge is everted and prolonged support provided without causing suture marks. (From Zitelli A, Moy RL: Buried vertical mattress suture. *J Dermatol Surg Oncol* 15(1):17–19, 1989.)

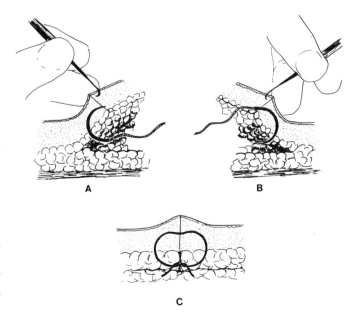

point in precise approximation of the wound edges. Consequently, closure with buried sutures alone provides a scar without the "railroad tracks" that percutaneous sutures produce at these sites (Figures C–117 through C–120).

For wound closure with buried sutures, use synthetic absorbable suture material; gut and chromic gut are obsolete. The older synthetic absorbable sutures were braided; polyglycolic acid (Dexon; Davis and Geck) and polyglactin (Vicryl; Ethicon) were the types used in the United States. Both have an in vivo half-life tensile strength of 2 weeks. Of the newer monofilament absorbable synthetics, polyglyconate (Maxon; Davis and Geck) has a half-life tensile strength of 3 weeks, whereas polydioxanone (PDS; Ethicon) has a 6-week half-life tensile strength. The monofilament synthetics produce less tissue drag but require more knots to hold securely. Maxon requires at least four throws, whereas six throws are needed for secure knots of PDS. PDS tends to curl; Maxon handles more easily than PDS. In addition to their longer in vivo half-life tensile strength, the monofilament sutures produce less foreign-body reaction. As expected, physicians vary widely in their preference. I have largely abandoned Vicryl, my former favorite, for Maxon when suturing the face or neck, and I use PDS when suturing the trunk. In general, I use 5-0 Maxon for the face, 4-0 Maxon for the neck and scalp, and 1-0 or 2-0 PDS for the trunk. Three individual buried vertical mattress sutures suffice for most skin wound closures. For small wounds, one or two sutures often are enough. For lengthy wounds, five to seven sutures are used.

For precise apposition of the wound edges, interrupted or running percutaneous sutures are used. These are removed in 3 to 4 days from the face and in 6 to 7 days from the trunk. When a return visit to remove stitches will be difficult or impossible, gut percutaneous sutures may be used. This is discussed in the next section in this chapter. On the face, however, monofilament nonabsorbent synthetic percutaneous sutures removed in a few days yield predictable, superior results.

Occluded wounds heal more rapidly than nonoccluded wounds. I use a combination of antibacterial ointment plus a piece of the suture wrapping to accomplish occlusion. Sutures are packaged in either metal foil or an impermeable cellophane-like material. Both kinds of packages are sterile and make excellent nonstick occlusive dressings for the first layer after application of the antibacterial ointment, which is then covered by gauze and affixed with tape. Any blood that escapes from beneath the edges of the foil is caught by the overlying gauze. This method provides less occlusion than adherent plastic dressings, but it is more occlusive than gauze or Telfa.

On the trunk, I generally close with buried sutures only. Following wound closure, Mastisol or spirit gum is painted up to the wound edges and a tape support is applied; over this is placed the foil and gauze dressing. The patient removes the foil and gauze dressing after about 2 days but leaves the tape support on for 1 week. The area may be gotten wet, because water will not dislodge the Mastisol or the spirit gum and tape.

WOUND CLOSURE WITH PERCUTANEOUS DISSOLVING SUTURES

Synthetic absorbable sutures are unsuitable for percutaneous wound closure, because they take many weeks or months to dissolve. However, gut can be used in certain situations. Plain gut sutures will dissolve in a few days to several weeks, depending on the location of the wound, the size of the suture, and individual variation. In general, gut sutures should not be used when there is significant tension or when cosmetic results are critical. Although some have advocated the use of chromic gut for skin sutures, I have abandoned it, because it may take 2 weeks or more to dissolve and frequently leaves railroad-track scars.

Wounds without any tension are ideal for closure with gut percutaneous sutures. I routinely remove scalp cysts through a linear incision without removing any of the overlying stretched skin. One or two sutures of 4-0 gut close these lesions without any tension, and the sutures usually fall out within 2 weeks (Figures C–32 through C–34). Nodular chondrodermatitis treated with cartilage removal alone leaves loose, somewhat redundant skin that can be closed with 6-0 plain gut, which generally falls out in 1 week. On the face, in wounds closed with buried vertical mattress sutures of absorbable synthetic, the skin edges can be precisely approximated using 6-0 fast-absorbing gut (Ethicon). Fast-absorbing gut is a specially heat-treated gut that disintegrates more rapidly than plain gut. In my experience, it has occasionally left fine suture-mark scars. However, 6-0 fast-absorbing gut is convenient when cosmetic results are not critical. I make use of this approach fairly frequently in older patients who have traveled some distance to have a skin cancer excised.

POSTOPERATIVE WOUND SUPPORT AND CARE

When closing a wound with only absorbable sutures—either buried mattress sutures alone or in combination with percutaneous gut—I apply a tape support directly over the wound after surgery. After wound closure and cessation of bleeding, I paint Mastisol or spirit gum on the wound edges up to the suture line. I use nonsterile fabric or flesh-colored paper tape, applied so as to "tent-up" the wound edges slightly and take tension off the wound. Over this, I place foil or other occlusive material, then add a gauze-and-tape dressing, which is removed in 2 to 3 days. The tape is to be kept in place 1 week or longer, if possible. The suture remnants usually come off when the tape separates. Follow-up care is detailed in the patient information sheet Care of Wounds Closed With Dissolving Stitches.

In hairy areas, prolonged tape support is not feasible. I do not use a dressing on the scalp after cyst removal and closure with percutaneous gut suture. I tell male patients to remove tape on the beard area gently when beard growth has loosened it and to leave the wound open.

ELECTROCOAGULATION OF SMALL BLOOD VESSELS

Vascular spiders can be treated by electrocoagulation using a bipolar current. The bipolar current is definitely superior to a monopolar current in treating these lesions. A small, pointed needle that can penetrate skin is required. Either a commercial epilating needle or a 30-gauge hypodermic needle is suitable.

In treating vascular spiders, adjust the apparatus for bipolar coagulation at a low-to-medium setting to produce a spark about 1 to 2 mm between the needle and the ground electrode. The patient then firmly grasps the ground electrode between his hands. With the current off, plunge the point of the needle several millimeters into the central part of the spider to the estimated depth of the vascular lesion. Then turn the current on briefly. The vessel should blanch. If it does not, increase the current intensity and repeat the treatment. Under no condition should there be any surface sparking or surface necrosis. Should surface sparking occur, it indicates the use of too strong a current or the patient is not adequately grounded.

The aim of this treatment is to produce a small, deep scar that destroys the blood vessel but is invisibly small. The bipolar current permits deep destruction with sparing of the epidermis. More than one treatment is often necessary. Sometimes it is impossible to eradicate a vascular spider in this manner. Until the physician becomes experienced with this technique, he or she should be very cautious and err on the side of too low current. The treatment can always be repeated.

Patients with myriads of small telangiectases—common in persons of Celtic ancestry and actinic damage—are probably best treated with one of the newer vascular-specific lasers. The flash-lamp pulsed tunable dye laser and the copper vapor laser selectively destroy blood vessels with minimal damage to surrounding tissue. These are expensive machines; however, in trained hands, they are capable of excellent results. Treatment of fine, multiple, very superficial vessels with electrodesiccation results in varying degrees of epidermal necrosis and some degree of scarring. It is also very tedious. Newer developments in laser technology may soon render electrocoagulation of cutaneous vessels obsolete.

REFERENCES

1. Bennett RG: *Fundamentals of Cutaneous Surgery.* St. Louis: Mosby, 1988
2. Roenick RK, Roenick HH Jr: *Dermatologic Surgery: Principles and Practice.* New York: Dekker, 1989
3. Epstein E, Epstein E Jr: *Skin Surgery,* 6th ed. Philadelphia: WB Saunders, 1987
4. Stegman SJ, Tromovitch TA, Glogau RG: *Basics of Dermatologic Surgery.* Chicago: Year Book Medical Publishers, 1982
5. Coleman WP, Colon GA, Davis RS: *Outpatient Surgery of the Skin.* New York: Medical Examination, 1983
6. Salasche SJ, Bernstein G, Senkarik M: *Surgical Anatomy of the Skin.* Norwalk CT: Appleton & Lange, 1988
7. Swanson NA: *Atlas of Cutaneous Surgery.* Boston: Little, Brown, 1987

Acne

Patient sheets pages P–5, P–57, P–87, P–113, P–127

5

ETIOLOGY

Acne, an inflammatory disorder of the sebaceous glands, is exceedingly common among teenagers and frequently continues into adulthood. The fact that innumerable remedies are advertised to the medical profession and the public indicates that none is satisfactory.

Certain drugs, notably the iodides and bromides, but also systemic corticosteroids, can produce acneiform eruptions. Acneiform eruptions may be caused or aggravated by externally applied fluorinated hydrocarbons, cutting oils, pomades, and other greasy materials.

DIAGNOSIS

The appearance of acne is distinctive, and diagnosis is usually easy. Rosacea (i.e., acne rosacea) has some resemblance to acne but lacks comedones, has patchy erythema, and preferentially affects middle-aged and elderly persons. The poorly understood syndrome known as perioral dermatitis has acneiform papules and pustules but, unlike adult acne, also has patches of low-grade dermatitis. Isolated deep inflammatory lesions—acne abscesses—may be indistinguishable from furuncles or inflamed cysts.

TREATMENT

Most textbooks make acne therapy sound simple and logical. It is neither. There are myriad treatments, each with champions and detractors. Although many dermatologists proclaim their success in treating acne, our patients are less convinced. It is common to encounter patients who are distressed because their continuing acne has not benefited from consultation with several dermatologists.

NONINFLAMMATORY ACNE LESIONS

Mechanical Removal

The therapy of noninflammatory lesions differs from that of inflammatory lesions. Comedones (i.e., blackheads) and closed comedones (i.e., whiteheads*) are noninflammatory lesions. They usually cause little distress. These lesions can be removed mechanically with comedo extractors and a fine needle or pointed blade to open closed comedones. Such maneuvers are temporary; new comedones form promptly. Many dermatologists believe—without proof—that mechanically removing comedones prevents the formation of inflammatory lesions. My belief is that mechanical removal is worthless.

I play down the significance of comedones to see whether patients are willing to ignore them. Most patients are content to live with blackheads once they understand that they are not caused by dirt and do not exacerbate their acne. I encourage women to conceal them with water-based makeup.

Topical Therapy

Some patients do request treatment for their open and closed comedones. The best agent is tretinoin (retinoic acid, Retin-A). Although it is effective, it acts slowly and is irritating. Start with the least irritating concentration of tretinoin, which is the 0.025 percent cream. Tretinoin should be applied sparingly at bedtime to the involved areas or to the entire face. Instruct the patient to initiate treatment by using the tretinoin cream every other night for 2 weeks. The aim is to produce minimal inflammation with little dryness and scaling. With time, the skin adjusts to treatment; after 2 weeks, the patient can try applying the tretinoin cream every night. If, after 2 or 3 months, the response is inadequate, the concentration of tretinoin can be increased to 0.05 percent, and ultimately to 0.1 percent.

Tretinoin is not an easy topical to use. The patient instruction sheet, Retin-A for Acne, is a great help, but there is no substitute for carefully going over these points with the patient in person. Because tretinoin is an irritant, other irritating acne agents, such as benzoyl peroxide preparations, astringents, or abrasive scrubs, should be avoided. Soap should be used sparingly. Tretinoin tends to make patients more sensitive to sunlight, but in my experience, the increase in sun sensitivity is mild.

Warn the patient of tretinoin's irritating potential, and counsel patience. Two to three months are usually required before there is significant improvement in the number of open and closed comedones. The effect of tretinoin is temporary; maintenance treatment is required for long-term control.

Topicals containing benzoyl peroxide are of proven effectiveness in reducing the number of comedones. Benzoyl peroxide is drying and irritating; many patients dislike using it. As with tretinoin, the frequency and concentration of benzoyl peroxide must be adjusted to produce only minimal irritation. Acne topicals containing benzoyl peroxide are available both over the counter and by prescription.

Abrasive scrubs and chemical peels using a wide variety of acids and other agents are widely touted as useful for limiting comedones and closed comedones. Unfortunately, these claims are not backed by controlled studies.

INFLAMMATORY LESIONS

The inflammatory lesions of acne—papules and pustules—are what really concern patients. The many therapies currently in vogue, and my assessment of their

---

*The term whitehead is used to describe two different lesions. Acne patients use whitehead to describe swollen sebaceous glands without the comedo plug visible on the surface. However, the term is also used by patients with milia, which are small cysts and have nothing to do with acne.

effectiveness, are summarized in Table 5–1. Except for isotretinoin, current acne therapies are of benefit only while they are being used. Consequently, they should be continued for months or years until the acne resolves spontaneously. Isotretinoin produces prolonged remissions, usually lasting for years.

The therapeutic measures outlined in Table 5–1 differ; some aim to hasten involution of established lesions, while the intent of others is to prevent new lesions. Intralesional corticosteroids, although subduing the lesions injected, do not prevent the development of new lesions. Effective systemic antibiotic therapy does suppress the formation of new inflammatory lesions—a result patients prefer.

Only systemic antibiotics, isotretinoin (13-*cis*-retinoic acid), and topical antimicrobials have been shown to be effective in suppressing acne. Of these three treatments, systemic antibiotics are by far the most useful. Isotretinoin, a vitamin A derivative, is almost always effective against severe nodulocystic acne that has failed to respond to systemic antibiotics. It has the additional advantage of prolonged improvement after therapy ends. However, because of its significant toxicity, it will not replace systemic antibiotics as the mainstay of acne therapy. Isotretinoin is a potent teratogen, frequently causes increases in serum lipids, and routinely produces cutaneous side effects, including cheilitis, nosebleeds, stomatitis, and xerosis.

Topical Therapy

Topical antibiotics combine proven effectiveness with cosmetic elegance. The currently available preparations are erythromycin (e.g., Akne-mycin ointment, A/T/S

Table 5–1. **SUMMARY OF TREATMENT OF INFLAMMATORY ACNE**

Treatment	Effectiveness
Topical Therapy	
Topical antibiotics in special formulations	+
Benzoyl peroxide	+
Tretinoin	+
Sulfur, resorcinol, and salicylic acid	?
Medicated soaps and cleansers	0
Abradant cleansers	0
Acetone, alcohol, and other degreasing lotions	0
Systemic Therapy	
Isotretinoin (Accutane)	+
Antibiotics	+
Corticosteroids	(+)sp
Sex hormones and antiandrogens	(+)sp
Vitamins	0
Office Procedures	
Acne surgery	(+)sp
Intralesional corticosteroids	+
Cryotherapy	?
Ultraviolet therapy	0
X-ray therapy	*
Miscellaneous	
Psychological factors	+
Sunshine	†
Diet	?
Skin hygiene	0
Nervous tension	?
Cosmetics	?

Abbreviations: +, effective; (+)sp, effective in special situations; ?, possibly slightly effective; 0, of no benefit.

*X-ray therapy has been proven effective in suppressing acne. In my opinion, its risks outweigh its benefits.

†Many, but not all acne patients benefit from sunlight.

lotion, EryDerm lotion, Erymax, T-Stat), clindamycin (Cleocin T lotion, solution, and gel), and meclocycline sulfosalicylate (Meclan cream). Topical clindamycin has caused rare cases of diarrhea and colitis; the other preparations are free of systemic side effects.

It is difficult to offer guidelines regarding which topical antibiotic to prescribe, because the field is continually changing, and there is a lack of adequate comparison trials. I use the topical antibiotics my patients like. Erythromycin solution and clindamycin solution have hydroalcoholic vehicles that most patients tolerate well. These two antibiotics are also available in gel forms, which some patients prefer. For patients with dry or irritable skin, I favor meclocycline cream; clindamycin lotion, which has a cream-type vehicle; or erythromycin ointment, specifically Aknemycin ointment.

Benzoyl peroxide is a widely used, potent antimicrobial. Many dermatologists swear by it. Benzoyl peroxide is available both by prescription and over the counter in a variety of creams, gels, and liquids. A distinct advantage of benzoyl peroxide is that it effectively reduces both inflammatory lesions and comedones. On the negative side, it tends to irritate the skin and occasionally causes contact allergy. Many patients have already tried benzoyl peroxide on their own before consulting a physician.

Sulfur, resorcinol, and salicylic acid are the classic old-time topical agents. The fact that none of these has ever been shown effective in controlled studies has not prevented their extensive use in both over-the-counter and prescription acne remedies. Topicals containing retinoic acid (tretinoin), of proven effectiveness in treating comedones and other noninflammatory lesions, are of less value in the therapy of inflammatory acne.

There is no evidence that special soaps, abradant cleansers, astringents, and similar products are of benefit in inflammatory acne. I tell patients they are a waste of money and advise ordinary soap and water for cleansing. Overenthusiastic use of acne cleansers may lead to low-grade facial irritant dermatitis.

Systemic Therapy

ANTIBIOTICS. Systemic antibiotics are the most common therapy for acne. The practical aspects deserve a detailed discussion. Start with tetracycline. Keep in mind that there is no standard dosage of tetracycline in acne patients, and that not all persons respond to tetracycline. A few patients do well on as little as 250 to 500 mg of tetracycline per day; however, the majority will require 1 g or more to show a satisfactory result. The response of acne to antibiotics is gradual; it takes 6 weeks to determine whether the medication is of benefit.

Tetracycline should be taken on an empty stomach; food significantly interferes with its absorption, as do calcium, iron tablets, antacids, milk, and other dairy products, all of which bind with tetracycline to form insoluble complexes that are not absorbed from the digestive tract. These substances must not be taken at the same time as tetracycline. Tetracycline has a significant clinical interaction with certain drugs, such as lithium. It also interacts with oral contraceptives; whether this interaction is clinically significant is doubtful. All of this information must be reviewed with patients; it is best to give them the patient sheet Tetracycline Treatment of Skin Disorders and then review it with them.

Despite occasional reports, the best current data indicate that tetracycline does not increase oral contraceptive failure. I continue to prescribe tetracycline for women taking birth-control pills, but for medicolegal reasons, I provide them with current information regarding the reports of oral contraceptive failure associated with tetracycline intake.

For patients not previously treated with systemic antibiotics, initiate therapy with a 6-week course of 1 g of tetracycline per day. Tetracycline is taken in two 500-

mg doses with water on an empty stomach, once on arising and once in the afternoon or evening; avoid bedtime dosing because it may cause esophagitis. Tell the patient not to consume dairy products within 1 hour of ingesting tetracycline. Mention the possibility of the occurrence of yeast vaginitis to women, and suggest that if this develops, they treat it with over-the-counter clotrimazole (Gyne-Lotrimin), miconazole (Monistat), or a similar preparation. At the 6-week follow-up visit, the patient's skin will be: (1) greatly improved; (2) partially but definitely improved; (3) unchanged or equivocal; or (4) worse.

The dramatically improved patient is a delight, but these are the minority. Improvement usually continues for another 6 to 8 weeks on the same dosage. After that, gradual reduction may be attempted. To find the smallest effective daily dose of tetracycline, have the patient decrease his or her daily ration by 250 mg at 6-week intervals. When the acne flares up, the patient should return to the dose that previously controlled the condition. This attempt to reduce the dose should be repeated. I generally prescribe a 4-month supply of tetracycline and ask the patient to return before the supply is exhausted. The patient instruction sheet, Long-Term Tetracycline Treatment, explains the details of this gradual decrease and allows the physician to write in a suggested schedule.

When the patient shows a partial response, I generally increase the tetracycline dosage to 1.5 g/day, usually as 750 mg taken twice daily. The patient is instructed to return in 6 weeks for another evaluation. If the response to the higher dose of tetracycline is satisfactory, I frequently have the patient continue on the same dose (1.5 g/day) for 2 to 3 months. If there is some response to tetracycline in 6 weeks, the same dose will usually produce additional benefit over the succeeding months.

When there is an equivocal response or failure, you have the arbitrary choice of trying a higher dose of tetracycline or changing to another antibiotic. Except during the summer months, I tend to use a higher dose of tetracycline. During the summer (i.e., tetracycline causes photosensitivity), or if the patient asks for another antibiotic, I use erythromycin.

When the patient's acne is worse after a trial of tetracycline, it should be explained that this was not the result of the tetracycline, but that the acne was in a spontaneously worsening phase. Antibiotics do not aggravate acne, except for the rare complication of gram-negative folliculitis.

The commonest complication of tetracycline therapy is yeast vaginitis. There are no hard data as to its frequency, but I estimate it occurs in about 10 percent of female acne patients receiving 1 g of tetracycline daily. Women should be routinely warned about it. The onset of genital itching and a vaginal discharge is an indication for specific anticandidal therapy; however, the tetracycline should be continued. If the vaginal symptoms do not clear rapidly, with an over-the-counter anticandidal agent, I advise the patient to consult her general physician or gynecologist for the proper pelvic examination. Not all cases of vaginitis are caused by yeast.

Phototoxicity is the second most common complication. Patients taking 250 to 500 mg daily rarely experience this complication. On 1 g a day, in sunny climates, many patients will sunburn easily. At 2 g daily, almost all patients will burn easily and must be warned to take appropriate sun-protective measures. I routinely provide them with the patient instruction sheet, Sunlight and Your Skin. The hands are frequently the site of sunburn, and photo-onycholysis—separation of the nail plate from its bed as a result of sunshine—is an occasional, distressing occurrence. Fortunately, this condition is reversible.

Gastrointestinal distress occurs occasionally. Usually it is temporary. Try having the patient divide the daily tetracycline ration into four doses rather than two. If there are still problems, start with one tetracycline capsule per day and see if this dose can gradually be increased. If the gastrointestinal distress persists, or if there is severe presternal burning or discomfort (i.e., heartburn), discontinue the tetracycline. Esophageal erosions may have occurred. Tetracycline taken at bedtime seems to be the common denominator in patients with this complication. It is a good idea to advise patients to take their tetracycline before bedtime with a full glass of water.

Blistering of the sun-exposed extremities and face, producing a porphyrialike clinical picture, is a rare complication. If this occurs, discontinue the tetracycline. Colitis as a complication of tetracycline therapy in otherwise healthy acne patients is exceedingly rare. However, if a patient complains that tetracycline gives him or her diarrhea, discontinue the drug.

Tetracycline should be discontinued if the patient becomes pregnant, because the drug is incorporated into the fetal bones and teeth. However, tetracycline does not cause birth defects. Tetracycline is contraindicated in children younger than 8 years of age, because it discolors the permanent teeth; however, acne is rare in this age group. In patients with inadequate renal function, tetracycline should not be prescribed. Some physicians periodically perform blood counts and urinalyses on patients taking long-term tetracycline. There does not seem to be any rationale for this practice.

ALTERNATIVE ANTIBIOTICS. If tetracycline fails, even when given in doses as high as 2 to 3 g/day, try another antibiotic. There is no rational way of choosing an alternative antibiotic; every physician has his or her favorites. I use erythromycin if tetracycline fails or produces annoying side effects. Erythromycin has been used for many years, is remarkably safe, and does not cause photosensitivity. Like other antibiotics, it may cause yeast vaginitis. It does have one major drawback: It frequently causes gastrointestinal disturbances severe enough to warrant discontinuing the drug. This happens so often that I give patients a 3- to 4-day supply of erythromycin from my office stock for them to try before having their prescription filled.

CAUTION. **Erythromycin interacts with a number of other drugs, especially theophylline, which is widely used in treating asthma.**

One salt of erythromycin, the estolate, may cause hepatic dysfunction and should not be used in the treatment of acne. Erythromycin base, stearate, and ethyl succinate are all safe for the treatment of acne.

If neither tetracycline nor erythromycin is effective, I prescribe minocycline. Start with 100 mg/day; if there is no response, cautiously increase the dosage to 150 or possibly 200 mg/day. The chief adverse effect of minocycline is dizziness. This side effect is dose-related and is rare on a daily dose of 100 mg or less. Very rarely, prolonged use of minocycline colors the skin gray or blue-black; this effect is reversible. Minocycline is well tolerated by the gastrointestinal tract and may be taken with meals. It is not a photosensitizer, but it is expensive.

Doxycycline is another tetracycline derivative effective in treating acne and is far less expensive than minocycline. The usual dose is 100 mg/day; some patients require 200 mg/day to respond. It may be taken with food or milk. Doxycycline is a significant photosensitizer; explicitly warn patients regarding this side effect. Gastrointestinal irritation is the other main side effect.

Failure of adequate doses of tetracycline, erythromycin, doxycycline, and minocycline to produce results is not uncommon. First, be sure you are not dealing with gram-negative folliculitis (discussed in the following section in this chapter). If patients fail to respond to these four low-risk antibiotics, a decision must be made whether to try antimicrobials with a riskier profile or proceed to isotretinoin. Three antimicrobials in this category are trimethoprim-sulfamethoxazole (Bactrim, Septra), clindamycin, and ampicillin. All have been shown effective in treating acne by controlled studies; all have significant drawbacks. Trimethoprim-sulfamethoxazole is one of the more effective antiacne agents, but its sulfonamide component may cause blood dyscrasia (obtain periodic blood counts) and the rare but serious allergic reaction known as the Stevens-Johnson syndrome. Clindamycin occasionally causes pseudomembranous colitis. Allergic reactions to ampicillin are not infrequent. The risks of using these agents should be clearly explained to the patient and weighed—by both the patient and physician—in deciding whether to use these agents or isotretinoin. In considering these alternatives, explain to patients that there is no guarantee that they will respond to one of these antimicrobials; however, isotretinoin almost always produces results.

GRAM-NEGATIVE FOLLICULLITIS. Gram-negative folliculitis is a complication that may occur in patients on long-term antibiotics. It may present either as worsening of previously controlled acne or as a sudden eruption of inflamed, pustular lesions. A variety of gram-negative organisms may be the cause; it is not clear from the literature whether multiple cultures are required to make the diagnosis.

Although antibiotic therapy with ampicillin or another agent directed at the causative organism may be effective, gram-negative folliculitis is usually an indication for isotretinoin. Isotretinoin generally eradicates both the gram-negative folliculitis and the underlying acne disorder. From a practical point of view, performing multiple bacterial culture and sensitivity studies on a patient with suspected gram-negative folliculitis may not be cost-effective. A single culture and sensitivity procedure costs more than $100, and one usually proceeds to isotretinoin treatment for antibiotic-resistant acne anyway; therefore, it is difficult to justify the expense of searching for gram-negative folliculitis.

ISOTRETINOIN. Isotretinoin (Accutane) revolutionized the therapy of severe, recalcitrant acne. The patient with severe, nodulocystic, draining acne who had unsuccessfully sought relief from numerous dermatologists can now be cured with isotretinoin. This benefit has a price; isotretinoin is a potent teratogen that has produced severe birth defects in infants born of mothers who are taking it. Isotretinoin acts differently than the antibiotics. Antibiotics suppress acne only while they are being taken; isotretinoin's effect generally lasts for 1 year or more posttherapy. Usually, isotretinoin requires 16 to 20 weeks to produce clearing. Isotretinoin's effect is gradual, and there is no improvement in the first month; in fact, some patients' acne worsens during the first 6 weeks of therapy. Usually by week 8 of therapy, improvement is apparent, and clearing continues.

Isotretinoin has varied biologic effects, including reduction of sebaceous gland activity. It causes many side effects [Table 5–2; refer to the patient instruction sheet, Isotretinoin (Accutane)]. Most minor side effects have been known since the first published studies on isotretinoin in 1979. Skeletal toxicity was first reported in 1983, and in 1986, the first report of abnormal retinal function associated with isotretinoin therapy appeared. Skeletal toxicity does not appear to be a problem with the short course of isotretinoin used in treating acne; however, the retinal changes were observed in acne patients.

The diversity and frequency of isotretinoin's side effects limit its use to treatment of acne that is unresponsive to other measures. Patients being treated with isotretinoin should be checked periodically, have appropriate laboratory work performed, and be asked about unusual side effects. The manufacturer's literature on isotretinoin emphasizes its restriction to patients with severe cystic acne; however, most knowledgeable dermatologists frequently use it for moderate acne that fails to respond to topical and systemic antimicrobials. As we have become better acquainted with isotretinoin, it is evident that although mild side effects are common, serious side effects are rare, except for the problem of birth defects. Consequently, increasing numbers of patients with chronic adult acne—especially women beyond childbearing age and men—are being treated with isotretinoin. Their delight is almost universal; after years of struggling with their unsightly blemishes, they finally have a clear complexion and no longer require long-term oral antibiotics.

Isotretinoin's most serious side effect—birth defects—is preventable. Women of childbearing age should be tested for pregnancy and told to use two methods of effective contraception for at least 1 month before starting isotretinoin and for 2 months after the duration of therapy. The manufacturer (Roche) has a pregnancy-

Table 5–2. **ADVERSE EFFECTS OF ISOTRETINOIN**

Type of Effect	Frequency* (%)
Common	
1. Cheilitis	100
2. Dry skin, desquamation of central face, pruritus, nonspecific symptoms related to dryness of nose and mouth, epistaxis	90
3. Conjunctivitis	40
4. Epistaxis	30
5. Hyperlipidemia	
a. Elevation of plasma triglycerides†	10–25
b. Elevation of cholesterol‡	3–7
6. Musculoskeletal symptoms	40
7. Thinning of hair	10
8. Rash	15
9. Peeling of palms and soles, skin infections, nonspecific gastrointestinal symptoms, headache, increased susceptibility to sunburn	5
Less Common	
1. Hematuria	
2. Liver function test abnormalities	
3. Depression	
4. Visual abnormalities, corneal opacities, abnormal retinal function	
5. Inflammatory bowel disease (association is not certain)	
6. Skeletal toxicity (associated with higher isotretinoin doses than generally employed for treatment of acne)	

*Compiled from manufacturer's data and other sources. Cheilitis, dry skin, or both occur in all patients taking isotretinoin

†Clinically significant triglyceride elevation occurs in fewer than 5% of patients with normal baseline values.

‡Clinically significant elevation of cholesterol is rare.

prevention program that includes reimbursing the patient for a gynecologic consultation. If contraceptive failure occurs, I believe an abortion is indicated. Fortunately, isotretinoin does not linger in the body; pregnancy is considered safe 2 months after therapy ends. Before starting isotretinoin therapy in a woman of childbearing age, I have her read and sign an informed consent form (Figure 5–1) agreeing to an abortion if she becomes pregnant while taking isotretinoin. The signed original is given to the patient; a photocopy is filed in the chart. Almost all patients have readily signed this form. A few have expressed reservations; for these, I have not prescribed isotretinoin.

A 16- to 20-week course of isotretinoin suffices in the treatment of acne. Until recently, there has been less agreement about the optimal daily dose. Originally, doses ranging from 1 to 2 mg/kg/day were recommended; however, later it was shown that lower doses, even as little as 0.1 mg/kg/day, produced almost equivalent clearing. Unfortunately, the relapse rate greatly increases with doses below 1 mg/kg/day. One study found that with doses of 1 mg/kg/day, only 10 percent of patients required retreatment, whereas 42 percent of patients required retreatment when treated with 0.1 mg/kg/day. With a 4- to 5-month course of 1 mg/kg/day, fewer than 10 percent of patients will suffer a significant relapse within 1 year. After that, however, the relapse rate gradually rises; within 6 years, approximately 40 percent of patients will have had a significant relapse.

It is a simple matter to adjust the dose, since isotretinoin is available in 40-, 20-, and 10-mg capsules dispensed in packages of 10. Although the package insert states that isotretinoin should be administered in two divided daily doses, it is just as effective—and much simpler—for the patient to take the entire daily dose with the evening meal. It is important that isotretinoin be taken with meals, as food enhances its absorption.

Laboratory monitoring involves a blood count, urinalysis, and an automated chemistry profile that includes triglycerides, cholesterol, and liver function tests. A

WARNING FOR WOMEN TAKING ACCUTANE (ISOTRETINOIN) FOR TREATMENT OF ACNE

Accutane has many adverse effects; one is serious. If Accutane is taken during pregnancy, serious birth defects will occur. Despite warnings, some women have become pregnant while taking Accutane and given birth to severely deformed and mentally defective babies. The birth defects resulting from taking Accutane during pregnancy are so serious that an abortion is necessary should pregnancy occur while taking Accutane. I will not prescribe Accutane to a woman who is not prepared to undergo an abortion should she become pregnant while taking Accutane.

It is mandatory that sexually active women use an effective method of birth control while taking Accutane and for 2 months after the end of Accutane treatment.

CONSENT FORM FOR WOMEN TAKING ACCUTANE (ISOTRETINOIN)

1. I understand that it is vitally important to avoid pregnancy while taking Accutane and have read the above warning regarding serious birth defects that will result if I become pregnant during Accutane therapy.

2. I certify that if sexually active, I will use two methods of contraception.

3. Should I become pregnant during Accutane therapy because of contraceptive failure or rape, I agree to have an abortion to end the pregnancy.

Signed: _____

Date: _____

The signed original of this information and consent form will be given to you. A photocopy of the signed form will be filed in your medical record.

FIGURE 5–1. Informed consent form.

baseline test battery should be performed before beginning treatment, and all samples should be taken while the patient is fasting so that the triglyceride studies are reliable. The package insert recommends such laboratory monitoring "at intervals"; I see patients and perform laboratory studies monthly.

Most of isotretinoin's side effects are uncomfortable nuisances. Dryness of the skin and cheilitis occur universally; their absence should lead you to question whether the patient is taking isotretinoin. Skin lubrication with white petrolatum and a bland lip pomade usually provides significant relief. Nosebleeds are a frequent problem; lubricating the nares with minute amounts of petrolatum is helpful. Because mild side effects of isotretinoin are universal, provide the patient with the information sheet Isotretinoin (Accutane), which describes how to deal with these problems.

It is not possible to provide rigid guidelines when more serious side effects occur (e.g., severe muscle pains; gastrointestinal problems; visual complaints; depression; abnormalities in triglycerides, liver function tests, or urinalysis). These situations require individual evaluation and careful judgment. If it is clear that the patient has an intercurrent illness, such as a viral disease, it is best to temporarily discontinue the isotretinoin to sort out causes of signs and symptoms. As isotretinoin becomes more widely used, additional side effects are revealed. Periodic review of the manufacturer's literature is essential; Roche has been conscientious in warning physicians regarding side effects and complications in medical journal advertisements and in the package inserts.

Relapses after isotretinoin therapy are managed in essentially the same way as other cases of acne. Minimal activity can often be controlled with topical antibiotics. With mild-to-moderate acne relapses, systemic antimicrobials can be tried. If these antimicrobials are ineffective, which is usual in my experience, another course of isotretinoin is the obvious choice. A 4- to 6-week repeat course of isotretinoin will often induce a remission lasting 6 months to 1 year or more. In healthy persons, laboratory monitoring is probably not necessary for such a short course, except that women of childbearing age should have a pregnancy test before beginning treatment. In some patients, repeating a standard 4- to 5-month course of isotretinoin with appropriate monitoring is necessary to deal with acne that recurs after one course of isotretinoin.

CORTICOSTEROIDS. Systemic corticosteroids temporarily suppress acne. The effect is rapid, and a *brief* course is invaluable when patients need prompt improvement in their acne because of an important social event, a wedding, a job interview, or a photographic session. A 7-day course of prednisone 20 mg/day taken in the morning is remarkably effective in producing prompt, although temporary, benefit. One dermatologist has aptly dubbed these "prom pills." I tell patients that this is a stopgap measure and not a substitute for long-term acne suppression with topical and/or systemic antimicrobial agents. Systemic corticosteroids must be used properly in treating acne; continuous, moderate to high doses may actually cause acne (i.e., steroid acne).

Systemic corticosteroids have been used in the past for treatment of a rare, severe, febrile acne, usually accompanied by arthralgias, that responds poorly to antibiotics but usually improves with systemic corticosteroids. It appears that combining systemic corticosteroids with isotretinoin is the best treatment of this rare form of acne.

Topical corticosteroids are without value in treating acne. Fluorinated corticosteroids may aggravate acne and should not be used on the face of a patient with acne. If seborrheic dermatitis coexists with acne—a fairly common combination—prescribe ketoconazole cream (Nizoral).

SEX HORMONES. Estrogens and estrogen-dominant birth-control pills are often beneficial in treating acne in women. It is not uncommon for acne to appear in adult women who have stopped taking an estrogen-dominant contraceptive. Whether cessation of the birth-control pill triggered the acne, or whether the hormone had been suppressing adult acne present all along, is unknown. Androgen-dominant birth-control pills may aggravate acne. In many women, oral contraceptives have no effect on acne. Estrogen therapy and birth-control pills have significant medical side effects. The risk-benefit ratio rarely justifies the use of oral contraceptives for treating acne.

ANTIANDROGENS. Spironolactone has been recommended for treatment of recalcitrant acne in adult women on the basis of its antiandrogen activity. There is no consensus among acne experts regarding its effectiveness, or even on what the appropriate dose should be. Spironolactone has numerous potential side effects, and patients must avoid pregnancy while taking it. Isotretinoin has a better benefit-risk profile than spironolactone.

VITAMINS. Vitamin A by mouth has had a long and undeserved vogue in acne therapy. It is without value. Because high doses may be toxic, it should not be used to treat acne. Vitamins are worthless in treating acne. Isotretinoin, a very effective antiacne drug, is a derivative of vitamin A. Patients undergoing isotretinoin treatment should not take vitamin A, because it increases isotretinoin's toxicity.

ZINC. In pharmacologic doses, zinc can suppress acne. Its effect is relatively weak—roughly equivalent to low doses of systemic antibiotics. We know nothing about zinc's long-term toxicity. Over the short term, there may be gastrointestinal irritation and ulcers. Although zinc is touted as a natural treatment for acne, I shun it. Systemic antibiotics are more effective, and we know that they are safe for long-term use.

OFFICE PROCEDURES

Acne Surgery

Acne surgery refers to several manipulative approaches, including removal of comedones, needling acne lesions, and incising acne lesions or abscesses with a small pointed blade. Incising fluctuant lesions for drainage used to be popular; with the advent of intralesional corticosteroids, incision is used less often. Incising a lesion may leave a small scar; injecting a corticosteroid does not. I incise only the rare, large, fluctuant acne lesions that do not respond to intralesional corticosteroids. When a large acne abscess requires drainage, after local anesthesia, make a 2- to 3-mm-long incision with a pointed No. 11 scalpel and gently scoop out the necrotic material with a 1-mm-diameter chalazion curette. The incision should be made parallel to the wrinkle lines of the face; if the procedure is cautiously performed, scarring is infrequent.

Many dermatologists express comedones and open closed comedones regularly. When these procedures are done gently, they do not produce scars. However, there is no evidence that they prevent inflammatory lesions. Many patients who have had such acne surgery elsewhere seem relieved if told that this procedure will not be performed.

Intralesional Corticosteroids

Intralesional corticosteroids are effective in treating acne. Injecting a diluted suspension of repository corticosteroid into a papulopustule leads to improvement within 1 or 2 days, with flattening of the lesion (Figures C–7 and C–8). Flat lesions are more readily camouflaged with makeup or a tinted acne lotion. When a 30-gauge needle is used, there is little discomfort. Triamcinolone acetonide suspension is the agent generally employed; use it in a dilution of 2 to 3 mg/ml. Higher concentrations may cause temporary skin atrophy and an annoying depression at the site of injection. Inject 0.02 to 0.04 ml at a depth of 4 to 5 mm (about one third the length of a 0.5-inch-long needle) as described in Chapter 1.

Diluted suspensions of triamcinolone acetonide are available from dermatologic supply firms (Appendix B), or you can prepare your own as follows: From a 30-ml vial of preservative-protected saline (i.e., labeled "multiple-dose saline"), remove and discard 10 ml of saline. Then add 5 ml of triamcinolone acetonide suspension, 10 mg/ml. This produces a 2 mg/ml suspension. Shake thoroughly before using. Intralesional therapy is useful as the sole method of treatment of intermittent acne. It is helpful as an adjunct when acne is not adequately suppressed with antibiotics.

Cryotherapy

Cryotherapy with dry ice or liquid nitrogen has been used for years for its peeling and desquamating effect. It reduces the number of comedones and closed comedones and may hasten the involution of existing papulopustules. Cryotherapy does not prevent new inflammatory lesions. Its action is dramatic: It stings considerably at the time of application, and redness persists 6 to 12 hours after treatment. I have found the benefits less dramatic and have abandoned it. However, many competent dermatologists consider cryotherapy an effective modality.

Ultraviolet Light Therapy

Ultraviolet sunlamps have enjoyed popularity because of the observation that sunlight benefits many acne patients. Sunlamps, however, do not produce light of the same wavelengths emitted by the sun; therefore, they fail to duplicate sunlight's beneficial effect. This does not prevent many patients and physicians from using ultraviolet lamps; there is no doubt that the tanning—and occasional burns—can be a potent placebo.

X-ray Therapy

Although superficial x-ray therapy will temporarily suppress acne vulgaris, such therapy may damage skin and in some persons, lead eventually to an increased tendency to form skin cancers. In my opinion, x-ray therapy for the treatment of acne is of historical interest only.

MANAGING THE PATIENT

PSYCHOLOGICAL FACTORS

Skillful psychological management rivals only systemic antibiotics in its importance as a treatment modality. It is hard for an adult to realize how distressing even trivial acne may be to teenagers. The physician must show sympathetic interest in the patient's problem and not deal with an acne patient as a nuisance to be gotten rid of as soon as possible. Granted, this is often difficult.

Discern the patient's expectations. A wise dermatologist used to ask new acne patients, "Do you expect me to cure your acne?" When they answered yes, he gently told them there was no cure for acne, but "I will help you." Be honest and admit the present unsatisfactory state of acne treatment; the patient will discover the truth soon enough.

Tell patients that treatment suppresses acne but does not cure it. Only nature and time will do this. Do not provide a timetable for patients to outgrow their acne; we see too many adults reassured by a previous physician that their teenage acne would disappear at an age they passed long ago.

Help the patient put his or her acne into perspective. Point out that when the patient looks at himself or herself in a mirror, he or she sees only unsightly pimples; when others view the patient, they see the entire person, and it is the looks of the whole package that count. Mention some physically attractive aspect—a woman's pretty hair or figure, a man's rugged physique. This support is all the psychotherapy most acne patients need.

Intralesional repository corticosteroid therapy is a useful crutch for acne sufferers. If a few pimples appear just before an important social or business engagement, intralesional repository corticosteroid injections usually subdue them in a matter of days. For more extensive acne flare-ups, a 1-week course of prednisone 20 mg each morning works wonders. Tell patients that rather than worry about a disfiguring crop of pimples just before an important job interview, date, or other stressful occasion, they can see you for the appropriate quick fix. Knowing that this emergency approach is available enables many patients to tolerate their acne better.

Many patients and their parents believe that acne is a result of some incorrect habit or cleansing method. You can lift this burden of guilt from patients' shoulders by pointing out that there is little patients can do, without a prescription, either to benefit or to aggravate their acne. I tell them that sunlight is the only effective nonprescription acne treatment. Patients are reassured that except for picking and eating a food that they find triggers acne flare-ups, they cannot make their acne worse.

Picking deserves special attention in patients with crusted, excoriated, or otherwise manipulated lesions (Figure C–9). This is more common in young women, and seems to be an outgrowth of misguided attempts to scrub away their pimples. Patients should be told emphatically not to pick, squeeze, or otherwise manipulate their pimples. When a crop of pimples renders a patient desperate, I advise him or her to hide them with flesh-colored water-based makeup or use a flesh-tinted acne lotion.

Treating acne is often discouraging for the physician as well as the patient. Many patients derive great benefit from the support of a sympathetic and concerned physician despite little objective improvement in their acne. Remember, time is usually on your side.

Sunshine benefits most acne patients. Some cases fail to improve with sunlight, and a small minority are even aggravated. Unfortunately, sunlight also causes gradual, irreversible skin damage; consequently, most dermatologists have mixed feelings about recommending sunbaths for acne. Short-term acne benefits must be weighed against the long-term risks of skin aging and skin cancer.

DIET

There are many opinions on the relation of diet to acne; however, little of it is supported by documented observations. Although chocolate has a notorious reputation for aggravating acne, attempts to show such effects have failed. A reasonable approach is to tell patients that foods do not cause acne, but that in some cases, certain foods may aggravate it. Chocolate, nuts, cola drinks, and root beer are the aggravators of acne most commonly cited by patients. I alert patients to these potential aggravators and suggest that they observe whether repeated flare-ups occur after they consume these foods. If so, they are asked to stop eating or drinking them. Occasionally, large quantities of milk aggravate acne; usually, this means 2 to 3 l/day. Patients consuming such large quantities of milk are asked to discontinue their milk intake for 3 to 4 weeks and then to resume it again as a test to determine its role in aggravating acne.

SKIN HYGIENE

Most acne patients have been indoctrinated in the importance of skin hygiene for care of their complexions. Many engage in lengthy, expensive, and sometimes irritating cleansing and scrubbing routines. This is worthless, and patients should be told that such cleansing does not help eliminate acne. Advise patients to wash with ordinary soap and water once or twice per day and to forget about such treatments as abradants, astringents, medicated soaps, and degreasing pads. Point out that it is not surface oil that causes acne but rather the oil that does not get to the surface. Stress that acne is not caused by dirt.

NERVOUS TENSION

It is easy to blame "nerves" for acne and thus subtly shift the blame for therapeutic failure from the physician to the patient. Emotional upsets and nervous tension may aggravate acne, just as emotional factors can worsen hypertension, diabetes, rheumatoid arthritis, and a host of other organic disorders. Reassure the patient that emotional stresses and worry sometimes aggravate acne but never cause it. Patients often feel guilty and responsible for their acne. The physician should relieve feelings of guilt, not add to them. Emotional stresses cause patients to become more aware of their acne and sometimes to excoriate or otherwise aggravate it physically. Explain this to patients and tell them gently but firmly not to pick, squeeze, scratch, or otherwise manipulate their pimples.

COSMETICS

The role of cosmetics in acne remains controversial. Certainly, some thick, greasy makeups can cause or aggravate acne.

Acne caused by makeup, lubricating creams, and moisturizing creams has been termed acne cosmetica. In this type of acne, noninflammatory lesions (i.e., open and closed comedones) tend to predominate. Often, the eruption has a uniform (i.e., monomorphous) appearance. Just what role acne cosmetica plays in the common adult acne of women remains unknown. When in doubt, it is best to have the patient discontinue use of all moisturizers, lubricating creams, and makeup preparations for 2 to 3 months. Lipstick, powder, and eye makeup are permitted.

Fortunately, most women will tolerate a water-based makeup without aggravation of their acne. They should wash makeup off thoroughly at night with water and a little soap. Moisture creams and lubricants should be avoided; if the patient insists on a "night cream" or has problems with dry skin, prescribe an acne topical in a cream formulation such as meclocycline (Meclan cream) or erythromycin in an ointment form (Akne-mycin ointment). Do warn patients that cosmetics, moisturizers, and sunscreens may cause acne flare-ups.

SUMMARY

The status of acne therapy is still unsatisfactory. Acne patients are full of concerns, questions, and misconceptions. Educating and counseling patients takes time; a patient instruction form is invaluable in managing acne. The instruction form Acne is tailored to my understanding of what represents effective acne therapy; you may wish to modify it. Treating acne is vexing but, when successful, enormously gratifying.

Acrochordon (Skin Tags)

Patient sheet page P–97

6

ETIOLOGY

Skin tags are benign, fleshy, sometimes pigmented outgrowths commonly found on the neck, armpits, and groin, especially in middle-aged and elderly people. They are often associated with seborrheic keratoses, and it is not uncommon to observe lesions intermediate between a flat, round seborrheic keratosis and the pedunculated fleshy skin tag. Showers of skin tags may appear in pregnant women.

The tendency to grow skin tags is genetically determined. Persons with numerous skin tags usually have at least one parent with the same problem, provided their parents reached middle-age. Some years ago, it was claimed that these common nuisances were a marker for colonic polyps. Further studies showed this to be a result of sampling errors.

Skin tags are often a nuisance. Those on the neck catch on clothing and jewelry, armpit skin tags interfere with shaving, and skin tags of the inguinal folds may be irritated by the elastic of undergarments. On occasion, trauma or irritation interferes with venous return, and these lesions become engorged, blue-black, and ultimately necrotic. This process usually leads to spontaneous cure of the skin tag—often at the price of considerable patient anxiety. Patients feel reassured if the swollen, blue-black skin tag is snipped off and submitted for histologic examination. Otherwise, there is no need to send typical skin tags to the pathologist.

TREATMENT

Skin tags are removed when they annoy patients. To forestall complaints that "the tags you removed all came back," explain that the patient will continue to grow new lesions. Liquid nitrogen freezing will remove these lesions without a trace. Equally satisfactory cosmetic results can usually be obtained by snipping them off with a fine scissors. Using a fine-toothed forceps to stretch the skin tag while snipping its base with a Gradle scissors is the technique I prefer. While I generally use Monsel's solution or aluminum chloride to stop bleeding, these agents occasionally produce minute scars. If cosmetic results are critical, use pressure or gelatin foam to control bleeding. The small scabs resulting from scissors removal heal in a few days and do not require special postoperative care or instructions.

The use of a local anesthetic before removing skin tags should be a matter of patient preference. From the physician's viewpoint, a local anesthetic permits slow and precise snipping off of each tag. If given a choice, most patients prefer a local anesthetic.

Electrodesiccation or cautery destruction of skin tags is recommended by most textbooks. Small, white scars frequently result (Figure C–116). Why use a technique that may scar, when liquid nitrogen or scissors snipping rarely leaves a trace?

Actinic Keratoses

7

Patient sheets pages P–9, P–41, P–99

ETIOLOGY

Actinic keratoses are the visible consequences of sunlight (actinic) damage to skin cells. They are restricted to the sun-exposed portions of the skin and are particularly common in the fair-skinned populations of sunny climes. I have never seen them in a dark-skinned black.

DIAGNOSIS

Diagnosis is usually straightforward; the scaly, often red, irregularly surfaced, sharply demarcated roughenings on the sun-exposed areas of fair-skinned persons are distinctive. The main differential diagnostic considerations are warts, seborrheic keratoses, Bowen's disease (i.e., intraepidermal squamous cell carcinoma), and basal or squamous cell carcinoma. Excluding malignancy is the most troublesome problem. When the lesion is infiltrated or moderately deep, precise clinical diagnosis is impossible, and tissue examination is required. Some diagnostic uncertainty regarding carcinoma always exists, even in superficial lesions. For this reason, any keratosis that recurs after treatment should be biopsied.

Coexisting dermatitis such as psoriasis or seborrheic dermatitis may be impossible to distinguish clinically from superficial actinic keratoses. In this situation, I treat the dermatitis vigorously with a topical corticosteroid for 2 to 3 weeks and then re-evaluate the patient's condition. The dermatitis usually responds to this regimen, whereas actinic keratoses undergo relatively little change.

TREATMENT

Patients usually seek treatment because they find the lesions unsightly or are concerned about potential malignancy. It is standard textbook advice to remove actinic keratoses because they are premalignant lesions that may degenerate into carcinoma. However, this is probably an uncommon event. Unfortunately, there is no data on whether removal of actinic keratoses is an effective method of preventing skin cancer.

When only a few keratoses are present, removal of all lesions is a realistic approach that reassures both patient and physician. However, it is not uncommon for patients to have lived for years with hundreds of actinic keratoses; to remove all of them is impractical. The patient with a myriad of actinic keratoses is best managed by periodic surveillance and removal of any enlarging or deeply infiltrated lesions. Patients should return between scheduled check-up visits if they observe unusual changes, growth, or bleeding in any lesion.

Most actinic keratoses are superficial; superficial destruction of the defective skin cells is all that is needed to treat these lesions. Treatments of choice are: (1) superficial surgical removal with curette, scissors, or rigid blade (i.e., tangential surgery); (2) liquid nitrogen freezing; and (3) topical 5-fluorouracil (5-FU). Treatment must be individualized.

Cosmetic results are best with topical 5-FU treatment because it selectively destroys actinically damaged cells. The second-best cosmetic results are achieved by superficial liquid nitrogen freezing. Cosmetic results after curettage are usually inferior to the other two methods, but if the curettage is carefully done, the scar is often invisible. I do not include electrodesiccation as a treatment because, although it is widely used, it frequently leaves unsightly scars.

Superficial surgical removal of actinic keratoses is readily accomplished by curettage as described in Chapter 4. Sometimes protuberant lesions, especially those on the hands, are best snipped off with scissors. Tangential surgery (see Chapter 4) with a rigid razor blade is an excellent way of removing deep lesions from the trunk and extremities. Tangential surgery provides the pathologist with an intact specimen of the entire lesion, enabling him to determine its depth and completeness of removal. Scarring after tangential surgery is more pronounced than with light curettage; reserve it for deep lesions of the extremities, trunk, and scalp. Caution patients who have had keratoses removed from the lower leg that healing will be prolonged.

The great advantage of superficial surgical removal is that it provides tissue for possible histologic examination (note that "possible"). When numerous keratoses are removed by curettage, it is unreasonable to submit all of them for histology. It suffices to submit the deep or questionable lesions. Sometimes the curette falls deeply into a lesion presumed to be superficial. This suggests malignancy; have the tissue examined by a pathologist. If in doubt, err on the side of getting tissue histology. Consider the current medicolegal climate.

Liquid nitrogen is particularly useful in patients who return repeatedly with crops of multiple actinic keratoses (Figures C–55 through C–59). If you don't use liquid nitrogen, I suggest you refer these patients to someone who does. The technique of liquid nitrogen treatment is described in Chapter 4; give the patient the postoperative instruction sheet Liquid Nitrogen Treatment. The main drawback of liquid nitrogen treatment is that the physician must rely entirely on a clinical diagnosis. Because actinic keratoses are sometimes indistinguishable from carcinoma, adequate follow-up is mandatory. If a keratosis does not clear up with liquid nitrogen treatment, biopsy it. This is best accomplished by superficial scissors or curette removal, which also cures benign lesions. With this limitation in mind, liquid nitrogen remains the best treatment for patients who continue to develop multiple actinic keratoses.

Topical 5-FU is the method of choice when there are many actinic keratoses on the face (Figures C–19 through C–21). It is an effective way of removing one or a few keratoses when they are superficial and the optimum cosmetic result is desired. As with liquid nitrogen, the treatment is based on clinical diagnosis without histologic control. Whereas liquid nitrogen destroys such superficial neoplasms as seborrheic keratoses and warts, topical 5-FU does not.

The selective toxicity of 5-FU for sun-damaged cells is the basis for its clinical usefulness; it destroys sun-damaged skin with little injury to normal tissue. Healing takes place by replication of the remaining epidermal and adnexal cells; effective 5-FU treatment requires significant skin destruction.

Skin destruction leads to the major complication of 5-FU treatment—patient noncompliance. Patients intensely dislike this treatment, because for 2 to 4 weeks, the treated area is raw and unsightly (Figure C–20). A second drawback to topical 5-FU therapy is the absence of a definite endpoint of treatment.

Allergy to 5-FU is an occasional complication in patients who have had multiple courses of topical 5-FU. It may be difficult to distinguish 5-FU allergy from an early or exaggerated pharmacologic response to 5-FU.

Topical formulations of 5-FU are available in the United States from Herbert Laboratories and Roche Laboratories. One firm produces a 1 percent solution and a 1 percent cream; the other, 2 percent and 5 percent solutions and a 5 percent cream. The choice of formulation is not critical. The solutions seem to work somewhat more rapidly—and also irritate normal skin more—than do the creams. Whichever formulation is used, the patient applies it until the physician has judged that enough destruction has occurred—usually when the lesions have ulcerated. Then the skin is allowed to heal. Often a lubricant aids patient comfort during this process.

Topical 5-FU produces raw, inflamed areas that are unsightly and often uncomfortable. This stage lasts 2 to 4 weeks and often leads to bitter complaints from patients. When informing patients about 5-FU therapy, be sure to show them photographs (Figures C–19 through C–21; also available from the manufacturers) of what happens during treatment.

Topical 5-FU, although effective in destroying actinic keratoses of the face, usually fails to remove keratoses of the hands and forearms. To overcome this handicap, different agents have been used in combination with 5-FU to potentiate its action. The best documented of these potentiators is tretinoin (Retin-A). Combined use of 5-FU and tretinoin will destroy actinic keratoses of the hands and forearms in many patients. Unfortunately, the erosions are frequently extremely painful, and patients may abandon the treatment. I have also found the results less predictable than on the face, where it is already difficult to get patients to complete an adequate course of 5-FU.

Step-by-step directions for using 5-FU follow. Although this is the technique I use, other schedules are equally effective.

1. Topical 5-FU is applied twice a day with the finger to the actinic keratotic areas of the face and massaged in well.

2. In most patients, the medicine is applied to the entire sun-damaged area—the forehead, cheek, or face—not just to individual keratoses. The reason for this is that topical 5-FU will destroy early keratoses that are not clinically evident. However, when patients have only one or a few keratoses, treatment directed only to the lesions is appropriate.

3. When applying 5-FU, the patient should avoid: (1) the eyelids; (2) the folds about the nose; and (3) the lips. 5-FU is irritating in these locations. Exceptions are made when specific lesions in these regions must be destroyed.

4. Have patients minimize sun exposure during treatment. Give them specific written instructions on the patient information sheet Actinic Keratoses, and inform them that in 3 to 5 days, the treated areas will become red.

5. The patient returns in 12 to 14 days.

6. At the follow-up visit, most patients have developed early erosions and should continue the medication for another 10 to 14 days, depending on how severe the reaction is. For patients using the 5 percent solution, 21 days of treatment usually suffice. The cream formulations usually require 1 week longer. Certain areas, notably the forehead and scalp, may need longer treatment than more sensitive areas, such as the lower cheeks and mouth. If at first there is little response, the patient continues the treatment and returns 1 week later. This is an unpleasant treatment; advise patients to return sooner if they are concerned about the severity of their reaction.

7. It is important that patients continue topical 5-FU until all keratoses are destroyed. This is easier said than done, because there is no definite treatment endpoint. I try to have patients continue treatment for 2 weeks after brisk erosions have appeared, and generally aim for a total course of 4 weeks of treatment. The erosions produced by 5-FU are unsightly and painful; patients often plead for a shorter course. It is important that they understand that a brief course of 5-FU will only irritate their keratoses and not destroy them. Considerable relief from the discomfort of 5-FU treatment can be achieved by frequent, thin applications of petrolatum.

8. The patient is given a definite end date for the treatment, which is written out for him. After 5-FU has been discontinued, white petrolatum should continue to be applied at bedtime to soothe raw areas while they heal. The patient returns after 6 weeks for final evaluation.

9. Some patients prefer to treat one area of the face at a time to minimize the extent of the cosmetic handicap. With an intelligent patient, this method usually works. I follow such patients through one area until it is completely healed, and then instruct them to proceed the same way systematically in other areas, pushing the treatment to rawness and then stopping. Emphasize that they are not to treat any area twice, and that you should evaluate any lesions that fail to respond to a single course of 5-FU. Ask these patients to return after they have completed their entire spot-by-spot treatment.

10. At the final follow-up visit, residual lesions should be destroyed. If you are confident that the lesions are benign (e.g., seborrheic keratoses are not removed by topical 5-FU) liquid nitrogen treatment is applicable. However, suspect any actinic keratosis that fails to respond to adequate 5-FU treatment as being a carcinoma; such a lesion is best treated surgically, and the tissue should be analyzed histologically. Remember that topical 5-FU is not an adequate treatment for skin cancer. It is a mistake to use a second course of 5-FU on lesions that failed to respond during the first treatment. On the other hand, it is both permissible and useful to retreat patients with topical 5-FU 1 year or more later if new keratoses appear.

Alopecia Areata

Patient sheet page P–11

8

ETIOLOGY

Alopecia areata is a fairly common skin disorder. A frequent familial pattern indicates that genetic factors play a role; however, the cause of alopecia areata remains unknown. The slightly increased incidence of thyroid disorders and vitiligo in patients with alopecia areata points in the direction of autosensitization. Textbooks and lay publications frequently stress the role of emotional factors; however, this is not a psychogenic disorder. Patients should not be made to feel responsible for their "nerves" causing the alopecia.

DIAGNOSIS

Diagnosis of typical cases is easy; the round, sharply demarcated patches of complete hair loss are characteristic. Keep in mind that alopecia areata is characterized by a defect in hair growth. At the onset, structurally defective hairs are usually visible on close inspection. The "exclamation-point hair," a short hair that is thinner at its base than at the top and represents the last gasp of a hair follicle prior to inactivity, is usually diagnostic. If hair at the edges of the patch pulls out easily and has clubbed ends, it helps to confirm the diagnosis and indicates that the process is active and the patch will enlarge.

The two chief differential diagnoses are tinea capitis and trichotillomania. In tinea capitis, scaling and inflammation of the scalp are often evident. Examination under Wood's (black) light and microscopy of KOH-cleared, broken-off hairs are useful in excluding tinea capitis. Unfortunately, both techniques are often misinterpreted; one must be careful not to interpret Wood's light fluorescence of debris, or the normal mild scalp fluorescence, as tinea capitis. Trichotillomania usually shows broken-off, normal-appearing, growing-stage hair. It is sometimes difficult to distinguish alopecia areata from trichotillomania except by observation over time or biopsy with appropriate sectioning.

Alopecia areata sometimes fails to produce the classic picture of patches of complete hair loss and instead shows diffuse, patchy, partial hair loss. This diffuse alopecia areata can be difficult to diagnose; keep in mind the moth-eaten appearance of the partial hair loss of secondary syphilis. A useful diagnostic pointer in evaluating hair loss is to look carefully for scarring. Alopecia areata does not produce a scar.

TREATMENT

Present-day treatment of alopecia areata only temporarily modifies its course. Fortunately, most cases are mild. Spontaneous hair growth frequently resumes after several months and progresses to complete regrowth. The patient information sheet, Alopecia Areata, has an optimistic tone, because it is intended for the majority of patients for whom alopecia areata represents a passing nuisance. Do not give this patient information sheet to a patient with severe alopecia, because the optimistic tone of the sheet is inappropriate.

Is there any effective treatment? Not really. Systemic corticosteroids will usually produce regrowth of hair. However, they probably do not affect the ultimate result, and in patients with severe alopecia areata, the new hair will promptly be shed when the corticosteroids are withdrawn. Because long-term corticosteroids invariably produce side effects, they are not justified. Some physicians do use systemic corticosteroids for several months in patients with severe alopecia areata. They believe this may favorably modify the course of alopecia areata. There is no objective evidence that this occurs. They are not doing the patient a favor, only postponing the time when he must make the difficult adjustment to the hair loss.

Topical corticosteroids do not penetrate sufficiently into the skin to promote cosmetically significant regrowth in alopecia areata. A useful approach—and often potent psychological boost—in limited areas of alopecia areata is the injection of repository corticosteroids. In about 75 percent of patients, hair will promptly regrow in the injected sites. Provided small amounts are injected, there is no significant systemic effect. The technique of intralesional injection is discussed in Chapter 1. In patients with alopecia areata, I use a concentration of triamcinolone acetonide of 10 mg/ml (undiluted Kenalog 10), inject about 0.05 ml per puncture at a depth of 5 to 7 mm, and space the punctures about 1 cm apart. When injecting, be sure that the needle enters the skin perpendicularly at a 90-degree angle, to minimize trauma and assure reproducible deposition of the corticosteroid at the necessary depth.

Inform patients that if the injection will stimulate hair growth, it will take about 1 month before that growth becomes visible. Explain that you injected a long-acting medicine that lasts 3 to 5 months; otherwise they'll be on your doorstep every few weeks. I advise patients to return for further injections only if new patches of hair loss develop, and if the test injections prove effective.

Uncontrolled studies with topical minoxidil (Rogaine) have claimed hair growth in alopecia areata. In this capricious, unpredictable disorder, controlled studies are imperative. Unfortunately, topical minoxidil produced no better results than a placebo in four different double-blind placebo-controlled trials.

Hair regrowth can be stimulated in alopecia areata by inducing skin inflammation. The inflammation must be prolonged and severe. Causing repeated bouts of contact dermatitis with dinitrochlorobenzene or diphenylcyclopropenone, two potent allergens, has been the most successful technique. Psoralen combined with ultraviolet irradiation has also been used. These approaches are still experimental, but may eventually result in a simple, practical treatment.

MANAGING THE PATIENT

For a significant minority of patients, the active phase of alopecia areata continues and causes extensive or recurring hair loss. Alopecia areata may extend relentlessly to complete baldness and even to loss of all body hair. In general, the earlier the onset, the worse the prognosis. Alopecia areata in young children distresses both patients and parents; in teenagers, severe alopecia areata can be an emotional disaster. Drastic personality disturbances may occur, especially in young women, because hair plays an important role in their sexual image. Sympathetic understanding and urging these patients to wear a wig as a temporary measure until hair regrows may help. On occasion, I have referred young patients to psychiatrists. For young persons with extensive alopecia areata, strike an optimistic note, and emphasize that the hair roots are merely "resting." Encourage distressed patients to contact the National Alopecia Areata Foundation (714 C Street, Suite 216, San Rafael, CA 94901) for support group information.

Even in extensive cases in which you can be fairly certain that the prognosis is bad, be optimistic. Sometimes the hair does regrow nicely, and when it doesn't, time helps patients to adjust. This grim discussion applies to the severe cases of alopecia areata, especially when it begins in young patients. Remember that in the majority of patients, events will justify your optimism. For those patients with extensive or total alopecia, a talented wigmaker often works miracles for patient morale and self-esteem.

Frequently, the newly regrowing hair in alopecia areata is white rather than the color of the surrounding, unaffected hair. This color change is usually temporary, but sometimes it is permanent. Be sympathetic; suggest that time usually corrects the color change, and encourage patients to tint their hair if they are distressed by this problem.

9 *Androgenetic Alopecia*

Patient sheets pages P–45, P–63

ETIOLOGY

Both men and women lose hair with aging. In men, this often leads to complete baldness. Hair loss in women is more subtle and rarely results in complete baldness. However, it is not unusual to see the scalp through the hair in women older than 70 years of age. Female hair loss often mimics male-pattern hair loss in its preference for the frontal and temporal areas and the crown of the scalp. This type of hair loss has been appropriately termed androgenetic alopecia to describe its etiology.

Androgenetic alopecia is a progressive disorder with ultimate destruction of the hair roots. Initially, the hair shaft gradually decreases in diameter—a useful diagnostic sign. In this early stage, the process may be reversible, as demonstrated by the hair regrowth that sometimes follows topical minoxidil (Rogaine) applications.

In men, the onset and progression of androgenetic alopecia vary greatly. Some men are bald by their late teens, whereas others have a thick head of hair in their 80s. It is not commonly appreciated that androgenetic alopecia in women (female-pattern alopecia) may also begin in the teens and 20s and follow a variable course. Early-onset female-pattern alopecia can produce distressing sparseness of hair in the patient's 20s.

DIAGNOSIS

The diagnosis is obvious in men who have the distinct pattern of hair loss in the frontotemporal areas and crown with sparing of the occiput. Most men present with their correct self-diagnosis, especially if there is a strong family history of early balding, and seek advice regarding treatment.

Diagnosis in women is straightforward if there is patterned hair loss, the woman is middle-aged or older, and close female relatives have the same problem. When these conditions are not met, a fairly detailed history, a physical exam, and laboratory tests will be required to rule out other disorders. Not infrequently, female-pattern hair loss is diffuse rather than patterned. In contrast to men, women with early-onset female-pattern alopecia rarely recognize their condition and it may be overlooked by professionals.

Androgenetic alopecia is usually a gradual, progressive process, although sometimes marked hair loss occurs in a period of months. Abrupt hair loss suggests a diagnosis, or the coexistence, of telogen effluvium—hair loss secondary to hair reverting to the resting phase. Physical stresses such as major surgery, high fever, rapid weight loss, or pregnancy may cause large numbers of hairs in the growing phase to revert to the resting (i.e., telogen) phase and be shed after a latent interval of a few months. When this occurs, light tugging releases numerous hairs with tiny, white, hair-root remnants at the end of the shaft. Telogen effluvium is common in women. It may coexist with female-pattern alopecia, and sorting out the respective roles of these conditions is difficult. If there are doubts, check carefully for the presence of hair with decreased diameter in the areas of hair loss, and tug at the hair to be sure you are not dealing with telogen effluvium. The scalp in patients with androgenetic alopecia should be normal, except perhaps for mild coexisting seborrheic dermatitis, which does not contribute to the hair loss.

Female-pattern alopecia may rarely be the result of androgen excess. If there are signs of virilism, such as hirsutism or voice changes, endocrine studies are indicated. If the index of suspicion is low, screening tests of serum testosterone and dehydroepiandrosterone sulfate (DHEA-S) are appropriate. If there is strong clinical evidence of androgen excess, which is a rare condition, evaluation by an endocrinologist is wise.

Androgenetic alopecia affects the scalp hair; if there is significant hair loss elsewhere, look for a systemic cause. However, the converse does not hold true; hair loss limited to the scalp does not rule out other causes. Thyroid disease, anemia, numerous drugs, certain physical stresses, vitamin A intoxication, and heavy-metal poisoning are among the many causes of scalp hair loss.

TREATMENT

GENERAL MEASURES

Advice for Both Women and Men

Androgenetic alopecia is a progressive disorder without a cure. Except for topical minoxidil, it is not possible to stimulate hair regrowth. Tell patients that such hair loss is not the result of lack of vitamins, poor scalp circulation, dandruff, or a host of other common misconceptions. It is important to reassure them that procedures such as tinting the hair, permanents, and frequent shampoos do not cause hair loss. Point out how difficult it is to inhibit hair growth, and that if we had a method to stop hair from growing, Western women could be liberated from their armpit- and leg-shaving routines.

This discussion of androgenetic alopecia focuses most attention on the treatment of male hair loss, because men raise this issue more often than do women. Hair transplantation is rarely practical for women, as only partial hair loss is the rule. Furthermore, women are usually willing to consider a wig or wiglet, whereas men rarely consider this an option.

In theory, it should be possible to ameliorate androgenetic alopecia by interfering with the androgens' adverse effect on the hair root. In women, systemic antiandrogens and high doses of estrogen improve female-pattern alopecia. Because these agents produce unacceptable side effects, the goal has been to find a topical antiandrogen that will act on the hair root without producing systemic effects. An antiandrogen affecting only the skin would also benefit patients with acne, another androgen-mediated skin disorder. Such a substance has been actively sought, without success, for several decades.

Because the natural history and treatment of androgenetic alopecia differ in men and women, different patient information sheets are provided: Hair Loss in

Men (Male-Pattern Alopecia) and Hair Loss in Women (Female-Pattern Alopecia). This is a complex subject. Have the patient read the information sheet before your discussion.

Advice Specifically for Women

For the middle-aged or older woman troubled by her sparse hair, a wiglet or wig is an excellent, socially acceptable solution. Since female-pattern alopecia usually leaves an adequate rim of hair, a skillfully designed wiglet that matches the existing hair is often undetectable. Other women happily wear a full wig. Explain that wearing a wig does not cause further hair loss.

You may wish to avoid the emotionally charged words "wig" or "wiglet"; instead, use the terms "hair replacement" or "hair addition."

Broken-off hair from excessive bleaching or too-strong permanents may cause patients to fear they are losing their hair. Point out that this is not true hair loss, but rather the result of hair breakage, and the remaining stubble will ultimately grow out.

Advice Specifically for Men

I encourage men to ignore their hair loss. Although we live in a narcissistic society, and looks are important, it is the overall effect that counts. Hair is just one facet of appearance, and many bald and balding men are successful in life and sexually attractive. The majority are satisfied when they learn that there is no simple, effective treatment for male hair loss, and it does not matter how often they shampoo or how long they wear their hair. For those who insist on treatment, options include topical minoxidil, surgical procedures, and wigs.

SPECIFIC MEASURES

Minoxidil

Topical minoxidil is not the magic treatment of androgenetic alopecia that advertisements suggest. There is agreement on the following facts:

1. Any hair-growing effect of topical minoxidil is temporary and lasts only as long as the minoxidil applications are continued. If minoxidil applications are discontinued, new hair growth is lost.

2. Cosmetically significant results are achieved in only about 10 percent of men; women appear to have an even poorer response rate.

3. In men, early hair loss at a younger age is more likely to respond than later hair loss at an older age.

4. In men, alopecia of the crown responds much better than hair loss in the frontotemporal area.

5. Topical minoxidil treatment appears reasonably safe, although rare systemic side effects from absorbed minoxidil have been reported. A few reports have described unwanted facial hair growth in women applying minoxidil to their scalp.

The main controversy is regarding how often minoxidil produces a satisfactory response. Do not believe publications enthusiastically describing 50 percent or better response rates. Usually funded by the manufacturer, these studies cite improvement in hair counts. Because we are treating a cosmetic disorder, it is visible improvement that matters, not whether the hair count has increased. Selection of patients and treatment site is significant. Most of the studies in men have dealt with alopecia of the crown of the scalp, which responds better than the frontotemporal hair loss that is of most concern to men. Statistics can also be boosted by treating only young men with early hair loss.

There is no quick test to determine whether minoxidil will be of benefit. It generally takes 4 to 6 months before any beneficial effect is apparent. One colleague has patients apply the minoxidil to one half of the scalp for 6 months and then ask a blinded observer, such as the patient's barber, if they detect any difference between the two sides.

Not infrequently, men and women with early hair loss ask whether minoxidil will prevent additional hair loss. "Possibly" is the only answer we can give. This question could be settled only by a large-scale, double-blind, placebo-controlled study involving thousands of persons over several years to allow for the variable and unpredictable progression of androgenetic hair loss.

Surgical Approaches

The surgical treatment of male-pattern alopecia was an outgrowth of an ingenious experiment performed in the 1950s by Norman Orentreich of New York. He decided to settle the question of whether frontal hair loss in male-pattern alopecia was the result of innate differences in the hair roots or a consequence of differences in regional blood supply. He took a small, full-thickness, punch skin graft from the occiput and transplanted it just behind the receding frontal hairline of men with early male-pattern hair loss. The hair-containing plug taken from the frontal scalp was transplanted to the occiput. Over the next few years, although the hairline continued to recede, the hair transplanted from the occiput grew vigorously, whereas the reverse transplant to the back of the head lost its hair.

Hair transplantation is an outgrowth of this experiment. Hair grafts are taken from the occipital scalp and transferred to the frontotemporal areas and crown. There have been many refinements to the technique. Smaller hair grafts are used to smooth out the hairline. Hair transplants may be combined with scalp reduction, in which bald areas from the crown are excised and primarily sutured. In addition, complex plastic surgical procedures involving large, hair-bearing flaps have been devised. Both skill and practice are needed for an artistic result; this is not a procedure to be done on a casual or occasional basis. The field has attracted its share of promoters and fee-gougers; I am careful to refer my patients to practitioners who are experienced in these techniques and use good judgment in selecting candidates for surgical treatment, as well as their level of fees.

Wigs, Hairpieces, and Other Artifices

Wigs and smaller hairpieces have improved dramatically over the years, and some men find them very satisfactory. A small minority of men augment their hair by hair weaving and similar techniques. Unfortunately, these need to be repeated at intervals and are expensive, because they require a good deal of operator time.

Periodically, charlatans promote the implantation of artificial hair. Individual synthetic hairlike filaments are inserted into the scalp skin and anchored in the subcutaneous tissue. All such attempts have ended disastrously, with severe foreign-body reactions and months to years of infection, purulent drainage, multiple surgical procedures, and scarring.

10 Aphthae (Canker Sores)

Patient sheet page P–17

ETIOLOGY

The cause of aphthae, or aphthous stomatitis, is unknown. In the great majority of canker sore sufferers, recurring crops of one or a few of these small, painful ulcers appear without apparent cause. Hereditary factors are significant; one parent or a sibling is usually affected. Textbooks emphasize that aphthous ulcers may occur secondarily to hematologic disorders, gluten enteropathy, or inflammatory bowel disease, but these associations are rare.

A minority of patients with oral ulcerations get severe, deep, necrotic, recurring lesions and are said to suffer from severe aphthosis. Along with severe oral ulcerations, genital ulcers and features of Behçet's disease may occur. This discussion and the patient information sheet, Canker Sores (Aphthae), do not apply to such severe or complex cases.

DIAGNOSIS

Diagnosis is usually obvious. Typically, the ulcers are small, punched-out, necrotic ulcers with a yellowish white dirty-looking base. The patient usually has a history of recurrent episodes of self-healing lesions over a period of years. Diagnosis can be a challenge in a young person without a preceding history of aphthae who develops multiple oral erosions and even more so in an adult who develops oral ulcerations. Herpetic gingivostomatitis is distinguishable from canker sores because of the blisters, extent of erosions, and the accompanying fever and systemic symptoms associated with herpetic gingivostomatitis. Coxsackieviruses (i.e., hand, foot, and mouth disease) can produce erosions, but these are usually smaller than aphthae and are accompanied by skin lesions on the hands and feet. Stevens-Johnson syndrome is distinguishable from canker sores because the disease process is more extensive, the skin is involved, and blisters are present in the syndrome. Aphthae appear as spontaneous ulcers; there is no blistering or vesicular phase. If a patient with oral ulcers has blisters anywhere in the mouth or on the lips, do not diagnose aphthae.

An adult presenting with necrotic oral ulcers without a history of preceding episodes of aphthae should be viewed with diagnostic skepticism. Pemphigus, cicatricial pemphigoid, and lichen planus can present as oral ulcers without other diagnostic features. While it is tempting to diagnose aphthae in these patients, resist making this diagnosis unless the lesions follow the typical course of aphthae: Prompt healing with asymptomatic intervals between attacks. The diagnosis of persisting oral ulcerations is often difficult.

There is a small subpopulation of patients with severe aphthosis who suffer from large, painful lesions that heal extremely slowly. These patients require careful study before the diagnosis of idiopathic severe aphthosis is applied.

TREATMENT

Emphasize that aphthae are not related to herpes simplex and are not contagious. Too often, I encounter patients who have been told by their personal physician that their canker sores are a herpes simplex infection, sometimes producing disastrous effects on their personal lives.

There is no cure for aphthae; the many recommended treatments indicate this unsatisfactory state of affairs. Only topical corticosteroids and tetracycline mouthwashes have been proven effective by double-blind, placebo-controlled trials. Do not be a therapeutic nihilist, however, because significant relief is usually possible. Different degrees of severity require different strategies; the simplest is protection.

PROTECTION

Application of Orabase, an over-the-counter ointment designed to adhere to the oral mucosa, can provide significant relief of discomfort while healing takes place.

TOPICAL CORTICOSTEROIDS

Frequent application of strong topical corticosteroids in the first 2 to 3 days will shorten the course of an ulcer, as well as relieve discomfort. The key to success is frequent use of small amounts of a potent or superpotent agent early in the course of the lesion and only for 2 to 3 days. The superpotent corticosteroids (see Chapter 1) are probably the most effective. These agents should be applied sparingly six to eight times a day for 2 to 3 days, then discontinued.

Most authorities prefer an ointment rather than creams, lotions, or gels; this is also my preference. Some studies have used a combination of topical corticosteroid and Orabase, with the aim of providing a stickier vehicle that will adhere longer to the ulcer. One such combination with triamcinolone is marketed as Kenalog in Orabase. There is no evidence that such mixtures are superior to the corticosteroid alone, and they are significantly more expensive. For patients with posterior pharyngeal ulcerations, anecdotal reports claim benefit from oral use of topical intranasal corticosteroid sprays used in the treatment of allergic rhinitis.

The topical corticosteroid suppresses the early, inflammatory stage of an aphthous ulcer. Because these agents actually interfere with wound healing, they must not be used for more than a few days in the early stages of an aphthous ulcer. This point is strongly made in the patient information sheet, Cortisone Ointments, and should be emphasized orally. The amount of superpotent corticosteroid should be carefully limited, with not more than 15 g used in 2 months.

TETRACYCLINE MOUTHWASHES

Tetracycline mouthwashes decrease the pain of established ulcers and help prevent the formation of new ones. Suspensions of 125 mg per 5 ml and 250 mg per 5 ml have been used. Four times daily, 1 tsp is swished around the mouth for 4 to 5 minutes and then spit out. Tetracycline mouthwashes can be used for 5 to 7 days for intermittent attacks, or for a month or longer to suppress chronically recurring ulcers. Explain that the tetracycline suspension has an unpleasant taste, but that there is no harm if a patient happens to swallow the medicine.

ORAL PREDNISONE

For patients who get occasional but multiple recurrent canker sores, suppression with a 3- to 4-day course of prednisone by mouth is often dramatically effective. As little as 2 days of prednisone sometimes suffices. Generally, a dose of about 40 mg/day is adequate. This dosage does not need to be tapered and is simply discontinued after 2 to 4 days. Repetition of such brief prednisone courses at intervals of about 1 month is reasonably safe in the absence of contraindications to a systemic corticosteroid.

TRIAMCINOLONE ACETONIDE INJECTIONS

Patients who have infrequent attacks of large, very painful ulcers can get immediate relief by sublesional injection of triamcinolone acetonide 2 to 5 mg/ml, with 0.1 to 0.2 ml injected beneath each ulcer using a tuberculin syringe and 30-gauge needle. The technique is described in the section on intralesional corticosteroid therapy in Chapter 1.

OTHER TREATMENTS

Frequently recurring crops of canker sores are the most difficult to manage. In addition to suppressing individual lesions with topical corticosteroids, the goal is to prevent or minimize recurrences. Long-term use of tetracycline mouthwashes is effective and safe.

Systemic antibiotics may be useful, but there is a lack of hard data. Tetracycline 1 g/day may decrease the frequency of recurrences. This is a safe, long-term treatment, as attested to by its wide usage in managing acne. Dapsone and colchicine have been described as effective in suppressing or minimizing recurrences of aphthae. Unfortunately, both these drugs have significant side effects, which limit their use to the most severe cases. The same is true for the systemic retinoid etretinate.

Numerous topical antimicrobials and antiseptics have been proposed for the treatment of aphthae, without any convincing evidence of effectiveness. For patients with multiple, painful lesions, topical anesthetics such as viscous lidocaine employed before meals may make eating more comfortable. The use of silver nitrate sticks and other caustics is to be condemned—these merely increase tissue destruction.

MANAGING THE PATIENT

A number of simple, safe strategies will provide significant relief for the majority of canker sore sufferers. Those patients with severe disease are best referred to a physician with special interest and expertise in treating oral disease.

Basal Cell Carcinoma
(Skin Cancer)

11

Patient sheets pages P–13, P–99, P–103

ETIOLOGY

Basal cell carcinoma is the commonest skin cancer. It results from sunlight damage to skin, although lesions are not always located on the areas of most intense sun exposure. Basal cell carcinoma may also occur decades after x-ray treatment. Unlike other carcinomas, basal cell carcinoma does not metastasize. When informing patients they have basal cell carcinoma, stress that it is only locally invasive and not a threat to general health. The patient instruction sheet, Skin Cancer (Basal Cell Carcinoma), is suitable only for basal cell carcinoma and should not be given to patients with other skin malignancies.

DIAGNOSIS

The appearance of nodular basal cell carcinoma is usually typical. The lesion has a pearly, sharply demarcated border and has blood vessels coursing over its surface. Sometimes, there is central ulceration. Variants of basal cell carcinoma are not diagnosed as easily; for example, superficial basal cell carcinoma often resembles a patch of dermatitis (Figure C–24), while an infiltrating, sclerosing basal cell carcinoma may resemble a scar (Figures C–10 and C–11). A tissue diagnosis is essential for proper treatment. Biopsy can be accomplished by using a punch or curette or by shaving off tissue with a scissors or scalpel blade.

    The chief differential diagnoses are squamous cell carcinoma, actinic keratosis, keratoacanthoma, and benign tumors such as nevi, molluscum contagiosum, seborrheic keratoses, and warts. Infiltrating basal cell carcinoma may perfectly simulate an old scar. In this type of lesion, thin strands of tumor can infiltrate the surrounding skin without producing grossly detectable changes (Figures C–17 and C–18).

TREATMENT

Treatment aims to destroy the tumor with optimal cosmetic results. Surgical excision, curettage and electrodesiccation, x-ray therapy, liquid nitrogen destruction, and chemosurgery are some widely used techniques. I consider conservative surgical excision the best method, because it provides an intact specimen for the pathologist to determine adequacy of removal, and cosmetic results are generally superior to those achieved by curettage and electrodesiccation or by irradiation.

The excision need not always be done in the standard ellipse or fusiform shape. Circular excisions using minimum 2- to 3-mm margins of normal tissue with partial closure of the defect are often useful, especially when the lesions occur on the nose. Round lesions can be removed with a punch. The majority of basal cell carcinomas do not penetrate significantly into the subcutaneous fat; therefore, standard conservative surgical excision usually provides adequate deep margins. The specimen should be marked on one margin—India ink works well—so that the pathologist can tell you the direction of any marginal extension of the tumor that he finds when examining step-level sections for adequacy of removal.

Ill-defined, large, or otherwise difficult lesions—especially if located near an eye or on the nose—are best treated by microscopically controlled excision (Mohs' micrographic surgery; Figures C–17 and C–18). In this technique, successive planes of tissue are removed until a microscopically tumor-free plane is reached. This specialized technique, invaluable for complex cases, is now available in most major United States medical centers and large dermatology practices.

Topical chemotherapy with 5-fluorouracil (5-FU) for superficial basal cell carcinomas has been advocated in advertisements. There are no guidelines as to how long to use 5-FU for this condition, and even in experienced hands, there is a significant failure rate.

COMPLICATIONS

Recurrence and scarring are the chief complications of basal cell carcinoma. Careful surgical excision minimizes both of these complications. Surgical excision requires more time and skill than curettage and electrodesiccation, but it provides superior cosmetic results.

MANAGING THE PATIENT

Patient education is essential. Have the patient read the information sheet, Skin Cancer (Basal Cell Carcinoma), and then discuss prognosis and treatment. Stress that basal cell carcinomas do not metastasize but do require treatment; otherwise, they continue to grow relentlessly.

Follow-up is an important part of basal cell carcinoma treatment. Traditionally, follow-up is emphasized for early detection of treatment failures. In the case of basal cell carcinoma, follow-up is more useful for the early detection of new basal cell carcinomas. Patients with one skin cancer are likely to develop others; of those with two or more basal cell carcinomas, about 40 percent will develop a new cancer within 1 year. Patients with skin cancers should be recalled for examination periodically.

Boils (Furuncles)

12

Patient sheet page P–15

ETIOLOGY

Furuncles are a common skin infection caused by the ubiquitous organism *Staphylococcus aureus.*

DIAGNOSIS

The most common differential diagnostic problem is distinguishing between a boil and an inflamed cyst; usually, patients with inflamed cysts are aware of a preceding asymptomatic subcutaneous lump. Other bacteria and fungi occasionally produce infections resembling the staphylococcal furuncle. If in doubt, a Gram stain and culture of pus obtained from the lesion will determine the diagnosis.

TREATMENT

Most boils are self-limited processes. This probably accounts for the standard textbook advice that the only treatment necessary for boils is gentle heat and possibly incision and drainage if the furuncle is fluctuant. A minority of boils do not follow this benign, self-healing course but develop into painful abscesses or lead to burrowing and multiple, carbuncle-type lesions. I find it impossible to tell which boils are going to behave aggressively, and consequently, I treat all early boils with systemic antibiotics. There is no point in treating a late, healing boil with systemic antibiotics, because it has been walled off, and systemic antibiotics will not penetrate into the infected core.

Systemic antibiotic treatment of boils should be given with the following points in mind:

1. Choose an antibiotic that is likely to be effective against staphylococci. In Western countries, most staphylococci are resistant to ordinary penicillin, tetracycline, and erythromycin. At present, the drug of choice appears to be semisynthetic, penicillinase-resistant, oral penicillins such as dicloxacillin. In patients allergic to penicillin, clindamycin (Cleocin) and minocycline (Minocin) are reasonable alternatives.

2. If the furuncle fails to respond, or if it is located in an area of concern (e.g., near an eye), drain and aspirate the boil, culture the pus obtained, and perform sensitivity tests.

3. A 5- to 7-day course of antibiotic usually suffices. The aim of the antibiotic is to stop the spread of the infection.

4. Antibiotics are not a substitute for surgical drainage if the boil contains a significant amount of pus.

Surgical drainage is indicated if pus is present or suspected. It is desirable to drain pus early, before further necrosis occurs. Although the presence of fluctuation indicates pus, its absence does not rule out the need for surgical drainage. Furuncles, especially if deep, may have a significant accumulation of pus without being fluctuant. Any persistently painful boil should be suspected to harbor pus in its depths.

For most boils, adequate surgical drainage can be established by a quick stab with a pointed No. 11 blade. Refrigeration analgesia with ethyl chloride or a similar spray makes the stab more tolerable. For larger incisions, a local anesthetic should be used. It is often difficult to anesthetize a boil adequately; superficial manipulation produces deep pain because of increasing pressure on the boil.

Epinephrine should not be included in a local anesthetic used prior to minor surgery of infected tissue. There is experimental evidence in animals that the vasoconstriction produced by epinephrine encourages an infectious process to spread.

Resting the affected part is helpful, especially if the boil is on an extremity. A sling works well to immobilize the arm or hand; furuncles of the legs may require rest at home with leg elevation.

Gentle heat is part of the traditional treatment of boils; specific directions are given in the patient instruction sheet Boils (Furuncles). It is probably wise to cover draining boils with a bandage. Boils are somewhat contagious, and covering draining boils with a bandage seems a reasonable measure to minimize spread of the *Staphylococcus*. Ask what the patient's occupation is; persons working in health-care facilities or restaurants should stay away from work until their boils have healed to prevent infecting others.

RECURRENCE

Recurring furunculosis is a therapeutic challenge. The majority of persons with recurring boils are otherwise healthy, although it is customary to obtain a urinalysis and blood count to rule out such underlying disorders as diabetes. It is easier to list what does not work to prevent recurring furunculosis than to describe effective measures. Long-term antibiotics usually prevent new boils, provided the *Staphylococcus* is sensitive to them. Unfortunately, in many cases boils return to plague the patient when the antibiotic is discontinued. Staphylococcal vaccines have been discredited. It is difficult to assess the value of any treatment, because recurring furunculosis often lasts for many months and then spontaneously disappears.

The approach I use is to reduce the population of staphylococci on the surface of the skin and from certain areas often colonized by them. This involves applying an antimicrobial ointment to the nares, armpits, and groin twice daily, in addition to applying an antiseptic to the entire skin. The antimicrobial ointment applied to the nares, armpits, and groin is designed to eradicate staphylococci from these common reservoirs. Mupirocin (Bactroban) ointment is the agent of choice; 1 week of treatment usually eliminates nasal carriage of staphylococci. The application of an antiseptic to the entire skin is intended to reduce the population of staphylococci on the skin, because a critical number of pathogenic organisms is necessary to produce a boil.

For "degerming" the entire skin, alcohol paintings are a simple method. Seventy percent ethyl or isopropyl alcohol is an effective antiseptic, although its action is transient. For a more prolonged effect, have the patient paint his or her skin once daily with an antibiotic solution of the type used in treating acne. Several brands of 2 percent erythromycin dissolved in a hydroalcoholic solution are available, as is 1 percent clindamycin. One caution regarding topical clindamycin: Small amounts are systemically absorbed, and there have been rare but well-documented cases of pseudomembranous colitis produced by topical clindamycin.

13 *Cysts*

Patient sheets pages P–23, P–107, P–109, P–111

ETIOLOGY

Skin cysts are benign neoplasms filled with keratinous debris. Depending on the structure of the cyst wall, they are classified as epidermoid or trichilemmal. Trichilemmal cysts are commonly found on the scalp and have a tough lining that permits them to be easily shelled out. Milia (whiteheads) are small, superficial cysts. Cysts are often attached to the overlying epidermis and may communicate with the surface through a thin stalk.

DIAGNOSIS

Diagnosis of milia and other superficial cysts is usually obvious; with deeper cysts, the diagnosis is presumptive until surgical incision. Lipomas, fibromas, pilomatricomas, and other subcutaneous tumors, as well as abscesses, may resemble cysts. Sebaceous gland hyperplasia produces yellowish nodules that are distinguishable from milia by their central indentation and lobulated periphery. Chronic actinic damage may cause comedones and yellowish nodules containing small cysts and degenerated connective tissue.

Two situations present difficult differential diagnoses. The first is that of an inflamed cyst versus a furuncle. The tip-off in favor of a cyst is a history of a small, asymptomatic lump, present for months to years, that slowly enlarged until it suddenly became inflamed. Sometimes the diagnosis of inflamed cyst is made only when a supposed boil is drained and fragments of cyst wall are obtained. The other differential diagnostic problem is the acne abscess, sometimes incorrectly termed an acne cyst. Acne abscesses are indolent, subcutaneous, fluctuant lesions resulting from rupture of a sebaceous gland; the resulting inflammatory response produces a pseudocapsule. Acne abscesses, unlike true cysts, do not initially possess an epithelial lining. Acne abscesses will respond to intralesional corticosteroids (Figures C–7 and C–8), whereas cysts require surgical removal of the wall. With repeated inflammation, acne abscesses may heal with formation of an epithelial lining. Patients with acne not uncommonly have both acne abscesses and true cysts.

There is no way to prevent cyst formation. Epidermoid cysts are often familial. Milia are common on the face at all ages, but are particularly a problem in elderly persons whose skin has suffered significant sun damage.

TREATMENT

Milia are readily removed by nicking the overlying skin with a hyperdermic needle and teasing out the small sac. Sometimes milia shell out easily; others require a

Shamberg comedo extractor or fine forceps and scissors to separate the sac from the surrounding tissue. Small milia can often be flicked out without using anesthesia. For larger or well-attached milia, however, injecting a local anesthetic prevents both pain and flinching. The small crusts produced by this procedure disappear without a trace in a few days.

Cysts are benign lesions; they are usually treated because the patient finds them a nuisance cosmetically or otherwise. Because a certain percentage of cysts become acutely inflamed, it may be reasonable preventive medicine to remove medium-to-large asymptomatic cysts. Not all subcutaneous lumps are cysts; often surgery is the only way to determine the diagnosis. Definitive treatment of cysts requires incising the skin and dissecting out the sac.

Before infiltration with anesthetic, mark the borders of the cyst and the proposed incision lines. Use epinephrine in the anesthetic and wait about 15 minutes for maximal vasoconstriction to occur so that there is a relatively bloodless field. Traditionally, surgeons are taught to remove the cyst intact. This requires an incision roughly as long as the cyst. I make a small incision, usually not more than 6 to 8 mm long, and deliberately rupture the cyst sac. After squeezing out the contents, I dissect the sac away from the overlying skin with the aid of forceps, hemostat, and a small curved scissors—the Gradle scissors is ideal. Good lighting is essential.

Close the defect with sutures; buried vertical mattress sutures of an absorbable synthetic material are ideal (see Figure 4–3). On the trunk and extremities, buried vertical mattress sutures often suffice for wound closure. Patients will be pleased by the absence of railroad-track suture scars. On the face and neck, buried vertical mattress sutures are usually augmented by percutaneous interrupted sutures to provide precise apposition of wound edges. The use of buried sutures permits early removal of the percutaneous sutures and avoids producing crosshatched suture scars.

Linear incisions are generally used to excise cysts on the face and neck. Because linear wounds of the trunk and extremities spread, some physicians prefer to remove cysts from these sites with a circular incision made by a 4-, 5-, or 6-mm punch. Some cysts are easier to remove than others. Those on the scalp are the simplest to remove, because they are superficial, firm-walled, trichilemmal cysts. On the other hand, cysts on the back often extend deeply down to the muscle and may require considerable dissection and significant enlargement of the original incision. I have learned to allow extra time when scheduling excision of a cyst on the back.

Scalp cysts are quickly and easily removed. Do *not* shave the scalp. Your patients will be most grateful. Keep long hair out of the way with hair clips or paper tape. After anesthesia, make a small incision through the stretched skin overlying the cyst down to the cyst wall. Incise the cyst wall, and squeeze hard on the cyst and surrounding tissue. This not only empties the cyst, but usually expresses much of the cyst wall, which you can then gently tug out with a hemostat. Some physicians do not suture the small wound; however, I prefer to place one or two sutures of 4-0 or 5-0 plain gut (Figures C–32 through C–34). With this technique, only a few drops of blood are lost. Postoperative care is simple. The patient is asked to wait 24 hours before shampooing and to comb the hair carefully so as not to snag the suture. The suture falls out in about 10 days.

For inflamed cysts, standard textbook advice advocates a two-step process for treatment. Upon presentation, the inflamed cyst is incised and drained or injected with intralesional corticoids. Some weeks later, when the inflammation has subsided, the cyst is excised in the usual manner. However, many physicians have learned that it is possible to treat inflamed cysts definitively in one step (Figures C–25 through C–31). After extensively infiltrating the surrounding tissues with local anesthetic and waiting for it and the epinephrine to take effect, incise the cyst mass with a No. 11 blade, with plenty of gauze available to absorb the free-flowing pus. Using a large chalazion curette, scrape out the pus and necrotic cyst wall. Then, using intense illumination, systematically explore the cyst cavity and remove cyst remnants using a forceps, hemostat, and either a Gradle scissors or a curved, serrated iris scissors. Frequent sponging with gauze inserted with a hemostat is essential. When the cyst cavity appears to be free of cyst wall and necrotic tissue, a dry dressing is applied, and the patient is instructed to change it once or twice a day as needed until the wound no longer oozes. Healing is by secondary intention, and usually, only a small scar is produced. This one-step procedure provides immediate relief of discomfort and, in my practice, a cure rate of over 80 percent. Patients prefer this one-step process.

A controversial point in this and other definitive methods of treating inflamed cysts is whether to use systemic antibiotics. Although bacteria are invariably present in these inflamed cysts, their significance remains a matter of debate. Usually, I do not employ systemic antibiotics. However, when there is a lot of redness in the surrounding tissues and I am impressed with the amount of purulent drainage, I "run scared" and prescribe a 4- to 5-day course of a systemic antibiotic.

Intralesional injection of a corticosteroid is a practical way of deciding whether the lesion is an acne abscess, boil, or cyst. If the lesion disappears, it was an acne abscess (Figures C–7 and C–8); if it does not, surgical treatment is indicated. Even with this precaution, a physician occasionally performs surgery on a presumed cyst and discovers only an acne abscess. When this happens, use a chalazion curette to scrape the cavity thoroughly, and suture the defect.

Cysts are benign; submitting a typical cyst to pathology is not always necessary. However, if in doubt, send the tissue for microscopic examination. Not infrequently, a solid tumor is encountered when performing surgery on a suspected cyst. In this situation, tissue examination is mandatory. If you encounter a solid tumor, try to dissect the lesion away from the surrounding tissue and deliver it intact. If you excise cysts by first rupturing the cyst wall through a tiny incision, removal of a solid tumor usually requires enlarging the incision.

The ease with which a cyst is separated from its surrounding tissue varies greatly. Trichilemmal cysts of the scalp shell out readily when pressure is applied against the skull. Cysts that have undergone inflammation may adhere to the surrounding skin; they can be difficult to remove. Avoid cyst destruction by electrocoagulation of the cyst wall and overlying skin. Such measures often fail and can produce ugly scars. Unfortunately, there is no substitute for surgical removal of cysts.

Atopic Dermatitis (Atopic Eczema)

Patient sheets pages P–19, P–27, P–39*

14

ETIOLOGY

Atopic dermatitis, also known as atopic eczema, is a genetically determined skin disorder often affecting characteristic sites. Although significantly associated with asthma, allergic rhinitis, and urticaria, atopic dermatitis is a genetically determined disorder and not an allergic disease.

DIAGNOSIS

Diagnosis of typical flexural eczema of the antecubitals and popliteals is easy. When only the face is involved, contact dermatitis—especially in a woman—is the major differential diagnosis. Contact dermatitis from an airborne agent (plants) and photosensitivity rashes may resemble atopic eczema. Atopic eczema tends to lessen with age. In later years, it commonly involves only limited areas such as the face, hands, or neck. The diagnostic tip-off is a history of atopic dermatitis in infancy or childhood. A family history of atopic dermatitis is also significant.

Atopic dermatitis in the infant usually does not show the typical flexural localization. It tends to be more diffuse and involves the trunk, face, and extremities. It may be difficult to distinguish infantile atopic dermatitis from seborrheic dermatitis. Sometimes, the family history is more helpful than the morphology of the eruption in the differential diagnosis. Although the treatment of most endogenous dermatoses in infancy is similar—essentially, topical corticosteroids—the prognosis is different. Infantile seborrheic dermatitis usually disappears within 1 or 2 years, whereas atopic dermatitis is often a chronic process.

The tendency of eczema in infants and children to clear spontaneously with increasing age is well known. Be cautious about reassuring parents that their infant will outgrow his atopic eczema soon. In many cases, eczema continues—sometimes intermittently clearing—into adulthood. The atopic diathesis is still present in these adults, and frequently manifests itself in later life in the form of localized eczema favoring the hands, neck, genital area, and face. Sometimes, such localized atopic dermatitis resembles psoriasis or the lichenified chronic localized dermatitis described as lichen simplex chronicus.

COMPLICATIONS

In the majority of cases, atopic eczema is a nuisance readily controlled by topical measures. Cataracts are an occasional complication of severe atopic eczema. Atopic

---

*Refer to the *Universal Medication Summary Sheet*, page xxi.

patients—especially infants and young children—are prone to secondary infection. A justly feared complication of atopic eczema is generalized infection with herpes simplex virus, referred to as eczema herpeticum. Eczema herpeticum can be a serious medical complication requiring specialized hospital care. Fortunately, acyclovir, a drug effective against the herpes simplex virus, is now available to treat this condition.

POPULAR MISCONCEPTIONS

Two widely held misconceptions interfere with the rational therapy of eczema. The first is that atopic eczema is an allergic diathesis requiring extensive (and expensive) diagnostic skin tests and therapy with dietary restriction and desensitization injections. Neither treatment is of value. Physicians treating atopic eczema with desensitization and diet therapy almost invariably prescribe topical corticosteroids as an adjunct. Because more than 90 percent of atopic eczemas clear with corticosteroids alone, the pointlessness of desensitization therapy is evident.

Dietary therapy is of no value in adult atopic eczema. I have yet to see an adult with atopic eczema whose rash consistently flared up when he consumed certain foods. Food allergy occasionally complicates atopic eczema in infants and children. Eggs, sometimes milk, and, less often, wheat, soy, nuts, seafood, and fish may be offending agents. When infantile atopic eczema fails to respond to topical management, have the parents eliminate eggs and milk from the child's diet for 3 to 4 weeks. If the eczema improves significantly, the child should be fed large, challenge amounts of the suspected food to see if the eczema flares up. If it does, the elimination and challenge should be repeated once to make sure these were not chance events—atopic eczema is prone to spontaneous remissions and flare-ups. Elimination-diet trials should be limited to 3 to 4 weeks, and dietary restrictions continued thereafter only if a causal effect can be demonstrated. A physician may occasionally encounter malnourished youngsters as a result of ill-advised, unnecessarily prolonged elimination diets. A recent study found that in severe childhood eczema, the outcome after 1 year was unaffected by diet, even though an elimination diet led to short-term improvement in some children.

The second common misconception is that atopic eczema is a nervous disorder or "neurodermatitis" to be treated by psychotherapy or with tranquilizers or sedatives. This treatment is cruel and inept: cruel because the patient is unjustly blamed for "nerves" causing the eczema, and inept because this assumption leads to inappropriate therapy with tranquilizers and sedatives. This is not to say that emotional upsets play no role in atopic eczema; they frequently worsen it. Furthermore, a significant number of atopic patients—and a significant number of the general population—have emotional disorders warranting psychotherapy. Atopic eczema is not a conversion reaction and needs appropriate dermatologic treatment, not psychotherapy. Sedatives and tranquilizers will make an itching patient more comfortable by dulling his or her sensorium; however, it is preferable to suppress the underlying skin disease.

TREATMENT

TOPICAL THERAPY

Topical corticosteroids will effectively control atopic eczema in well over 90 percent of patients. Their use is discussed in Chapter 1. Keep in mind that: (1) significant systemic absorption may occur when large areas of eczematous skin are treated with topical corticosteroids; and (2) potent corticosteroids should not be used on the face or skin-fold areas. Show patients how to apply the corticosteroid and give them the patient instruction sheet Cortisone Ointments.

If topical corticosteroids fail to provide adequate control, add coal tar to the regimen. A tar-oil bath additive produces a mild tar effect. Lotions, creams, gels, or ointments containing crude coal tar applied thinly at bedtime achieve a more potent tar effect. Details of the use of coal-tar preparations are given in Chapter 34.

Bacterial infection often complicates eczema, and subclinical infection may significantly aggravate atopic eczema. Although systemic antibiotics have been the treatment of choice in the past, mupirocin (Bactroban) ointment applied twice daily is just as effective. In patients with crusted eczema or eczema that is responding poorly, it is worthwhile to try a 7- to 10-day course of mupirocin ointment applied twice daily while continuing once-daily corticosteroid applications at a different time. Please note that this endorsement applies only to mupirocin. Older topical antimicrobials, such as neomycin and bacitracin, are ineffective and may sensitize the patient. Do not use them.

Coal tar is irritating to some persons and occasionally sensitizes the patient, causing contact dermatitis. It is best to initiate coal-tar therapy by having the patient apply it to only a small area for 1 week as a therapeutic trial.

Other topical agents are best avoided. Topical antihistamines, older topical antibiotics, and anti-itch preparations are worthless and may sensitize the patient.

Patients frequently aggravate their dermatitis with inappropriate self-treatment. Instruct your patients not to apply anything to their skin except as you direct. Clinically, it is difficult to distinguish a spontaneous flare-up of atopic eczema from eczema aggravated by irritation or allergic contact dermatitis. Consequently, try to exclude the likelihood that a topical medicament is aggravating the eczema.

Hand dermatitis as part of atopic eczema may be a stubborn problem. Treat hand dermatitis according to its severity as outlined in Chapter 15.

INTRALESIONAL CORTICOSTEROIDS

Intralesional injection of repository corticosteroids is a neat way of treating stubborn, localized atopic eczema. The technique is described in Chapter 1.

SYSTEMIC THERAPY

Systemic corticosteroids are occasionally necessary for treating severe atopic eczema. Usually a 1 to 2 week course will suffice. Use prednisone given as a single morning dose. Begin with 60 to 80 mg/day for an adult, and decrease the dosage by 5 to 10 mg/day as soon as improvement occurs. The aim of systemic corticosteroids is to relieve the inflammation and swelling to a point where topical steroids can control it. If proper topical therapy is initiated, it will rarely be necessary to use systemic corticosteroids for more than 2 weeks. If more than 2 weeks of systemic corticosteroids are required, the patient should be switched to every-other-day prednisone and weaned off it gradually. When prolonged systemic corticosteroids are required to control atopic eczema, search for a complicating contact dermatitis. Sometimes, what appears to be recalcitrant atopic eczema is actually atopic eczema that is complicated by contact dermatitis, usually caused by a topical medicament.

Systemic antibiotics are indicated when atopic eczema becomes infected; this is not an uncommon occurrence. I prefer to prescribe either erythromycin or an oral semisynthetic penicillin such as dicloxacillin. A 5- to 8-day course usually suffices. It is sometimes difficult to determine whether oozing and crusting are part of the eczematous process or represent secondary infection. A Gram-stained smear of intact pustules is a more reliable test for infection than a culture. Cultures may be misleading, because dermatitic skin is frequently colonized by pathogenic bacteria without resultant disease. Cultures cannot distinguish between colonization and infection. Because subclinical infection is a well-known aggravator of atopic eczema, it is wise to err on the side of overtreatment. There is little harm in a short course of an oral antibiotic. If you are reluctant to prescribe an oral antibiotic, a 7- to 10-day course of topical mupirocin is an effective alternative.

OTHER MEASURES

Patients with eczema invariably have dry skin. They will benefit from systematic lubrication as explained in the patient instruction sheet Dry Skin (Asteatosis, Xerosis). Stress that they are to use only the lubricants and procedures that you recommend.

Atopic eczema is frequently worsened by nervous tension, contact with rough woolen clothing, cold weather, or extremely hot weather. Stress and nervous tension are part and parcel of life; however, the other aggravating factors can be avoided or minimized. Woolen garments should not be worn next to the skin; this also holds true for any roughly textured synthetic fabric. The deleterious effect of wool on atopic skin results from mechanical irritation, not allergy.

Cold weather, with its low humidity, desiccates atopic skin and leads to fissuring and dermatitis. To counteract this drying effect, have patients lubricate their skin more frequently and intensively during winter. The use of humidifiers in the patient's home may help.

Hot weather is notorious for producing severe atopic flare-ups. Sweating is defective in dermatitic skin; tell the patient to minimize severe heat stress. Air-conditioning is the appropriate remedy. If only one room can be air-conditioned, it should be the bedroom.

Hand Dermatitis

Patient sheets pages P–19, P–29, P–31, P–33

15

Hand dermatitis is common. It causes patients anguish, can be seriously disabling, and is frustrating to physicians. The classical method of dermatologic diagnosis—evaluating morphology and distribution of the rash—often fails in hand dermatitis. Most hand eczemas (the words *eczema* and *dermatitis* are used interchangeably) tend to look alike even though their etiologies differ. Hand eczema is often chronic; a doctor often sees new patients whose hand eczema has plagued them for years while they made the rounds of local physicians. Hand eczema is a clinical entity in its own right. Although there is often hand involvement in atopic dermatitis or psoriasis, it is not referred to as hand eczema, but rather as atopic dermatitis or psoriasis of the hands. Usually, the cause of hand eczema is not obvious. Most hand dermatoses are the result of nonspecific irritation in a person predisposed to develop dermatitis (Figures C–35 and C–36). Fortunately, the therapy for nonspecific hand dermatitis is the same as for atopic or psoriatic hand dermatitis.

There is a rational way to approach the diagnosis of hand dermatitis. Furthermore, most hand eczemas are well treated with topical corticosteroids, systematic lubrication, and minimizing exposure to irritants. Successful treatment hinges on using measures appropriate to the site and severity of the dermatitis. Both treatment and hand protection require meticulous attention to detail; the patient instruction sheets Hand Protection for Hand Dermatitis, Overnight Plastic Occlusion for Hand Dermatitis, and Hand Dermatitis Treatment are invaluable in managing hand dermatitis.

The majority of patients with hand dermatitis do well when provided with proper advice and a topical corticosteroid. Precise treatment directions are given in the patient instruction sheet Hand Dermatitis Treatment; general care of the hands is detailed in the patient instruction sheet Hand Protection for Hand Dermatitis. If you prefer to treat only mild hand dermatitis and refer the severe cases, proceed to the topical therapy instructions.

Those wishing to wrestle with the more difficult hand dermatoses should study the sections on etiology and diagnosis. Severe hand dermatitis, although relatively infrequent, is a major therapeutic headache. Successful treatment requires scrupulous attention to detail, and the necessary information cannot be condensed.[1]

ETIOLOGY

Hand dermatitis mainly results from the skin's inability to cope with local noxious influences. To varying degrees, endogenous and exogenous factors are involved in its causation. These factors, summarized in Table 15–1, interact in subtle and complex ways; for discussion purposes, they are treated separately.

Table 15–1. ENDOGENOUS AND EXOGENOUS FACTORS INVOLVED IN HAND DERMATITIS

Endogenous
Atopic dermatitis (i.e., constitutional eczema)
Psoriasis
Psoriasiform disorders
    Vesiculopustular disorders of hands (e.g., dyshidrosis, pompholyx, acral pustulosis, pustular bacterid,
      pustulosis palmaris et plantaris)
Nummular eczema (i.e., discoid eczema)

Exogenous
Irritants
    Chemicals (e.g., solvents, alkalies, soaps, detergents, acids)
    Dry, cold air
    Friction
Allergens (i.e., contact allergy): vast number of possible allergens; of particular significance in chronic
    hand dermatitis are topical medicaments

ENDOGENOUS FACTORS

Atopic Dermatitis

Atopic dermatitis frequently involves the hands. Only the hands may be involved in an adult or teenager who had typical flexural atopic eczema as a small child. A history of previous atopic eczema in a person with hand dermatitis is strong evidence that the condition is atopic hand eczema. A history of atopic dermatitis in close relatives suggests that atopic factors may be significant in producing the dermatitis.

Psoriasis

Psoriasis causes many chronic cases of hand dermatitis (see Figures C–60, C–103, and C–104). There may be little or no psoriatic involvement elsewhere. In many cases, involvement of the soles and/or perianal area or a plaque on the scalp will tell you that you are dealing with psoriasis. Psoriasis in close blood relatives should alert you to consider psoriasis as a possible cause.

Psoriasiform Disorders

Several curious disorders affecting the hands and/or feet are characterized by recurring grouped vesicles or pustules and a chronic course. The pustules are sterile. Dermatologists do not agree on their nomenclature; they are varyingly diagnosed as dyshidrosis, pustulosis palmaris et plantaris, acral pustulosis, pustular bacterid, or acrovesiculatio recidivans. These psoriasiform disorders are suppressed by corticosteroids, psoralen-ultraviolet A (PUVA) therapy, ultraviolet B therapy, etretinate, and methotrexate. The only topical agents of proven value are corticoids, ultraviolet B therapy, and topical PUVA. In many such cases, there is psoriasis on some part of the body. I group these conditions together because they respond similarly to treatment.

EXOGENOUS FACTORS

Irritants

Irritants such as acids, strong alkalies, and detergents act nonspecifically to inflame skin. We are all exposed to irritants, but we do not all have hand dermatitis. One factor is the level of exposure to irritants; for example, more homemakers, waiters, and nurses have hand eczema than do accountants. Because endogenous factors are also significant, not all homemakers have hand eczema. Wet work is a notorious cause of hand dermatitis. Frequently overlooked is the irritating effect of dry, cold air as a cause of chapping and dermatitis. Friction from holding a tool, gardening, or even handling paper is often a significant irritant. Irritants aggravate any hand dermatitis, irrespective of underlying causes, and must be carefully avoided. Irritants are the most important exogenous causes of hand dermatitis.

Allergens (Contact Allergy)

Allergic contact dermatitis can either be a primary cause of hand dermatitis or aggravate a pre-existing hand eczema. In a few cases, contact allergy is the sole cause of hand dermatitis. It is important to ferret out these cases; they are curable. In industrial workers, the chance that a specific allergen is the cause of dermatitis must be carefully considered. Inquire carefully about the nature of the patient's work, substances encountered at work, and relationship of the dermatitis to vacation periods. Pinpointing the specific contactant requires patch testing by a specialist, because reliable patch testing with industrial materials is difficult. In homemakers, contact allergy is rarely the primary cause of hand dermatitis. However, allergy to topical medicaments and rubber gloves not infrequently complicates all types of hand dermatitis. Unfortunately, even allergy to the corticosteroids used in treatment may occasionally occur.

IMPORTANT. In men and women with hand dermatitis of varying etiologies, 10 to 20 percent have superimposed contact dermatitis from a topical medicament used to treat the primary rash. Superimposed allergy to a topical medicament—including topical corticosteroids—is often unsuspected, because it does not present as an acute contact dermatitis, but rather as a dermatitis that fails to improve. This is another reason to patch-test patients whose hand dermatitis fails to respond to treatment.

MAKING THE DIAGNOSIS

The steps in diagnosing hand eczema are outlined in Table 15–2. Search for endogenous factors by inquiring about a past history of eczema, especially atopic eczema

---

Table 15–2. **DIAGNOSTIC STEPS IN EVALUATING HAND DERMATITIS**

1. History
   a. Time of onset
   b. Occupation
   c. Time relationship to work—effect of vacations and travel
   d. Previous and current topical therapy
   e. Chemicals, detergents, medicaments, lubricants, cleansers, and rubber gloves used or encountered at work, home, or in hobbies
   f. Dermatitis at sites other than hands
   g. Previous dermatitis
   h. Dermatitis, eczema, or psoriasis in close blood relatives
2. Examination
   a. Hands
      Dorsal versus volar involvement
      Nail pitting with normal paronychial tissues
      Palmar vesicles or pustules
   b. General
      Ideally, examine entire skin
      Feet and perianal areas are especially significant

Adapted from Epstein E: Hand dermatitis: Practical management and current concepts. *J Am Acad Dermatol* 10:395, 1984

in infancy and childhood. Determine whether the patient's close blood relatives have hand eczema, psoriasis, or other chronic skin problems. A commonly seen pattern, especially in women, is that of atopic eczema in infancy that clears up in childhood only to recur as hand eczema in the teens or 20s.

Note whether the rash is primarily volar or dorsal. Hand dermatitis limited to the palms is usually endogenous. The dorsal skin is more sensitive to external irritants or allergens and is usually involved when exogenous factors are significant. Symmetry—especially if only the palms are involved—also favors endogenous causes. These are guidelines, not absolute rules.

Look carefully at the nails. Pits or marked dystrophic changes with normal cuticles are good evidence of psoriasis (Figure C–105). If the posterior nail fold is involved in dermatitis, the nails will show dystrophic changes irrespective of the cause of hand dermatitis; this is why pitting is significant only when the nail folds are normal.

Examine the patient's entire skin, paying particular attention to the feet and perianal area. Dermatitis on other parts of the body is strong evidence of an endogenous component of the hand eczema. Often the only evidence of a psoriatic factor in hand dermatitis is typical psoriasis involving the perianal skin and gluteal cleft. Many patients deny having any rash other than on their hands, only to have the examination contradict their statement. Look carefully at the patient's feet. If the feet and hands both have dermatitis, this is strong evidence of an endogenous cause.

EXOGENOUS FACTORS

The two most important areas of questioning are: (1) the patient's occupation; and (2) what the patient has been applying to his hands as lubricants and medication. Persons with certain occupations, such as homemakers, dishwashers, and waiters, are heavily exposed to irritants and encounter relatively few potential allergens. In other occupations, one must think of an allergen as a possible cause, especially if the patient handles such well-known allergens as epoxy glues, chromate-containing materials, or formaldehyde. What happens to the patient's rash when he or she goes on vacation? If there is strong suspicion of an occupational allergen, the patient should be referred to a specialist experienced in patch-testing. Do not attempt patch-testing unless you have had special training in it; otherwise errors of execution and interpretation of the patch-test are likely.

Previously used lotions, creams, and medicaments—both over-the-counter and prescription—frequently aggravate hand dermatitis. Have the patient list everything he or she has been applying to the hands and ask him to bring in all topical medicaments at the next visit. You may be surprised at the number and nature of topicals employed, and how many the patient forgot to mention when you took the history.

These steps will give you an idea of the respective roles of endogenous and exogenous factors and help you formulate treatment. Conversely, the treatment results will influence your diagnosis. Most hand dermatoses clear rapidly with treatment and do not require sophisticated investigation. A recalcitrant process may require repeated, detailed questioning regarding contactants, a variety of therapeutic approaches, and, possibly, patch-testing.

DIFFERENTIAL DIAGNOSIS

The catch-all label of hand eczema is usually appropriately applied by most physicians. There is one disorder that occasionally misleads even the wary—tinea manum. Tinea manum is frequently unilateral, affects mainly the palms, and is sharply demarcated; frequently, there are dystrophic changes in one or more finger-nails. The feet invariably have tinea pedis, but this is not particularly helpful, as tinea pedis is common in the general population. Finding the organism on KOH-cleared scrapings or on culture is diagnostic; you will not find it unless you suspect a fungus and look for it. Tinea manum usually clears when treated with systemic antifungals but often relapses.

Bowen's disease (intraepidermal squamous cell carcinoma) often looks like eczema. Its unchanging nature and failure to respond to treatment should lead to biopsy and the correct diagnosis. Other disorders, such as lichen planus, drug eruptions, and subacute lupus erythematosus, may involve the hands. Usually, these processes involve other parts of the body in addition to the hands; examination of the entire skin may indicate the correct diagnosis.

The trichophytid, or "id," reaction on the fingers associated with fungus of the feet is a definite entity, but it is not as common as was formerly thought. An id hand eruption is a hypersensitivity process triggered by tinea pedis. Before the advent of griseofulvin, it was a common explanation for vesicular eruptions of the fingers and palms. The id reaction is rarely the sole cause of a hand eruption. Only occasionally is it possible to clear a hand eruption by vigorous treatment of tinea pedis with internal griseofulvin and the newer topical fungicides. Most patients previously diagnosed as having ids have chronic vesicular hand eruptions that are aggravated in a nonspecific way by activation of their tinea pedis.

TREATMENT

ELIMINATING CAUSES

Two aims should be kept in mind in managing hand dermatitis: (1) elimination of the cause or causes; and (2) suppression of the dermatitis with active therapy. Eliminating the cause or causes is more easily said than done; usually, there are multiple causes, only some of which can be altered. Endogenous factors (i.e., a constitutional tendency toward eczema) cannot be changed. Of the exogenous factors, irritants are the most common. Systematic protection of the hands is essential. Every patient with hand dermatitis should be given the patient instruction sheet Hand Protection for Hand Dermatitis. Go over the significant points, and ask the patient to read the instructions daily for 1 week. For many patients, such as homemakers, nurses, or dishwashers, it will be impossible to follow the hand protection instructions precisely. Stress that they are a goal to be aimed at. Over-the-counter hand creams and lotions and various self-treatment routines are frequently irritating; insist that the patient apply only what you have prescribed.

It is harder to eliminate contact with possible allergens than to avoid irritants; irritants are usually easily identified. The most commonly identified allergen aggravating hand dermatitis is a topical medicament. Benzocaine and other topical anesthetics, mercurial antimicrobials, and neomycin are common offenders. Do not prescribe these preparations; be sure the patient is not using any such product he bought over the counter, obtained from a friend, or received from a previous physician.

Eliminating contact with other possible environmental allergens is a challenge. The physician must establish that the patient has a relevant contact allergy—that he is allergic to something that the hands touch. This can entail prolonged, involved studies; fortunately, they are usually unnecessary. The vast majority of hand dermatoses resolve nicely with careful hand protection and appropriate topical therapy and do not require patch-testing.

In treating hand dermatitis, therapy does not simply follow diagnosis; there should be continuing interaction, because diagnosis is influenced by the response to treatment. The common housewife's hand dermatitis usually responds well to protective routines and topical corticosteroids. When it does, it's assumed to be basically an irritant process. When a hand dermatitis does not respond to therapy, a continuing search for causes should be undertaken. Sometimes, only prolonged observation clarifies the diagnosis. This is especially the case in psoriasis of the hands, which may begin insidiously as a nonspecific-appearing hand dermatitis.

STRATEGIES FOR IRRITANT AVOIDANCE

Hand protection consists of contact avoidance and/or the use of protective gloves. Barrier creams usually fail to protect the hands. However, frequent lubrication of the hands helps to counteract the effect of detergents and is critical in preventing the chapping and fissuring that occur under conditions of cold, wind, and low humidity.

Protection from wet work requires impermeable gloves. Rubber gloves are effective. Unfortunately, because rubber gloves occasionally sensitize, vinyl gloves are preferable. Although household-weight rubber gloves are sold in every supermarket, vinyl gloves suitable for household chores are not widely available. Excellent heavy-duty vinyl gloves are available under the trade name of Allerderm from Allerderm Labs (see Appendix B). For the convenience of patients, ask some nearby pharmacies to stock these gloves. Even vinyl gloves may cause allergy, although rarely.

Most textbooks advise the wearing of cotton gloves under waterproof gloves. Usually, this is neither necessary nor practical. Although the cotton gloves absorb some sweat, they do not change this from an occlusive environment. It is difficult enough to get busy homemakers and wet workers to don one set of gloves. However, some persons tolerate waterproof gloves only when wearing cotton gloves underneath them.

Thick household-type vinyl gloves—like household-type rubber gloves—are unsuitable with many wet materials or solvents. Disposable, thin vinyl (not latex) gloves give highly effective protection from water and detergents and offer some protection from paints and other solvents. They are inexpensive and suitable for delicate tasks. Many specialized protective gloves are available for industrial applications; industrial hygienists are a good reference source.

While most patients are aware of the inimical effects of contact with detergents or paint solvents, few know how much damage the physical factors of friction and dry air can do. Repetitive friction from a hammer, screwdriver, wrench, or other tool may activate dermatitis. Gardening requires leather gloves to protect the hands from contact with soil. While earth is not an irritant per se, the soil particles exert a powerful abrasive effect. Add to that the soap-and-water scrubbing required for cleanup, and you can see why leather rather than fabric gloves should be worn when gardening.

Low humidity is a potent cause of dermatitis—and not just on the hands. Hand dermatitis is frequently worse in winter, after a trip to a windy climate, or after prolonged exposure to the low humidity of an airplane. Wearing leather gloves is extremely beneficial. Fabric gloves are unsuitable; the aim of the gloves is not warmth but to provide a barrier against the low-humidity air.

It pays to quiz patients about their protective measures, especially if their hand dermatitis fails to improve or if recurrences are frequent. Do they have a pair of vinyl gloves in each bathroom and the kitchen? If the gloves are not readily available, they will not be used. Are gloves discarded when a puncture is discovered? Are leather gloves worn when gardening? What gloves are used when painting? Do they protect their hands from cold dry air with leather gloves?

Active therapy can be summarized in one word: Corticosteroids. Despite the bewildering array of diagnostic designations applied to hand dermatitis (e.g., atopic eczema, homemaker's hand dermatitis, pustulosis palmaris, dyshidrosis, pompholyx, nummular eczema, psoriasis of the palms), they all respond to corticosteroids and virtually nothing else. The following discussion is restricted to the use of corticosteroids and reflects the severity and location of the dermatitis rather than esoteric diagnostic terms. Because most hand dermatoses require prolonged therapy, the emphasis is on topical corticosteroids. Treating hand dermatitis with corticosteroids is simple, safe, and quite rewarding.

Systemic Corticosteroids

In acute, severe, blistering hand dermatitis, a brief course of systemic corticosteroids is of dramatic benefit. The aim of the systemic drug is to render the dermatitis susceptible to topical corticosteroids; when there is edema and blistering, topical corticosteroids will not penetrate deeply enough to be effective. Usually, a 4- to 7-day, tapering course of steroid suffices. Prednisone is the drug of choice, given as one dose in the morning. Systemic corticosteroids should be used only for severe processes; therefore, prescribe enough of the drug: 60 to 80 mg of prednisone the first day, decreased by 10 to 20 mg each day thereafter. Begin topical corticosteroid therapy when there is some decrease in blistering and swelling.

Avoid systemic therapy with injections of long-acting repository corticosteroids such as triamcinolone acetonide. Not only do these preparations cause prolonged adrenal suppression, but the patient observes that for the next few weeks his hands remain improved regardless of behavior, and he never learns the technique or the effectiveness of proper topical therapy. When, 3 to 6 weeks later, the hand eczema flares, the patient returns for another "magic" shot.

Other Systemic Therapies

When bacterial infection is present or suspected, systemic antibiotics are indicated: either erythromycin or a semisynthetic penicillin (e.g., cloxacillin) taken by mouth. In the presence of hand infection, it is preferable to prescribe a systemic antibiotic and a topical corticosteroid rather than rely on topical applications of an antibiotic-corticosteroid combination.

Antihistamines, sedatives, and tranquilizers do not improve dermatitis, but only dull the patient's sensorium. There are rare exceptions; a highly anxious patient may need a few days of support with a tranquilizer or mild sedative taken at bedtime.

TOPICAL THERAPY

General Principles

Topical corticosteroids and lubrication are the mainstays in treating hand dermatitis. Although acute vesicular dermatoses may benefit for a few days from tap-water soaks, most hand dermatitis is dry and scaly and requires lubrication. White petrolatum is an ideal lubricant from a medical viewpoint, but it is too greasy for most patients to tolerate. Commercial hand creams are often not greasy enough; some contain lanolin and other potential sensitizers. Unfortunately, most corticosteroid creams are not lubricating enough, and corticosteroid ointments are unacceptably greasy. Furthermore, if a moderately potent or stronger corticosteroid is used, frequent applications are unnecessarily expensive and may predispose the patient to skin atrophy.

Separating the corticosteroid and lubricant effects by once- or twice-daily applications of a mild or stronger corticosteroid combined with frequent lubrication with an indifferent lubricant is a rational approach. However, it may be hard to find a suitable daytime lubricant and to adhere to a routine involving two products. I have also found it advantageous to avoid the use of over-the-counter lubricants, as patients tend to experiment with supermarket specials or samples that come in the mail. Compliance is more precise when the patient is specifically instructed to apply only medications prescribed for him.

My compromise has been the use of hydrocortisone cream augmented by white petrolatum. This method of treatment is based on the observation that 15 to 20 percent white petrolatum can be incorporated into a cream base without a perception of greasiness. This medicated hand lubricant serves as both a lubricating agent and a corticosteroid vehicle. Patients like it and will use it on a long-term basis, both as a lubricant and to control mild flares of dermatitis. The formula of this medicated hand lubricant is: hydrocortisone ointment 2.5 percent (petrolatum base) 20 g; hydrocortisone cream 1 percent qs 120 g. Hydrocortisone ointment 2.5 percent rather than petrolatum is used to prevent dilution of the hydrocortisone concentration. Actually, this formula yields a hydrocortisone concentration of about 1.2 percent, which is appropriate because 1 percent is close to the threshold of effectiveness for hydrocortisone. Have the pharmacist put the prescription in two jars. Homemakers should keep one jar in the kitchen and the other in the bathroom for frequent use after handwashing. For those working outside the home, one of the containers should be kept at work.

The choice of topical corticosteroid therapy depends on the location and severity of the dermatitis. Dermatitis of the backs of the hands responds much more readily to topical corticosteroids than does palmar dermatitis. The effectiveness of topical therapy can be increased both by using more potent steroids and by using plastic occlusion. Plastic occlusion increases corticosteroid penetration roughly 10 times. If there is significant volar dermatitis, plastic occlusion will usually be required.

Occlusion exerts a beneficial effect independent of its enhancement of corticosteroid penetration. Occlusion alone has been demonstrated to improve plaque-type psoriasis. In hand dermatitis, occlusion leads to rapid healing of fissures and often dramatically improves psoriasiform and atopic hand dermatitis.

Plastic occlusion increases the unwanted as well as the desirable effects of corticosteroids. Highly potent corticosteroid formulations may cause skin atrophy; plastic occlusion markedly accentuates this complication. Clinically, such atrophy appears as thin, irritated skin with easy fissuring. The patient usually complains of sensitive, easily injured skin. Sometimes atrophy is mistaken for a flare-up of the dermatitis and is made worse by more vigorous treatment with high-potency corticosteroids.

Generally, 1 percent or 2.5 percent hydrocortisone ointment will prove adequate when used with occlusion. If a more potent corticosteroid is necessary, I prescribe desonide ointment (Tridesilon) with instructions for occlusion. Rarely is occlusion with a stronger product warranted.

CAUTION. Avoid the use of superpotent corticosteroids with occlusion in treating hand dermatitis.

Occlusion of the hands is best accomplished by wearing thin, pliable, properly fitting plastic (not rubber) gloves overnight. This practice is uncomfortable, but after a few days, the benefits become so obvious that patients usually cease their complaints. Be sure the gloves are not too tight; fit the patient with the proper size and give him one or two extra pairs. The brand is unimportant, but it is important that the gloves be pliable, slightly elastic, and readily available.

To avoid atrophy, use the minimum amount of occlusion and the least potent corticosteroid needed to control the dermatitis. For long-term treatment, 1 percent hydrocortisone is best, because it does not cause hand skin atrophy. Patients vary greatly in their tolerance of highly potent corticosteroids; although some patients tolerate corticosteroids for years, others show undesirable atrophy after a few weeks of use (Figure C–5). Hand dermatitis treatment should be tailored to location and severity to produce adequate suppression with minimal risk of atrophy.

This system of managing hand dermatitis centers on a treatment instruction sheet that provides precise directions for the use of topical corticosteroids. All patients are given the hydrocortisone-containing medicated hand lubricant described previously to use many times during the day. This will suffice for a mild dermatitis. For moderate dermatitis, this regimen is augmented by applying a moderately potent corticosteroid at bedtime. For more severe dermatoses, this basic lubricant regimen is augmented by: (1) a single bedtime application of a more potent corticosteroid; or (2) overnight occlusion using a low- or moderate-strength corticosteroid.

After history and examination, the following steps should be taken in the treatment of hand dermatitis:

1. Provide the patient instruction sheets Hand Dermatitis Treatment and Hand Protection for Hand Dermatitis.
2. Briefly review the instructions and tell the patient to read both sheets daily for 1 week to become familiar with them.
3. Write a prescription for the medicated hand lubricant.
4. For more severe dermatitis, augment the lubricant with a bedtime application of a more potent corticosteroid.

This method of treatment is simple, and it works. If you do not want to get involved with occlusion and high-potency corticosteroids, treat mild or moderate dorsal dermatitis and refer severer cases to dermatologists specializing in this condition.

Specific Details

MILD DORSAL DERMATITIS. The majority of hand dermatoses seen in homemakers and others exposed to heavy use of irritants show mainly dorsal involvement; erythema and scaling dominate. Occlusion is not needed. Prescribe the medicated hand lubricant, which the patient should apply to the entire skin of both hands many times a day.

The patient returns for follow-up in 1 to 2 weeks. If you are on the right track, there will be dramatic improvement. Go over the long-term aspects of treatment and specifically explain to the patient how to reduce the frequency of application gradually. Explain that treatment is a long-term process and that the prescription for the medicated hand lubricant is refillable. The occasional patient with mild dorsal dermatitis who does not respond should be treated as described in the following section of this chapter.

MODERATE DORSAL DERMATITIS. In moderately severe dorsal dermatitis, I use a moderate- or high-potency corticosteroid at bedtime without occlusion. The hydrocortisone-containing medicated hand lubricant is used during the day. As the patient improves, the potent corticosteroid is gradually phased out. This approach requires two minor changes in the patient instruction sheet Hand Dermatitis Treatment. In the first sentence, underline "cortisone cream" and draw an arrow away from it and then write "medicated hand lubricant." This indicates to the patient that the medicated hand lubricant is the basic cortisone. At the bottom of the page, add a sentence directing the patient to apply the highly potent corticosteroid sparingly to the rash at bedtime. Direct the patient to phase out this part of treatment by using it every other night, then every third night as the skin improves, and discontinuing use of the high-potency corticosteroid at bedtime when the rash clears.

When the dermatitis has cleared, the patient continues the lubricating treatment during the day on a long-term basis. Recurring dermatitis is an indication for resuming nightly use of the high-potency corticosteroid.

If a highly potent corticosteroid is applied once daily, either with or without occlusion, it makes little difference whether 1 percent hydrocortisone or a bland emollient is used for skin lubrication. The potent corticosteroid completely overshadows any effect of the hydrocortisone. Nevertheless, my preference is to use the hydrocortisone-containing medicated hand lubricant as a basic skin lubricant even when a highly potent corticosteroid is used simultaneously. After the high-potency corticosteroid has been phased out, the hydrocortisone-containing lubricant usually controls recurrences. Treatment is simplified, because the patient uses only one preparation (i.e., the topical hydrocortisone) to control minor flare-ups.

HAND DERMATITIS WITH SIGNIFICANT VOLAR INVOLVEMENT. When there is significant involvement of volar surfaces and/or severe dermatitis of the dorsa, overnight occlusion should be added initially to frequent daytime corticosteroid or lubricant applications. The overnight occlusion should be considered a booster treatment. A moderate- to high-potency corticosteroid should be employed for overnight occlusion only. The daytime medication should be either a bland emollient or the hydrocortisone-containing hand lubricant I favor, because the patient will use it as a lubricant.

Depending on the severity of the dermatitis, use either 2.5 percent hydrocortisone in petrolatum or a more potent corticosteroid, preferably in a petrolatum base, for occlusion treatment. Stress that the occlusion should be confined to the rash and not used on the entire hand. If the eruption is limited to the palms, cut the fingers off the plastic gloves. When the dermatitis involves only fingers, the patient is to cut the appropriate fingers off the plastic glove and hold them in place overnight with nonirritating "paper" tape.

Have the patient return 7 to 10 days after initiating treatment; if the dermatitis is better, ask him to use occlusion only every other night. If the patient does well on every-other-night occlusion, instruct him at the next visit to use it only every third night; after an additional 2 weeks, see if occlusion can be discontinued. With care, it should be possible to withdraw overnight occlusion when the dermatitis is better, before clinically obvious atrophy occurs.

IMPORTANT. Provide only a small amount of high-potency corticosteroid so the patient cannot continue treatment for months on his own.

Most patients can be weaned away from occlusion, although some find it necessary to use it once or twice per week indefinitely. Long-term occlusive treatment with a potent corticosteroid is usually safe when used not more than twice per week. It may be possible to shift the patient to hydrocortisone or an intermediate-strength corticosteroid, with occasional occlusion as the situation demands.

Variations

These treatment methods can and should be modified. Volar dermatitis affecting only the fingers frequently responds to nightly use of a high-potency corticosteroid without occlusion. Patients who object to overnight occlusion may successfully treat their hands by wearing the plastic gloves for 3 or 4 hours while awake. If the patient objects to petrolatum as a lubricant, prescribe something less greasy. Be willing to modify your treatment to suit your patients; the medicament or lubricant will work only if they comply with the treatment program.

Intralesional Therapy

Intralesional corticosteroids are useful in treating hand dermatitis when there is a small but active area of dermatitis (Figure C–60) and when there is extensive vesicular volar dermatitis that responds poorly to occlusion with potent corticosteroids. The technique and problems of intralesional therapy are described in Chapter 1. Intralesional corticosteroid injections in the hands should be used reluctantly, as infection occasionally follows.

REFERENCE

1. Epstein E: Hand dermatitis: Practical management and current concepts. *J Am Acad Dermatol* 10:395, 1984

16 *Seborrheic Dermatitis*

Patient sheets pages P–19, P–35*

ETIOLOGY

This common skin disorder is misnamed; seborrheic dermatitis has nothing to do with the sebaceous glands. It is a genetically determined skin dysfunction; the mechanism is unknown. The ubiquitous organism *Pityrosporum ovale,* the cause of tinea versicolor, may often be a contributing factor.

DIAGNOSIS

Typical cases are easily diagnosed, because seborrheic dermatitis commonly favors certain areas: (1) the scalp and scalp margins; (2) the glabella, eyebrows, and eyelid edges; (3) the skin about the nose; (4) the ears and retroauricular folds; (5) the presternal area and mid-upper back; and (6) the skin folds—inguinal, gluteal, axillary, and inframammary.

The scalp is the commonest location; ordinary dandruff† is seborrheic dermatitis of the scalp. Frequently, the rash spreads onto the forehead and lateral scalp margins. The rash of seborrheic dermatitis is red and scaly, except in skin-fold areas, where it usually takes on a smooth, red, glazed appearance.

Psoriasis is the chief differential diagnosis. On the scalp, seborrheic dermatitis tends to form diffuse, scaling areas with mild redness, whereas psoriasis produces sharply demarcated, infiltrated, often crusted plaques. Frequently, it is impossible to be sure what disease is present, and some physicians express their diagnostic uncertainty by using the term seborrhiasis. Not uncommonly, a patient will have typical seborrheic dermatitis of the scalp that gradually worsens over the years, becomes recalcitrant to therapy, and finally presents as typical psoriasis.

In skin-fold areas, seborrheic dermatitis and psoriasis frequently have the same red, glazed appearance. Candidiasis and dermatophytosis (ie., tinea cruris) must be differentiated from and can sometimes coexist with seborrheic dermatitis. Stubborn diaper rash is usually seborrheic dermatitis, sometimes with superimposed candidiasis, and frequently with irritation from topical therapy. Cradle cap is seborrheic dermatitis of the scalp in infants. Always consider psoriasis when managing patients with seborrheic dermatitis.

---

*Refer to the *Universal Medication Summary Sheet*, page xxi.

†Possibly an oversimplification. One current view is that mild, noninflammatory dandruff represents the physiologic desquamation of the scalp known as pityriasis capitis. Patients with dandruff show a spectrum of severity of scalp scaling. In mild cases, it is usually impossible to decide whether the process should be considered physiologic (pityriasis capitis) or a mild form of disease (seborrheic dermatitis). From a practical viewpoint, such considerations are immaterial; the treatment for pityriasis capitis is the same as that for mild seborrheic dermatitis.

TREATMENT

Be sure your patient understands that treatment is a matter of control rather than cure. Failure to accept this will invariably lead to patient dissatisfaction. Although seborrheic dermatitis is a chronic, recurring condition, it usually responds nicely to topical therapy. Secondary infection, manifested by oozing, pustules, and crusting, occurs occasionally, especially about the ears. A 5- to 7-day course of erythromycin or a semisynthetic penicillin by mouth generally resolves the secondary infection. Systemic corticosteroids are not indicated unless there is a superimposed severe contact dermatitis.

Corticosteroids, certain antifungals, tars, sulfur, and salicylic acid are the preferred topicals for treating seborrheic dermatitis. Antifungal agents effective against *Pityrosporum ovale* [e.g., selenium sulfide, imidazole derivatives (miconazole, clotrimazole, and others), zinc pyrithione, topical ketoconazole] are frequently beneficial. The antifungal agent ketoconazole is highly effective in suppressing seborrheic dermatitis. On the face and scalp, 2 percent ketoconazole cream is as effective as 1 percent hydrocortisone cream. For more severe dermatitis, ketoconazole applications can be alternated with a topical corticosteroid, thereby reducing the frequency of topical corticosteroid applications. Treatment of seborrheic dermatitis depends on its site as well as its severity and is discussed in this chapter on a regional basis.

SCALP

Mild dandruff is most easily controlled by frequent shampooing. Ask the patient to shampoo, if practical, whenever he or she showers. Dandruff medications added to shampoos vary in their effectiveness. The best are 2.5 percent selenium sulfide (a prescription item), 2 percent zinc pyrithione, and ketoconazole (a prescription item). Tars, sulfur, and salicylic acid are of less benefit. A 2.5 percent selenium sulfide shampoo should be used only once every 2 weeks; in between, any other shampoo is acceptable. The other medicated shampoos may be used every day. Tar shampoos may cause a yellowish discoloration of white or gray hair. Patients need to find out which shampoo routine works best for them. If you have samples, have the patient try them and pick his or her favorite. Stress that daily shampooing is safe and does not cause hair loss (a common misconception).

If frequent medicated shampoos fail to control scalp seborrhea, topical corticosteroids, topical ketoconazole, or tars are indicated. It is more difficult to deliver medications to the hairy scalp than to smooth skin. Creams and ointments cannot be used. For moderate seborrheic dermatitis, prescribe a corticosteroid gel or liquid to be applied sparingly 2 or 3 times weekly and massaged in well. These are clean, elegant preparations that neither stink nor stain. Ketoconazole cream applied 2 to 4 hours before shampooing, or overnight before a morning shampoo, is another effective treatment. Currently, topical ketoconazole is available in the United States only as a cream; ask patients to apply it with wet fingers, which converts it into a lotion.

Tars are the next step if frequent shampooing, topical ketoconazole, and a topical corticosteroid fail to provide adequate control. Coal-tar solutions (TGel scalp solution), coal-tar gels (Psorigel, Estar gel), or coal-tar and oil topicals (Balnetar, TDerm tar emollient) may be applied sparingly to the scaly areas 3 to 8 hours before shampooing. Warn patients that tars can photosensitize skin and predispose to sunburn of the scalp.

If the combination of frequent shampoos, a topical corticosteroid, and ketoconazole or a tar applied before shampooing fails to control seborrheic dermatitis, the patient almost certainly has psoriasis.

EARS AND SCALP EDGES

A fluorinated corticosteroid gel, cream, or ointment applied once or twice daily usually produces dramatic control. Write on the prescription, and also instruct the patient, that the medication must not be used on the face. For the scalp edges, gels and lotions are preferable. On the ears, a greasy corticosteroid ointment applied at bedtime is usually very effective. Ketoconazole cream is also effective; I like to alternate it with a topical corticosteroid.

FACE

Start with 2 percent ketoconazole applied twice daily. If control is inadequate, add a daily application of 1 percent or 2.5 percent hydrocortisone cream. Avoid using stronger corticosteroids on the face. Stubborn facial seborrheic dermatitis often yields to 2 percent sulfur and 2 percent salicylic acid incorporated into 2.5 percent hydrocortisone cream.

EYELIDS

Seborrheic blepharitis, which produces crusting and itching eyelid edges, is a common, chronic problem. Eyelid crusting often responds to diluted Johnson's baby shampoo (no other brand) applied to the edges of the lids with a cotton-tipped swab. Ophthalmologists are fond of treating seborrheic blepharitis with topical antimicrobials such as sulfacetamide ointment. In my experience, an antibiotic-hydrocortisone ointment combination is superior to either alone. Unfortunately, these combinations have been virtually withdrawn from the United States market. Often, plain 1 or 1.5 percent hydrocortisone in ophthalmic ointment base suffices. If this treatment is not adequate, have the patient use the hydrocortisone topically in the morning and an antibiotic at bedtime, applying each thinly. Tetracycline and erythromycin are safe for long-term topical use; avoid potentially sensitizing antibiotics such as neomycin.

CAUTION. Glaucoma is a possible complication of topical corticosteroids used in the eyes. The fluorinated corticosteroids seem to be more troublesome in this regard than hydrocortisone. The patient should be instructed to apply a tiny amount of hydrocortisone ointment to the eyelid edges with the eyes closed and to keep it out of the eyes. Patients should also be told to interrupt their eyelid hydrocortisone application if they develop herpes simplex, because of the danger of developing herpetic keratitis. Periodic ocular pressure checks are a prudent precaution for those patients requiring continuous use of topical corticosteroids to control severe seborrheic blepharitis.

CHEST AND BACK

Combination therapy with ketoconazole cream used once daily and a moderate-potency corticosteroid used once daily at different times is usually effective. The moderate-potency corticosteroid may be a cream, gel, or ointment, depending on the hairiness and dryness of the skin. Hydrocortisone tends to be relatively ineffective in these areas. Be sure that the moderate-potency corticosteroid is labeled "Do NOT use on face or skin-fold areas." For stubborn seborrheic dermatitis that responds poorly to this combination regimen, add tetracycline or a tetracycline-class antibiotic by mouth in the same dose as that used for treating acne. The response is often dramatic, although the mechanism is not understood.

Seborrheic intertrigo (i.e., skin-fold dermatitis) is best treated using both 1 percent hydrocortisone cream and a cream having antiyeast as well as antibacterial effects, such as ketoconazole cream or econazole cream. The hydrocortisone and antimicrobial cream can be applied at the same time or in an alternating pattern; either approach seems to work. Instruct the patient to use only water in cleansing skin-fold areas, because soap is an irritant. If there is a poor response, increase the potency of the hydrocortisone to 2.5 percent or possibly switch to one of the low- or moderate-strength corticosteroids such as desonide. Long-term use of these agents may cause skin thinning; make it clear to the patient that the drug should be used only for a short period of time until the dermatitis improves. Follow this short-term treatment with 1 percent hydrocortisone. Do not use strong corticosteroids in the armpits, groin, or inframammary folds because of their notorious tendency to cause skin thinning and striae when used in skin-fold areas. Traditional antiseborrheic dermatitis remedies such as tar and sulfur are poorly tolerated in the armpits and groin; if you do prescribe them, do so in a concentration of 1 percent or less. These cautions apply to the armpits and groin, but not to seborrheic dermatitis of the retroauricular fold. The skin behind the ears tolerates moderate-potency corticosteroids, as well as topical sulfur, tars, and salicylic acid.

17 *Dermatofibromas*

Patient sheets pages P–37, P–61

ETIOLOGY

Dermatofibromas (histiocytomas) are firm, benign skin tumors whose cause is unknown. Left alone, dermatofibromas persist for decades. Some believe they represent a peculiar reaction to trauma, possibly insect bites. This theory offers a useful explanation for patients, who may be told "It is a scar reaction, possibly from an old insect bite."

DIAGNOSIS

The typical dermatofibroma is a smooth, hard, dome-shaped papule with a pink-to-violaceous-to-brownish color. These lesions occur in the dermis and give the epidermis a stretched appearance. They favor the extremities, especially the legs, and are more common in women than in men (Figures C–43 through C–45).

The history and appearance of dermatofibromas usually permit a clinical diagnosis. The principal differential diagnosis is that of a nevus (Figure C–42), especially if lesions are enlarging or inflamed (Figures C–37 and C–38). As with any pigmented lesion, melanoma enters the differential diagnosis. Other malignancies, such as basal cell carcinoma, squamous cell carcinoma, or even fibrosarcoma, should be considered if the lesion is enlarging or atypical. It is sometimes impossible to distinguish a keloid or hypertrophic scar from a dermatofibroma.

TREATMENT

Reassurance is all the treatment that is needed unless you are unsure of the diagnosis or the patient is annoyed by the lesion. If the diagnosis is in doubt, or if reassurance is required, a 1.5- or 2-mm-diameter punch biopsy provides a tissue diagnosis with little visible scarring. Women often object to the protrusion of dermatofibromas, especially on the legs, where they interfere with shaving.

Dermatofibromas extend deep into the dermis; permanent removal requires full-thickness skin excision. Because these lesions are usually found on the extremities or trunk, the scar following excision is usually more prominent than the original dermatofibroma. I no longer excise dermatofibromas. When treatment is required, I use liquid nitrogen, usually preceded by a small punch biopsy to provide histologic confirmation. This is a neat and histologically controlled way of treating annoying dermatofibromas (Figures C–37 through C–41 and C–43 through C–45).

After injecting a local anesthetic, use a 1.5- or 2-mm-diameter punch to take a deep biopsy from the center of the lesion. Pack the wound with Gelfoam, or a similar tissue-neutral hemostatic. Freeze the dermatofibroma thoroughly; moderately deep freezing is required. Apply a Band-Aid dressing and provide the patient instruction sheet Liquid Nitrogen Treatment for postoperative care.

Explain to the patient that the biopsy is to confirm the diagnosis and the liquid nitrogen freezing will flatten the growth. Sometimes, a second or third freezing is needed to produce satisfactory flattening. Rarely, a dermatofibroma will recur after several years. If so, it can be frozen again. The patient instruction sheet Dermatofibromas explains the options.

18 *Dry Skin (Asteatosis, Xerosis)*

Patient sheet page P–39

ETIOLOGY

Dry skin is a common patient complaint. It occurs at all ages but becomes more of a problem with advanced age. Many older patients chronically complain of dry, itchy skin. The legs are the most common site, but any body part may be affected.

Dry skin describes a clinical problem whose etiologic factors are incompletely understood. Skin moisture plays a central role; anything that causes the skin to lose moisture results in a tendency to dryness and chapping. The drier the air, the more rapidly skin moisture is lost. Consequently, dry skin is a particular problem in cold, winter climates where the warm indoor air is low in humidity. Removal of lipids and other skin components by soaps, detergents, and excessive bathing contributes to the damage. Dry skin begins with scaling and chapping; if it is not checked, eczematous changes supervene and dominate the clinical picture. Frequently, the patches of eczema are round and fairly sharply demarcated—the so-called nummular eczema. These round patches may be mistaken for ringworm. The patient may aggravate them by vigorous scrubbing or by applying irritating remedies.

DIAGNOSIS

Diagnosis is usually easy in the early stages, which mostly are characterized by dryness, chapping, and low-grade erythema. Ichthyosis is the chief differential diagnosis. Ichthyosis is differentiated by its constant presence, its uniform morphology, and often, a positive family history. When eczematous changes are present, it may be difficult to decide whether you are dealing with a primarily eczematous disorder associated with dry skin, or whether the eczematous changes are secondary to irritated, dry skin. Dry skin is almost invariably present in patients with atopic eczema and is a common accompaniment of psoriasis.

From the standpoint of treatment, it makes little difference whether the condition is a primarily eczematous disorder with associated dry skin or eczema superimposed on dry skin, because eczematous skin is treated similarly, irrespective of the underlying problem. The prognosis, of course, is different: It's much more favorable if one is dealing simply with eczematous changes superimposed on dry skin.

TREATMENT

The treatment of dry skin is dependent on its severity. Mild dryness and chapping respond well to skin hydration and lubricating measures. When dermatitis supervenes, topical corticosteroids should be added. When there is extensive, severe dermatitis, a 3- to 5-day tapering course of prednisone provides dramatic relief.

SKIN HYDRATION AND LUBRICATION

When only dryness and chapping are present, minimizing the use of soap and simple measures to hydrate the skin are usually enough. Bathing adds moisture to the skin; apply a lubricant immediately to diminish water loss. The greasier the lubricant, the better. Petrolatum (Vaseline) applied thinly is an excellent lubricant, but most patients find it messy. My preference is to have patients apply mineral oil *thinly* to the wet skin after bathing. Instead of toweling dry, the patient allows the water to evaporate. This lubricating routine is best carried out at bedtime, because then the residual slight oiliness affects only the bedclothes. Mineral oil is inexpensive and universally available. It is preferable to baby oil, which contains perfumes and other additives. This simple, highly effective mineral oil lubricating routine is detailed in patient instruction sheet Dry Skin (Asteatosis, Xerosis).

Patients with dry skin are frequently told to decrease the frequency of bathing; this isn't necessary unless the patient is bathing more than once daily. What is essential is that they not apply soap directly to their dry skin and that they lubricate their skin immediately after showering or bathing. Diluted soap running down the body with shower water is permissible.

For those preferring a tub bath, bath oils are a simple and effective way of achieving total body lubrication. Bath oils consist of oil, surfactants, perfumes, and dyes. One or two tablespoons are added to the tub, and the patient should soak for at least 10 to 15 minutes. Soap is to be avoided; the emulsifier-oil combination acts as a cleansing agent. The patient gently pats himself dry so that some of the oil film remains on the skin. Because bath oils make the tub dangerously slippery, I avoid their use with the elderly. Mineral oil, baby oil, and other oils are not suitable as bath additives, because they lack the emulsifiers that allow bath oils to mix with water.

Salad oil or hydrogenated vegetable cooking fats are sometimes recommended as inexpensive skin lubricants. They are safe and effective but give clothes, pajamas, and towels an unpleasant, rancid odor. Mineral oil and plain petrolatum do not do this.

Commercial skin-lubricating lotions or creams can also be applied after bathing. Most of these products are mainly water; consequently, they are highly acceptable to patients. However, as lubricants, they are inferior to mineral oil or petrolatum. Used by themselves, these lotions and creams are a reasonable approach for treating mild or localized skin dryness.

Many lubricating lotions contain additives, such as urea, vitamin E, and aloe vera, which may irritate or sensitize the patient's skin. One exception is ammonium lactate, available as a 12 percent prescription lotion (Lac-hydrin 12). This product has been shown to be superior to a control lotion in improving dry, scaly skin. Occasionally, Lac-hydrin 12 causes unacceptable stinging. Ammonium lactate is also available as a 5 percent nonprescription lotion (Lac-hydrin 5); whether this lower concentration provides similar benefits is not clear.

Although commercial lubricants are usually well tolerated by patients with nothing more than dry skin, be reluctant to use these products when dermatitis is present. Many lubricants are irritating or contain potential sensitizers such as lanolin, perfumes, and preservatives. When there is dermatitis, play it safe and stick to mineral oil or petrolatum.

CORTICOSTEROID THERAPY

When eczematous changes are present, a topical corticosteroid should be applied sparingly one or two times per day. Ointments are usually more effective than creams or lotions. If an ointment is applied sparingly and massaged in well, it is not too messy. For fastidious patients, a useful compromise is to prescribe a cream or lotion for use during the day and a greasy corticosteroid for use at bedtime. If you do not wish to burden the patient with the expense of purchasing two medications, have him apply plain petrolatum at bedtime after thoroughly massaging in the corticosteroid cream.

Systemic treatment is needed only in rare, severe cases of dry-skin dermatitis. A brief, 2- to 5-day, tapering course of prednisone provides dramatic relief and is more practical than whole-body application of topical corticosteroids. Start with 40 to 60 mg of prednisone taken in one dose on the first day, and then decrease the dose by 10 to 20 mg per day over the next 2 to 4 days. Antihistamines and other so-called antipruritics are of no value in treating dry skin. At best, they sedate the patient so the itching is less worrisome. It is preferable to treat the cause.

MANAGING THE PATIENT

Success in managing dry-skin dermatitis requires compliance and the patient's understanding that lubricating measures may be required for a long time. The patient instruction sheet Dry Skin (Asteatosis, Xerosis) will help get this message across. Stress that dry-skin dermatitis tends to recur, and that the patient should resume the hydrating and lubricating measures at the first sign of dry skin.

Fragile Skin Bleeding

Patient sheets pages P–43, P–99

ETIOLOGY

Senile purpura is the standard term for the tendency to ecchymoses and purpura of the dorsa of hands and forearms that annoys many older persons. Substitute the phrase fragile skin bleeding for the pejorative senile purpura, because the condition is not a result of senility but comes from solar damage to the connective tissue of the skin. As a result of these degenerative changes in the connective tissue, even trivial shearing may cause an extensive ecchymosis.

DIAGNOSIS

The diagnosis is obvious at a glance, because the bleeding is limited to the dorsa of the hands and forearms and usually spares the volar aspects of the forearms and the remaining skin. Purpura and ecchymoses secondary to connective-tissue damage sometimes occur in systemic disorders such as rheumatoid arthritis and may also be seen as a result of prolonged corticosteroid administration. Differentiate such conditions by the history and by examining the legs, because the purpura of rheumatoid arthritis and corticosteroid damage usually affects the legs, whereas the purpura of solar damage generally spares the lower extremities. Systemic corticosteroids worsen the fragile skin bleeding caused by solar damage.

TREATMENT

Fragile skin bleeding is permanent; there is no effective treatment. Do reassure patients that the condition is the result of localized skin damage and not a sign of a blood disorder or other serious illness. It usually suffices to tell patients that the bleeding is a result of sun damage to the skin and ask them to read the patient information sheet Fragile Skin Bleeding for further details. The patient information sheet encourages patients to minimize future sun damage; also give them the patient information sheet Sunlight and Your Skin.

20 *Herpes Simplex*

Patient sheet page P–47

ETIOLOGY

Herpes simplex infections are caused by the herpes hominis virus, which has two distinct strains: HSV 1 and HSV 2. Genital herpes is usually caused by type 2 virus, and the type 1 strain is responsible for most facial infections.

The initial infection with herpesvirus, or primary herpes simplex infection, generally produces a painful, marked, local reaction along with systemic symptoms such as fever and malaise. Type 1 primary herpes simplex infection usually occurs in children as an inflammation of the oral mucosa and gums. It sometimes occurs in adults as well. The typical grouped blisters of herpes may not be evident in primary herpetic gingivostomatitis, and new, isolated vesicles can continue to erupt for days. The primary attack of genital herpes is painful and associated with systemic symptoms, especially in women, in whom it may produce severe vulvovaginitis. Primary genital herpes is mostly a disease seen in adults, because it is usually acquired through sexual intercourse.

Following the primary infection, the virus establishes residence in a nerve root ganglion and may periodically travel down the nerve to the skin to produce recurrent disease. These recurring groups of blisters, herpes simplex recurrens, are the most common clinical presentation of herpes simplex.

DIAGNOSIS

Primary herpes simplex is often misdiagnosed as an infection (Figures C–49 and C–50), cellulitis, insect bite, or even contact dermatitis. Herpes simplex recurrens is usually readily diagnosed; crops of blisters on an erythematous base appear in approximately the same area with each attack. Most patients with recurrent herpes appear with their own correct diagnosis and want treatment. In the early stages, before significant blistering occurs, and in the later phases, when only erosions or crusts may be present, diagnosis can be difficult, and herpes may perfectly resemble a nonspecific dermatitis or a pyoderma. Extensive herpes simplex recurrens may resemble herpes zoster or an acute vesicular contact dermatitis. Herpes simplex presenting in more unusual locations, such as the fingers, may be misdiagnosed because of failure to consider the possibility of herpes in the differential diagnosis.

Herpes simplex recurrens of the genitalia is often atypical in its appearance and may present diagnostic difficulties. The clinically diagnosable stage of grouped vesicles may be transient or may not appear at all. Any recurring erosion, rash, or sore in the genital area should be suspected of being herpes simplex.

Herpes simplex is essentially a clinical diagnosis. The virus can be cultured from active lesions; this specialized procedure is available in most urban areas. The new immunofluorescent methods are rapid and highly specific. The cells at the bases of the vesicles of herpes simplex, herpes zoster, and varicella show alterations in morphology. Cellular material can be obtained by unroofing a blister and gently scraping the base with a clean blade after absorbing the blister fluid with sterile gauze. The cellular debris is smeared thinly on a slide and stained with Giemsa or Wright's stain.

Herpes simplex, herpes zoster, and varicella produce identical cellular changes, consisting of huge, multinucleated giant cells many times the size of an epidermal cell, as well as nuclear inclusion bodies. When present, the virally caused giant cells are obvious.

COMPLICATIONS

Primary herpes simplex infection of neonates and young infants is serious and may be fatal. In patients with eczematous disorders, both primary and recurrent herpes may become generalized, a disorder called eczema herpeticum. Some of these patients become very ill. Patients on immunosuppressants may develop progressive, atypical herpes infections.

Ophthalmic herpes simplex is justifiably dreaded because it may cause corneal ulcerations that can progress to scarring and blindness. Topical corticosteroids aggravate herpetic eye disease and are contraindicated in ophthalmic herpes. A deleterious effect of topical corticosteroids has been documented only for ophthalmic herpes. No clear-cut effect—either beneficial or adverse—has been shown for corticosteroids applied to cutaneous herpes.

An occasional complication of recurrent herpes simplex is erythema multiforme. This hypersensitivity reaction usually appears a few days after the onset of the herpes. It may be severe enough to overshadow the herpetic infection completely. Erythema multiforme responds dramatically to systemic corticosteroids.

The yellow, crusting stage of herpes simplex is sometimes mistaken for a bacterial infection and treated with topical or systemic antibiotics. Bacterial superinfection of herpes appears to be rare; usually, petrolatum lubrication during the crusting stage is all that is needed in terms of treatment.

CONTAGION

Herpes infections are contagious to those who have not previously been infected. Few individuals escape type 1 infection during childhood. Contagion of type 1 herpes is uncommon among adults; however, the genital, type 2 virus is epidemic among sexually active adults. The traditional advice that this disease is contagious only when lesions are present is incorrect; both men and women may shed virus when free of visible lesions. Consequently, it is possible to infect sexual partners in the absence of lesions. This concern regarding contagion often causes severe anxiety in sexual partnerships.

TREATMENT

Acyclovir given internally effectively suppresses herpes simplex. Oral acyclovir shortens the course of primary and recurrent herpes simplex. It is critical to initiate acyclovir treatment early in the course of the disease. The manufacturer's recommended dose of 200 mg five times daily is both cumbersome and suboptimal. Initiate treatment with 600 to 800 mg and continue treatment with 400 mg three times daily. Generally, 3 to 4 days of therapy is adequate for treating recurrent herpes, and a 7- to 10-day course is effective for treating primary herpes. Acyclovir does not accelerate the healing of established lesions; it inhibits the spread and development of new lesions. Acyclovir is well tolerated by the patient; mild gastrointestinal side effects are infrequent.

Recurring herpes simplex is best managed by treating each attack. It is critical that the patient have a supply of acyclovir on hand in order to start therapy at the first sign of an attack. Patients usually recognize the early stages of an attack when they note erythema accompanied by itching or burning. This is the optimal time—before blisters appear—to initiate acyclovir therapy. Patients suffering one attack after another will benefit from chronic suppressive therapy with acyclovir, using dosages that range from 400 to 800 mg daily; 400 mg twice daily is being used in a number of studies. Although the manufacturer recommends a maximum of 1 year of continuous suppression therapy, many have used it longer. Unfortunately, physicians continue to prescribe the expensive but ineffective acyclovir ointment.

NOTE. The safety of acyclovir treatment during pregnancy has not been determined.

Topical therapy, even topical acyclovir, is of no value in cutaneous herpes simplex. For ocular herpes, topical antiviral agents are of definite benefit.

Herpes simplex recurrens may occur at varying intervals; with one attack succeeding another for months, and then, without apparent reason, the victim is spared further episodes for 1 year or more. Equally unpredictable is the severity of individual attacks. An episode of herpes may be mild, with a few small evanescent blisters that disappear within days, or it may be severe and involve much of the lips, with huge blisters and crusts that make the patient miserable for more than 2 weeks.

COMPLICATIONS OF TREATMENT

Complications of treatment are invariably the result of inappropriate treatment. Irritant dermatitis from over-the-counter remedies is fairly common. Allergic dermatitis from a topical antibiotic applied to treat supposed secondary infection occurs occasionally. Because of the risk of herpetic keratitis, topical corticosteroids should never be used to treat herpes of the eye.

MANAGING THE PATIENT

Acyclovir will lessen the patient's discomfort and shorten the attacks of both primary and recurrent herpes simplex. Acyclovir is not a cure; the virus persists in the nerve ganglion. Topical therapy should be limited to bland agents.

During the acute vesicular stage, tapwater compresses will soothe the blisters. Dryness and painful fissuring when crusts have formed are relieved by sparse applications of petrolatum. Discourage the use of the many over-the-counter cold-sore remedies. Many of these products are irritating, some can cause allergic dermatitis, and all are worthless.

Herpes of the lips and face is often triggered by sunlight. Sun-protective lip pomades, described in the patient information sheet Sunlight and Your Skin, benefit patients whose herpes appears after a skiing trip or a beach outing.

Recurrent herpes of the genitalia is particularly trying for the patient; often, the friction of sexual intercourse triggers an attack. Abstinence is not a satisfactory solution. Use of lubricants during intercourse sometimes helps avoid a recurrence. As noted earlier, a course of maintenance acyclovir usually provides a symptom-free interval. Explain to patients that attacks of genital herpes may eventually become less frequent and finally cease.

21 *Herpes Zoster (Shingles)*

Patient sheet page P–49

ETIOLOGY

Herpes zoster results from the activation of varicella (chicken pox) virus dormant in the body. The mechanism of activation is unknown; the majority of patients with herpes zoster are otherwise healthy. Although textbooks stress the association of shingles with lymphomas, other neoplastic disease, and immunosuppressants, a thorough search for systemic disease in healthy-appearing persons with herpes zoster is usually not warranted. However, zoster may be the first sign of the immunosuppression that occurs in AIDS.

When herpes zoster is accompanied by widespread, disseminated lesions, a search for underlying disease is indicated. Widespread dissemination (i.e., an accompanying varicella) is often the consequence of damage to the patient's immune system. A few disseminated lesions may be disregarded; it is not uncommon to see a few vesicles at a distance from the neural distribution of herpes zoster.

DIAGNOSIS

Only a glance is required for diagnosis of the linear patches of grouped vesicles on an erythematous base stopping sharply at the midline. Difficulties in diagnosis may be encountered in the early stages of herpes zoster, before blistering has become evident, when the red, infiltrated, sharply demarcated, sometimes painful patches may suggest bacterial cellulitis, an insect-bite reaction, or even a fixed drug eruption. The appearance of blisters in the next 1 or 2 days usually allows the correct diagnosis to be made. Herpes zoster in the blistering stage is occasionally misdiagnosed as a severe contact dermatitis. Linear herpes simplex may closely resemble herpes zoster, but the presence of intense burning or pain favors the diagnosis of the latter.

The neuralgia of shingles may precede the skin eruption by 1 week or more. Patients may complain of a painful "strained back" preceding herpes zoster of the trunk. Sometimes, the history of marked burning or pain in the affected area before the rash breaks out is useful in the differential diagnosis of early herpes zoster. Although recurrent herpes simplex is sometimes preceded by tingling or itching in the affected area, usually such symptoms are mild and are present less than 1 day before the rash appears.

CONTAGION

Patients with herpes zoster should be considered as contagious as if they had varicella. They are potentially contagious to infants and small children who have never had varicella, as well as to any adult whose immune system has been altered by illness and/or drugs. In particular, patients must scrupulously avoid anyone with malignancies or those taking long-term corticosteroids or immunosuppressants (e.g., kidney transplant patients, systemic lupus erythematosus patients).

TREATMENT

For the acute phase, prescribe acyclovir in adequate doses. Acyclovir, which is effective in treating herpes simplex infections, has significant antivaricella activity, although much higher doses of acyclovir are needed to suppress zoster. The standard oral dose for acyclovir treatment of herpes zoster is 800 mg every 4 hours while the patient is awake, for a total of 4 g in each 24-hour period. Acyclovir is available in 200-, 400-, and 800-mg pills. The 800-mg size taken five times daily is much more acceptable than asking the patient to swallow four of the 200-mg capsules at each dose. Excessive blood levels of acyclovir may cause the drug to be precipitated in the renal tubules and result in kidney damage. The oral dose of 800 mg every 4 hours is safe in patients with normal kidney function. Instruct patients to take each dose with a full glass of water.

NOTE. Acyclovir is also used intravenously to treat serious herpes simplex and herpes zoster infections. Because acyclovir is poorly absorbed from the gut, safe intravenous doses of acyclovir are much lower than oral doses.

High doses of oral acyclovir will stop the progression of zoster in 1 or 2 days. Generally, 5 to 8 days of treatment suffice; the absence of new lesions and healing of old lesions are useful end points. Acyclovir treatment benefits the skin lesions; it also reduces the short-term severity of postzoster neuralgia. Unfortunately, acyclovir does not appear to reduce the frequency or severity of *chronic* postzoster neuritis.

Dilute acetic acid (i.e., white vinegar) compresses are a simple, inexpensive treatment for blisters and crusts. The technique is described in the patient instruction sheet Herpes Zoster (Shingles). Dryness and fissuring during the later healing stages are relieved by sparse applications of white petrolatum (Vaseline).

NEURALGIA

The neuralgia of herpes zoster is the real therapeutic challenge. The pain may be excruciating and may continue after the skin eruption has healed. The neuralgia of shingles tends to be more severe in older persons. In younger patients, the neuralgia is usually mild and transient.

Treatment of the neuralgia requires adequate analgesics. I usually use aspirin or acetaminophen (Tylenol) for mild pain. For moderate pain, I combine 30 to 60 mg of codeine with these agents or prescribe Vicodin, a combination of acetaminophen and hydrocodone bitartrate. Very severe pain requires oral meperidine (Demerol). In most patients, severe pain is short-lived; I prescribe narcotic analgesics if they are necessary to provide relief.

Systemic corticosteroids are of no value in the prevention of postzoster neuralgia. Earlier studies claiming this effect were flawed; better-designed trials have failed to demonstrate any effect of systemic corticosteroids on the frequency of postzoster neuralgia.

In addition to adequate analgesics, patients often benefit from a mild sedative at bedtime. Barbiturates should be avoided; preferred drugs are promethazine (Phenergan), hydroxyzine (Vistaril, Atarax), chlordiazepoxide (Librium), diazepam (Valium), or similar mild, nonbarbiturate sedating agents.

A number of different psychotherapeutic agents sometimes help patients with chronic postzoster neuritis. Among these drugs are amitriptyline (Elavil), carbamazepine (Tegretol), and chlorprothixene (Taractan). These medications have complex actions and many potential side effects. They are potent drugs and should be tried only after analgesics and time have failed. I refer patients with chronic zoster neuralgia to neurologists who are experienced in the use of these drugs.

COMPLICATIONS

Zoster sometimes leaves scars. On the skin, scars are usually mild and only a modest cosmetic handicap; in the eyes, scars can prove disastrous. Ophthalmic herpes zoster is a serious emergency requiring ophthalmologic consultation. Zoster of the eyelid does not necessarily mean that the eye is involved. If, however, the patient reports pain in the eye itself, or if the bulbar conjunctiva is inflamed, ophthalmologic consultation is imperative. Sometimes, severe swelling of the eyelid makes it difficult to evaluate the condition of the eye; when this occurs, I prefer to have an ophthalmologist see the patient. Early and adequate doses of acyclovir appear to prevent significant ophthalmic zoster.

Although zoster is usually limited to the sensory nerves, motor nerves may be involved, with disturbances of urination, muscle weakness, or paralysis. These effects are usually localized, limited, and clear spontaneously.

Postherpetic neuralgia can be a distressing and lengthy complication—it may go on for years. The psychotherapeutic drugs mentioned previously, as well as others, may be effective in treating postherpetic neuralgia. Nerve blocks and even neurosurgery have been recommended; I have had no experience with these procedures. Sometimes, reassurance and analgesics are all the physician can offer. Because postherpetic neuralgia is often a long-term problem, bear in mind the habituating effects of potent analgesics and strong sedatives. At times, the unrelenting pain warrants referral to a specialized pain control center.

Hives (Urticaria)

Patient sheet page P–51

22

ETIOLOGY

Acute urticaria is a common problem, and it usually responds dramatically to medications. The patient information sheet Hives (Urticaria) is designed for those with acute urticaria. Chronic urticaria is an infinitely more complex problem that cannot be covered in a routine patient information sheet. The discussion in this chapter is limited to acute urticaria.

Urticaria is a nonspecific vascular reaction of the skin. Patients and physicians tend to equate hives with allergy. However, many cases of urticaria have a pharmacologic basis; certain foods (e.g., strawberries) or drugs (e.g., codeine) have an innate urticariogenic action. Cholinergic urticaria, with its small papules triggered by heat or physical or emotional stress, is an endogenous pharmacologic phenomenon. Exogenous physical factors such as cold, heat, pressure, or light can cause urticaria.

Urticaria may be related to an underlying disease such as infections, collagen diseases, or neoplasia. If a patient with acute urticaria reports malaise or systemic symptoms, an underlying infectious process must be ruled out. Urticaria itches but usually does not cause other significant symptoms.

DIAGNOSIS

Urticaria is defined as transient wheals; the transient nature of the lesion is an important part of the definition. Individual hives usually develop and recede within a few hours. Often, the diagnosis is made from the history; the hives may be absent at the time of examination. When hivelike lesions persist for more than a few hours, the eruption is not true urticaria.

From the standpoint of therapy, it is important to limit the diagnosis of urticaria to lesions lasting only hours. True urticaria usually responds to antihistamines and epinephrine. The fixed erythemas, such as erythema multiforme, are usually unaffected by antihistamines and require corticosteroids for suppression. Not infrequently, patients report wheals that persist for 12 hours or more and show a clinical picture intermediate between true urticaria and the classic fixed erythemas. Such intermediate forms have been termed erythema-group reactions; they resemble fixed erythemas in that they respond to systemic corticosteroids but not to antihistamines.

TREATMENT

Assuming that you have asked the patient to discontinue any suspected drugs or foods and have ruled out an underlying infectious process, treatment consists of suppressing the eruption with drugs. Discontinuing "any suspected drug" is easier said than done when you encounter patients who are taking numerous drugs for serious illnesses. In this situation, eliminate all nonessential drugs (e.g., barbiturates, aspirin), treat the patient with urticaria suppressants, and hope for the best.

Patients with urticaria should not take aspirin or aspirin-containing medicines. Allergy to aspirin may cause hives. Even in those patients who are not allergic to it, aspirin tends to aggravate hives pharmacologically.

Antihistamines are the best drugs for suppressing urticaria. The traditional antihistamines, such as chlorpheniramine (Chlor-Trimeton), diphenhydramine (Benadryl), and hydroxyzine (Atarax, Vistaril), are sedating. Three nonsedating antihistamines are available in the United States: terfenadine (Seldane), loratadine (Claritin), and astemizole (Hismanal). Astemizole is not suitable for the treatment of acute urticaria because of its delayed onset of action and slow elimination, with a half-life of more than 1 week. Terfenadine and loratadine are excellent drugs for treating acute urticaria.

CAUTION. Terfenadine interacts with ketoconazole and erythromycin to produce cardiac arrhythmias. It should not be given concomitantly with either drug. Doses higher than the recommended 60 mg twice daily have also been associated with cardiac arrhythmias. Additional short-acting, nonsedating antihistamines are available in Europe and are expected to become available in the United States.

Of the traditional antihistamines, the alkylamines, such as chlorpheniramine, brompheniramine (Dimetane), and triprolidine (Actidil), are tolerated for daytime use by most patients. These agents are inexpensive and available without a prescription in the United States. Diphenhydramine is also popular and available over the counter, but it is so sedating that I consider it suitable only for bedtime use. Hydroxyzine, promethazine (Phenergan), and cyproheptadine (Periactin) are other examples of effective antihistamines that are potent sedatives and best used at bedtime.

When two antihistamines are employed, they should be from different chemical classes. It is neither necessary nor desirable to employ many different antihistamines. Limit yourself to one or two antihistamines from each of these groups, and become familiar with them.

CAUTIONS

1. Antihistamines may cause drowsiness. To varying degrees, the traditional antihistamines are sedating. Warn patients that it may be dangerous to drive or perform similar tasks requiring alertness, and tell them not to consume alcohol while taking antihistamines.

2. Antihistamines may increase intraocular pressure. Ask patients if they have glaucoma.

3. Antihistamines may cause urinary retention in older men.

Keep two points in mind when prescribing antihistamines.

1. Patients with urticaria may require two to three times the usual adult dose of traditional antihistamines. However, such *increases are not safe with the nonsedating antihistamines terfenadine, loratadine, and astemizole*, in which the manufacturer's recommended dose should not be exceeded. For terfenadine, the recommended dose is 60 mg twice daily. The recommended dose for loratadine is 10 mg daily. Astemizole has a delayed onset of action and is not suitable for treatment of acute urticaria.

2. Antihistamines vary in their central nervous system side effects. It is not uncommon to encounter patients who are unable to work or drive safely because treatment of their acute urticaria was initiated with stiff daytime doses of the more sedating antihistamines, such as diphenhydramine, hydroxyzine, promethazine, and cyproheptadine. These agents preferably are used at bedtime.

I initiate treatment with daytime use of terfenadine 60 mg twice daily, loratadine 10 mg once daily, or one of the less-sedating over-the-counter antihistamines. In the near future, other nonsedating, short-acting antihistamines should be available as alternatives for daytime use.

When patients tolerate daytime use of the less-sedating, over-the-counter antihistamines such as chlorpheniramine, brompheniramine, or triprolidine, I initiate treatment with one or two tablets taken three times daily with meals—a convenient reminder. If this dose provides only partial relief, it is gradually increased until the hives are controlled or side effects appear. The patient instruction sheet Hives (Urticaria) reflects the need for adjustment of the antihistamine dose. It may be necessary to increase the antihistamine dose to four or five tablets taken three times daily; a surprising number of patients tolerate such doses. Do not use long-acting tablet forms for daytime treatment of acute urticaria. Their delayed onset and cumulative effect make dosage adjustment difficult.

At bedtime, I frequently have the patient take a more sedating and/or longer-acting antihistamine; I prefer 25 or 50 mg of hydroxyzine. Promethazine, 12.5 or 25 mg at bedtime, is also very useful. The popular antihistamine diphenhydramine (Benadryl) is available over the counter in 25-mg capsules. A dose of 100 to 150 mg at bedtime safely utilizes diphenhydramine's potent sedative effect. If the urticaria is mild, the daytime antihistamine given at bedtime usually suffices. The long-acting tablets of chlorpheniramine or brompheniramine can be used at bedtime to keep the patient comfortable overnight.

When control of hives is achieved, the patient should continue the same dose for an additional 2 or 3 days before gradually decreasing the antihistamines. This schedule is arbitrary and must be individualized, but generally, it is wise to allow a 5- to 7-day period of gradually decreasing the antihistamine dose before discontinuing the drug. Any urticarial flare-up while tapering the antihistamine requires an increase in dosage.

I generally employ two antihistamines in treating acute urticaria; written directions lessen patient confusion. The treatment schedule in the patient information sheet Hives (Urticaria) takes only a minute to complete and provides three options. Category A is for nonsedating antihistamines and has a warning for antihistamines in which the recommended dose must not be exceeded (e.g., terfenadine). Category B details dosage adjustments for the mildly sedating antihistamines (e.g., chlorpheniramine, brompheniramine, tripolidine). Category C provides directions for the more sedating antihistamines, which I prescribe only for use in the evening or at bedtime (e.g., hydroxyzine, diphenhydramine, cyproheptadine).

Epinephrine, 0.3 ml of a 1 : 1000 dilution injected subcutaneously or intramuscularly is an effective immediate treatment for severe acute urticaria. It is preferable to avoid the use of epinephrine in patients with hypertension or cardiac disease. Epinephrine may produce a hypertensive crisis in patients taking beta-blockers. A beneficial effect is usually evident in 30 to 40 minutes. Patients who respond well to epinephrine usually do well on antihistamines. Those who fail to respond to epinephrine will usually require corticosteroids to control their wheals.

Other sympathomimetic drugs, such as ephedrine or pseudoephedrine (Sudafed), may be given by mouth. For severe urticaria, I occasionally prescribe them in addition to antihistamines. As these agents often cause jitteriness, they should be taken only at breakfast and lunch. The dose of ephedrine is 25 to 50 mg, and the dose of pseudoephedrine is 30 to 60 mg. Fixed combinations of antihistamine and pseudoephedrine are available over the counter and are convenient.

Although urticaria generally responds better to antihistamines than to corticosteroids, sometimes corticosteroids are necessary to suppress hives. If wheals last more than a few hours, if joint swelling accompanies urticaria (i.e., serum sickness syndrome), or if there is no response to epinephrine, systemic corticosteroids usually will be required.

Prednisone is the corticosteroid of choice, and, because it is relatively short-acting, it initially may be required twice daily before the patient switches to the usual once-daily morning dose. Start by prescribing enough corticosteroid to suppress the hives; usually, between 40 and 80 mg of prednisone are required initially. Once control is achieved, taper the dose by 5 to 10 mg per day over a 10- to 12-day period.

Corticosteroids should be used reluctantly, and only if antihistamines fail. Not only may corticosteroids mask an underlying disease process, but they interfere with the body's anti-infection mechanisms. Before using corticosteroids, rule out an infectious process; a blood count, urinalysis, and sedimentation rate are the minimum necessary laboratory tests. If more than 2 weeks of corticosteroids are required, a thorough medical reassessment is indicated.

Hyperhidrosis

Patient sheet page P–53

23

ETIOLOGY

Excessive sweating localized to the axillae, palms, and soles is a common complaint in healthy persons. It usually first becomes evident at puberty. A strong familial tendency is often evident. Localized hyperhidrosis has been referred to as "mental" or "emotional" sweating, because it is triggered by a wide variety of emotional and physical stresses. However, these are not psychiatric disorders or conversion reactions; these persons suffer from an exaggeration of a physiologic response common to all humans.

Hyperhidrosis can be a significant social handicap. Severe axillary hyperhidrosis soaks through dress shields, sweaters, and coats. Hyperhidrosis of the fingers and palms makes hand shaking a wet and slippery embarrassment. Constantly wet hands may smudge writing, ruin documents, and interfere with many manual tasks. Hyperhidrosis of the soles often leads to overgrowth of microorganisms and a foul odor.

Hyperhidrosis of the soles may result in tender, elevated, red plaques termed symmetrical lividity of the soles. The maceration of the thick stratum corneum of the soles often leads to a white appearance mistaken by patients for athlete's foot. This soggy stratum corneum is an ideal substrate for the growth of microorganisms, which leads to odor and an irregular, pitted appearance referred to as pitted keratolysis (Figure C–51).

DIAGNOSIS

The diagnosis of localized functional hyperhidrosis is usually correctly made by the patient. A handshake and a look at the palms suffice in the case of palmar hyperhidrosis. A physician with a sensitive nose will often suspect plantar hyperhidrosis on entering a room, especially if the patient has removed his shoes. The soggy appearance of the soles, sometimes with bluish red plaques and/or keratolysis, makes hyperhidrosis of the soles an easy diagnosis. In axillary hyperhidrosis, skin changes are usually absent; look at the patient's clothing. When there is significant axillary hyperhidrosis, the blouse or shirt will be soaking wet. Examination of the patient's clothing will enable you to distinguish between a fastidious patient who objects to slight excessive sweating and one whose axillae produce torrents of fluid.

TREATMENT

With the exception of axillary sweating, there is no cure for hyperhidrosis; treatment is a matter of suppression. Axillary sweating can be cured by resecting a sufficiently large segment of axillary skin to significantly reduce the number of sweat glands.

SYSTEMIC THERAPY

Anticholinergic agents (atropinelike drugs) have been used systemically for many years to control sweating. Unfortunately, such side effects as dry mouth, blurred vision, tachycardia, and urinary retention have limited their use. There is clinical evidence that some anticholinergics are better than others at controlling sweating. Systemic therapy is best reserved for young persons who find it important to periodically control their sweating—for a dance, a job interview, or other stressful but important social or business engagement. I prescribe glycopyrrolate (Robinul), beginning with 1 mg taken three times daily. This dose may be increased to 2 mg three times daily if the response is inadequate. Warn the patient about potential side effects, especially blurred vision, and remind him to reserve this treatment for special occasions.

TOPICAL THERAPY

Aluminum chloride hexahydrate in absolute ethanol is the most practical topical therapy available. Do not confuse this preparation with the usual commercial aluminum salt–containing "antiperspirants," which actually are effective deodorants but worthless as antiperspirants. In the United States, 20 percent aluminum chloride hexahydrate in anhydrous ethanol is available by prescription under the trade name of Drysol. An over-the-counter preparation containing 13 percent aluminum chloride hexahydrate in alcohol is sold as Certain Dri. Aluminum chloride topicals are used differently on the thin skin of the axillae than on the thick skin of the palms and soles. The patient instruction sheet Hyperhidrosis provides separate directions for these sites.

Axillae

Treatment should be initiated with the aluminum chloride topical applied at bedtime and rinsed off in the morning. If irritation—a common problem—occurs, daytime use of 1 percent hydrocortisone cream (nothing stronger) may provide sufficient control for continued use of the aluminum chloride. Once axillary hyperhidrosis is brought under control, the patient gradually reduces the frequency of treatments to a level that adequately controls it. If sweating is not controlled after 10 to 14 days of overnight use of aluminum chloride, its effect can be potentiated by covering the area overnight with a thin plastic film. This option is described in the patient instruction sheet Hyperhidrosis.

If aluminum chloride fails to provide relief or produces unacceptable irritation, surgical removal of sweat glands is effective. In the simplest technique, a fusiform segment of axillary skin with its sweat glands is excised. Removal of sweat glands by liposuction or by dissection of sweat glands from the underside of skin flaps have their advocates. Liposuction removal of sweat glands avoids the large scar associated with other surgical techniques and may prove to be the treatment of choice.

Palms and Soles

On the thick skin of the palms and soles, an aluminum chloride topical is usually well tolerated. A trial of overnight applications is the first step. If 10 to 14 days of open applications are ineffective, try plastic occlusion. For the palms, plastic gloves are ideal; for the feet, a plastic bag works well. The patient instruction sheet Hyperhidrosis provides details. When control is achieved, the frequency of treatment is reduced to a maintenance level.

Malodorous feet are a special situation. Aluminum chloride is an antimicrobial, and this action, combined with its suppression of sweating, may be all that is needed to eliminate odor. Treat persistent odor with morning applications of an antibiotic solution, such as the clindamycin solution designed for acne. Some patients prefer morning applications of an antimicrobial powder such as Zeasorb powder. Smelly shoes that were worn before the start of therapy should be discarded.

ELECTROPHORESIS

What if topical aluminum chloride fails or is not tolerated? Often, these agents produce partial reduction in sweating, and supplemental systemic treatment with glycopyrrolate at times of special stress provides reasonable control. If not, electrophoresis with tapwater may be tried; it is claimed to be an effective way of controlling excessive sweating, often for weeks on end. Battery-operated instruments are available for home use (General Medical Corporation). Although some patients like them, others find them inadequate.

24 *Impetigo*

Patient sheet page P–55

ETIOLOGY

Impetigo is a superficial cutaneous coccal infection. The relative roles of streptococci and staphylococci remain controversial and are mostly of academic interest. Impetigo usually responds to erythromycin, a penicillinase-resistant penicillin such as dicloxacillin, or cephalexin.

Impetigo can occur at any age; in North America, it is predominantly a disorder of children. It is customary to inquire about staphylococcal or streptococcal infections (e.g., impetigo, furuncles, strep throat) among family members and playmates in an attempt to discover a source of infection. Such sources should be examined and treated; usually, no contagious source is found.

DIAGNOSIS

Diagnosis of typical cases of impetigo is easy. The enlarging lesions with actively blistering or crusted borders and central clearing (Figures C–46 and C–47) resemble few other disorders. Inflammatory tinea corporis (i.e., ringworm) caused by zoophilic fungi contracted from a pet or farm animal can produce a clinical picture that morphologically resembles impetigo. Usually, tinea develops more slowly than impetigo. In bullous impetigo, blisters persist (instead of rupturing early and leaving crusts) and other vesicular disorders must be considered. Herpes simplex, herpes zoster, varicella, and severe blistering contact dermatitis are occasionally mistaken for impetigo.

Impetigo is by definition a superficial bacterial infection of the skin. Deeper pyodermas, termed ecthyma, are not impetigo. Considerable confusion has arisen regarding treatment and complications of impetigo, because some studies have failed to make this distinction.

CONTAGION

Impetigo contagiosa is indeed contagious. Children with this disorder should be kept home from school for 1 or 2 days after initiating treatment. Parents should be advised about contagiousness and simple hygienic measures instituted as outlined in the patient instruction sheet Impetigo. Usually, the crusting, contagious stage of impetigo clears up within 2 days of therapy with systemic antibiotics.

TREATMENT

SPECIFIC THERAPY

Impetigo is a delight to treat; the response to effective topical or systemic antibiotic therapy is dramatic. Formerly, topical antibiotics were inferior to systemic antibiotics, but the advent of mupirocin ointment (Bactroban) has changed that. Mupirocin ointment applied three or four times per day is equally as effective as appropriate systemic antibiotics.

For localized impetigo, mupirocin applications appear to be the treatment of choice. Mupirocin acts as rapidly as appropriate systemic therapy and does not cause systemic side effects. Mupirocin rarely sensitizes the patient's skin—its chief drawback is its expense. Other topical antibiotics, such as bacitracin, neomycin, and gentamicin, are not effective for treating impetigo.

When there is extensive impetigo, systemic antibiotics are indicated (Figures C–47 and C–48). Also, if there is evidence of bacterial infection elsewhere (e.g., in the throat, ears, or nose), systemic antibiotics appear to be the approach of choice. Formerly, ordinary penicillin was as effective as erythromycin. Impetigo is increasingly being caused by penicillin-resistant strains; among the appropriate antibiotics are erythromycin, a penicillinase-resistant penicillin such as dicloxacillin, and cephalexin. Minocycline and doxycycline are effective, well-tolerated antibiotics for patients who are allergic to penicillin and whose gastrointestinal tracts are upset by erythromycin. A 5- to 7-day course of antibiotic usually suffices; I make the prescription refillable once and tell the patient that if the impetigo does not completely clear, he or she should have the prescription refilled and take a second course. Emphasize the importance of taking the entire supply of antibiotic and not stopping after 1 or 2 days when the lesions are better. Is there an advantage to combining mupirocin topically with systemic antibiotics? Probably not, and mupirocin is expensive.

NONSPECIFIC TOPICAL THERAPY

Gentle removal of crusts is important, especially when impetigo is treated topically. Lukewarm water works well for this purpose. Soaking is discontinued when crusts no longer form.

When impetigo is treated systemically, the healing lesions tend to dry out and fissure. Consequently, I suggest that patients apply a relatively nonsensitizing antibiotic, such as bacitracin or a bacitracin-polymyxin combination, thinly three or four times per day until healing is complete. These inexpensive preparations are available over the counter. When there are crusts, the ointments should be applied after the crusts have been soaked off. It is possible that ordinary petrolatum (Vaseline) or some other bland emollient may work as well. Avoid the use of neomycin, because it is a significant sensitizer.

Impetigo clears up in 1 week. Patients should be told to return if impetigo has not resolved by then. Failure to clear in 1 week can usually be traced to several causes: (1) failure to take the antibiotic; (2) a wrong diagnosis; or (3) superimposition of the impetigo on another process (e.g., contact dermatitis) which is still present.

COMPLICATIONS

Streptococcal skin infections, like streptococcal infections elsewhere, may result in glomerulonephritis. The incidence of glomerulonephritis depends not only on the presence of nephritogenic strains of streptococci, but on how long the pyoderma had been present before treatment. Nephritis as a complication of impetigo is rare in North American private practice. Reports showing relatively high incidences of glomerulonephritis have usually dealt with children raised in poverty-stricken surroundings with neglected lesions. Often, conditions reported as "impetigo" actually represent long-standing, deep pyodermas. I see no point in needlessly alarming patients and parents by mentioning the possibility of kidney disease.

Keloids

Patient sheet page P–59

25

ETIOLOGY

Keloids are tumors of excessive scar tissue. Obvious skin injury (e.g., surgery, an accidental cut, an insect bite, a pimple) usually precedes keloid formation. Occasionally, the initiating injury is so trivial it escapes notice; these are "spontaneous" keloids. Keloids are more likely to occur in dark-skinned persons and in certain areas of the body, especially the upper chest and upper back. For additional details, a comprehensive review[1] is recommended.

DIAGNOSIS

The smooth, sharply circumscribed, elevated tumor is usually diagnostic, especially if there are multiple lesions. A history of preceding trauma supports the diagnosis. Sometimes tumors, either benign (e.g., dermatofibroma) or malignant (e.g., infiltrating basal cell carcinoma), may resemble keloids. If in doubt, do a small punch biopsy. Distinction between hypertrophic scars and keloids, put forward by some texts, is probably not realistic, because there is no demarcation between hypertrophic scars and keloids.

TREATMENT

Patients seek treatment of keloids because of their appearance or because of discomfort. Keloids, especially those on the trunk, may cause significant, persistent burning, discomfort, or pain. Textbooks correctly describe the treatment of keloids as unsatisfactory. It is easier to list what not to do. Surgery usually is best avoided; a new and larger keloid is often the result, especially on the trunk and upper arms. However, even this generalization has exceptions; simple surgical excision will cure over one half of the keloids of the ear lobes.

Intralesional repository corticosteroids constitute the best current treatment (Figures C–52 through C–54). They usually are promptly effective in eliminating keloidal pain and discomfort, but flatten the keloid only slowly. Multiple treatments are usually necessary. Explain to the patient that the injections will not eliminate the keloid, but will make it flatter and less noticeable. Even successful treatment leaves a flat, shiny scar.

Local anesthesia before the intralesional injection is recommended unless the keloid is tiny. Triamcinolone acetonide suspension is the repository corticosteroid most widely used. Start with the 10 mg/ml concentration (Kenalog-10). The corticosteroid should be injected fairly deeply (i.e., 5 to 8 mm) into the keloid. This requires considerable pressure on the plunger of the tuberculin syringe, which should be equipped with a Luer-Lok device to prevent separation of the needle from the syringe. Inject 0.1 to 0.2 ml of suspension at 5- to 10-mm intervals along the keloid. Limit the amount of triamcinolone acetonide injected to less than 20 to 30 mg.

The patient should be re-evaluated in 6 to 8 weeks. The repository corticosteroid acts for about 3 months and works slowly. At the follow-up visit, injections can be repeated, using the 40-mg/ml concentration (Kenalog-40) if there was no response to the 10-mg/ml dose.

CAUTION. The 40-mg/ml concentration increases the risk of skin atrophy. Inject no more than 0.1 ml at a site, and inject it at least 5-mm deep. With careful, repeated, intralesional corticosteroid injections, most keloids cease causing discomfort and gradually flatten. Sometimes, months or years after a keloid has successfully yielded to intralesional corticosteroids, it recurs and may be injected again.

Intralesional corticosteroids may cause undesirable local and systemic side effects. The injected drug is absorbed; large amounts may cause significant adrenal suppression. Cutaneous atrophy, depigmentation, telangiectasis, and even ulceration may occur as a result of the atrophy-promoting effects of corticosteroids. Local side effects are more likely with higher concentrations and if the drug is injected intradermally. Intralesional corticosteroids should be injected subdermally at a depth of 5 to 8 mm.

Other treatments for keloids include radiation, pressure, topical tretinoin (Retin-A), and freezing with liquid nitrogen or dry ice. None of these treatments is as simple and effective as intralesional corticosteroids. Some workers combine a destructive method, such as liquid nitrogen freezing, with intralesional corticosteroids. There is no documented benefit of this dual approach.

Prolonged application of silicone gel sheeting appears to flatten keloids. Many months of treatment are required, and the gel must cover the keloid for at least 12 hours daily. We lack controlled studies and, therefore, do not know either the optimum application technique or the existence of any significant differences in the results achieved using the different brands of silicone sheeting. If you decide to treat a large, stubborn keloid with silicone sheeting, please review the current literature because any textbook advice will be out of date in this rapidly changing field.

Controlled studies have shown that one or two daily applications of 0.05 percent or 0.1 percent tretinoin cream are of modest benefit in reducing keloids. I use topical tretinoin as an adjunct to intralesional injection of keloids. In addition to tretinoin's effect on the keloid, there is the psychological benefit of involving the patient in his treatment. Because tretinoin tends to irritate the skin, have the patient start by using it only once every other day. As the skin hardens, gradually increase the applications to twice daily.

PREVENTION

Is it possible to prevent postoperative keloids in those prone to form them? Radiation, while effective, requires a significant dose, about 1500 to 2000 rad. Most physicians, and patients, are opposed to radiation for benign conditions. Intralesional corticosteroids may prevent postoperative keloids. At surgery, a fairly dilute (5- to 10-mg/ml) suspension of triamcinolone acetonide is injected into the wound edges. Additional steroid is usually injected 2 to 4 weeks postoperatively. Because corticosteroids inhibit wound healing, caution is necessary.

1. Rockwell WB, Cohen IK, Ehrlich HP: Keloids and hypertrophic scars: A comprehensive review. *Plast Reconstr Surg* 84:827, 1989

26 *Molluscum Contagiosum*

Patient sheet page P–71

ETIOLOGY

Molluscum contagiosum is characterized by small skin tumors caused by a poxvirus. While more common in young persons, it may affect persons of any age. Molluscum contagiosum is becoming an increasingly common sexually transmitted disease affecting the genitalia, abdomen, thighs, and buttocks.

DIAGNOSIS

Molluscum lesions (Figures C–85 and C–86) are shiny, white-to-flesh-colored, dome-shaped lesions with a firm, waxy appearance. When well developed, they have a diagnostic central indentation or umbilication. The tiny, early lesions often lack this feature. Most molluscum lesions are smaller than 5 mm, although lesions occasionally are larger.

Molluscum lesions may undergo spontaneous inflammation which may be mistaken for a bacterial infection. At times, a low-grade rash surrounds molluscum lesions; with removal of the lesions, the rash clears.

Molluscum lesions are most commonly misdiagnosed as warts. Unlike warts, however, they are smooth, and careful observation with low-power magnification will reveal the diagnostic central pit. It is easy to misdiagnose a solitary molluscum lesion, especially when it is inflamed. Pyogenic granuloma, inflamed cyst, keratoacanthoma, inflamed wart, and basal cell carcinoma are errors I have made. Superficial biopsy provides the correct diagnosis, because histology reveals the characteristic molluscum bodies within the lesion.

TREATMENT

Locally destructive measures are the only effective treatment, because there is no systemic anti–molluscum virus agent. Fortunately, molluscum lesions respond nicely to a variety of destructive therapies. Molluscum lesions are easier to treat than warts.

Application of the blistering agent cantharidin is a gentle, painless treatment and my first choice. Cantharidin is commercially available dissolved in flexible collodion under such trade names as Cantharone and Verr-Canth; these agents may be purchased from firms specializing in dermatologic supplies (Appendix B). A minute drop is applied to each lesion with a pointed stick; a toothpick is ideal.

Allow at least 5 minutes for thorough drying. The patient must not touch the treated site during this time. Failure to wait at least 5 minutes for thorough drying causes spreading of the cantharadin and horrendous blisters. After applying the cantharadin, I instruct the patient not to move until I return; then I leave the room to make a phone call or briefly see another patient. On return, I caution the patient to expect a blister or irritation at each site. The patient can get the treated areas wet; no special precautions are needed. Have the patient return in 10 to 14 days, at which time most of the molluscum lesions will have disappeared. Repeat the cantharidin painting. Usually, 2 to 4 treatments suffice.

CAUTION. The genitals are sensitive to this blistering agent. Use minute amounts of cantharidin in treating the genitalia, and be certain that the patient remains still for 5 minutes to ensure drying. The same caution applies to small children.

In some patients, cantharidin works poorly. Its effect can be potentiated by covering treated sites after drying with an occlusive tape such as Blenderm tape. It is critical that at least 5 minutes be allowed for thorough drying before tape application; otherwise the cantharidin spreads under the tape and produces a huge blister. Blenderm tape is translucent; when blistering occurs, the tape should be removed and the site left open. Cantharidin is an ideal treatment—it is painless, does not scar, and is almost invariably successful. However, precise application to the treated site and thorough drying are critical.

If cantharidin is not available, almost any superficial destructive measure can be used to remove molluscum lesions. The lesions can be lightly curetted or superficially snipped off with a sharp scissors. They can be slit open with a small, sterile hypodermic needle and the contents squeezed out with a comedo extractor or a forceps. Liquid nitrogen freezing can be used. However, the various proprietary irritant wart topicals often fail to clear molluscum lesions.

Molluscum lesions tend to disappear spontaneously. In some patients, such as an uncooperative small child with lesions on the eyelids, it is best to explain this tendency toward natural cure, and do nothing.

27 *Nevi and Melanoma*

Patient sheets pages P–67, P–69, P–103, P–107

Moles are mainly cosmetic nuisances. The problem they pose is to distinguish a harmless mole from a melanoma. The only certain way is by histology; because we cannot excise every mole, we must rely on clinical criteria in deciding when to biopsy. This unit focuses on the clinical diagnosis of melanoma.

Melanoma is the eighth most common cancer, and its incidence worldwide is increasing more rapidly than that of any other malignancy. The current estimated lifetime frequency of melanoma is 1 per 100 persons. Although earlier diagnosis and treatment have improved the cure rate, deaths from melanoma are outstripping the therapeutic gains.

This chapter discusses the challenges facing the clinician in the following sections:

- Etiology of nevi
- Etiology of melanoma
- Types of melanoma
- Prognosis of melanoma
- Clinical diagnosis
- How—and when—to biopsy a suspected melanoma
- Histopathologic diagnosis of melanoma
- Treatment of nevi
- Treatment of melanoma.

ETIOLOGY OF NEVI

The word nevus is used in two ways. In a general sense, nevus refers to any circumscribed, persistent, genetically determined skin malformation. More often, it is used in a restricted way to describe a tumor or aggregation of melanocytes (nevus cells). The lay term mole usually corresponds to nevus cell tumors. Other forms of nevi (e.g., hemangiomas, organoid nevi, connective-tissue nevi) are usually referred to as birthmarks in lay terminology. The congenital melanocytic nevus, which is present at birth, is usually called a birthmark rather than a mole.

CONGENITAL NEVI

The number and location of melanocytic nevi are largely genetically determined. Parents with moles tend to have children with moles. The common nevus is rare at birth. It appears as a flat brown spot during infancy or childhood and gradually becomes more prominent. Often, melanocytic nevi appear in crops, or showers, especially in late childhood and during adolescence. Sunlight stimulates the formation of new moles and causes changes in existing nevi.

The congenital melanocytic nevus, although composed of melanocytes, differs from the usual melanocytic nevus. Congenital nevi, present at birth, enlarge in proportion to the growth of the infant and child. Unlike usual nevi, congenital nevi have a significant potential for transformation into malignant melanomas (Figures C–63 and C–64). The larger the congenital nevus, the greater the risk of transformation into a malignant melanoma. Although everyone agrees that giant congenital nevi have a significant incidence of malignant transformation, it is not known how often smaller congenital nevi become malignant.

Pathologically, nevi are classified by the location of the melanocytes. A nevus with melanocytes found at the dermo-epidermal junction is called a junctional nevus. Melanocytes restricted to the dermis form a dermal nevus. A nevus formed of both junctional and dermal cells is a compound nevus. When nevus cells are deep in the dermis, the mole has a bluish black color and is called a blue nevus (Figure C–82).

The patient instruction sheet Moles refers to the benign melanocytic nevus.

DYSPLASTIC NEVI

In recent years, much has been written about the unusual-appearing moles called dysplastic nevi or atypical moles. Awareness of these atypical or dysplastic moles resulted from observations of patients with multiple primary malignant melanomas and those with familial melanomas. These patients often had multiple, unusual-appearing nevi that showed dysplastic changes on microscopic examination. However, dysplastic nevi also occur in patients with nonfamilial melanoma and in a significant portion of the general population. Atypical moles are not malignant, and it is not necessary to remove them unless melanoma is suspected. However, the presence of atypical moles is a marker indicating an increased risk for developing a melanoma. This is true not only for melanoma kindreds but also for the general population.

The issue of dysplastic nevi is confused, because the clinical diagnosis of a dysplastic nevus correlates poorly with the histologic findings. To compound the confusion, pathologists disagree as to what constitutes dysplastic changes. It has been suggested that the term atypical mole be used for these unusual, flat moles with indistinct, irregular borders, often showing reddish tones. Atypical mole is purely a clinical, descriptive term that implies no particular histological changes. Unfortunately, a more rational descriptive term does not help the clinician manage these lesions.

It is agreed that atypical or dysplastic moles are not malignant; the problem is distinguishing them from melanomas. Irregular border and color variation are two of the best criteria for clinically suspecting a melanoma, but these are also characteristic of the atypical mole. Experienced clinicians also consider the background mole pattern when evaluating an unusual mole. An atypical nevus in a patient with dozens of such lesions (Figure C–81) merits only observation, whereas a similar lesion in a patient with only a few ordinary nevi warrants removal.

There is no question that persons with atypical moles are at increased risk for developing a melanoma. Furthermore, the more numerous the atypical nevi, the greater the melanoma risk. However the emphasis on dysplastic nevi as markers and precursors of melanoma may be excessive. Many of the publications on melanoma originate from melanoma clinics at university centers. Familial melanoma cohorts gravitate to these centers and then are subjected to intense case finding studies, which may lead to a skewed melanoma population.

ETIOLOGY OF MELANOMA

The definitely identified etiologic factors for melanoma are: (1) skin pigmentation; (2) genetic predisposition; and (3) sun exposure. Melanoma is rare in blacks. It is more common in fair-skinned people of Celtic ancestry than in those with dark hair who tan easily.

The genetic factor is clearly illustrated by families with a predilection for melanoma, in which melanomas are found in multiple persons over several generations. Having a first-degree relative with melanoma significantly increases the risk of developing it.

The role of sunlight is evident both from the protective effect of pigment against developing melanoma and from the greater prevalence of melanoma in sunny climates. For most melanomas, sunlight plays a different role than it does in causing basal cell and squamous cell carcinomas. Basal cell and squamous cell cancers result from cumulative sun exposure and therefore tend to occur in people with outdoor occupations such as farming, construction, and fishing. These tumors are usually found on areas of maximal sun exposure: nose, ears, face, lips, and neck.

With the exception of lentigo maligna melanoma, melanoma is *not* related to cumulative sun exposure. Melanoma is most commonly seen on the back and lower extremities, and it tends to occur in indoor workers who have had intermittent, intense sun exposure. Sunburns during childhood or youth appear to be most significant. Studies on melanoma frequency in immigrants to Australia and Israel indicate that those who came as small children showed the high melanoma prevalence of Australia or Israel, whereas adult immigrants continued to have the lower melanoma prevalence of their countries of origin.

This etiologic information allows identification of persons at increased risk for developing melanoma. The following are generally agreed-upon risk factors:

1. Melanoma in a first-degree relative.
2. A "large" number of nevi, exceeding 50, 80, or 100, depending on the study. The more nevi, the greater the risk.
3. Multiple atypical or dysplastic nevi.
4. Fair skin that always burns and never tans.
5. A history of multiple severe sunburns in childhood.

The first three risk factors are far more significant than the last two. The risks are additive. Anyone with two of the first three risk factors probably has a 10- to 30-fold increased risk of developing melanoma and must be alerted to this danger. Periodic, careful self-examination and examination of the entire skin by a trained physician have been advised for such high-risk persons.

TYPES OF MELANOMA

It is customary to classify melanomas into four clinicopathologic categories: (1) superficial spreading; (2) nodular; (3) lentigo maligna melanoma; and (4) acral lentiginous melanoma. Although the distinctions between these types are sometimes blurred, the classification is clinically useful.

Superficial spreading melanoma features prominent epidermal involvement. Superficial spreading melanomas have biphasic growth—they enlarge both horizontally and vertically. Lateral spread of these melanomas is referred to as the radial growth phase. Most superficial spreading melanomas remain in the thin, radial growth phase for months or years, but ultimately, vertical growth supersedes radial growth, with a drastic worsening of prognosis. This is the most common type of melanoma (Figures C–67 through C–69).

In nodular melanoma, the malignant cells grow downward without a visible radial component. This melanoma is justifiably feared, because prognosis is related to depth of invasion (Figures C–65 and C–66).

Lentigo maligna melanoma differs from other melanomas in a number of ways. It is clearly related to cumulative sun exposure and tends to affect the sun-exposed areas of skin in older, fair-skinned individuals. Initially, it resembles the lentigines that are common in such people. It evolves slowly from a precursor lesion, the lentigo maligna, a flat, irregularly bordered, unevenly pigmented spot (Figures C–76 through C–78). As long as the atypical melanocytes remain in the epidermis, the lesion is considered a lentigo maligna. When the atypical melanocytes invade the dermis, the lesion is called a lentigo maligna melanoma. Clinically, the appearance of nodules in a lentigo maligna indicates dermal invasion has occurred and and the lesion has changed from a precursor to a fully malignant melanoma.

Acral lentiginous melanoma consists of irregularly shaped, irregularly pigmented macules affecting the palms, soles, subungual, and periungual areas, as well as mucosal surfaces (Figures C–70 through C–72). The term palmo-plantar mucosal melanoma has been suggested to describe this group of tumors. Histologically these tumors are characterized by a horizontal growth phase with extensive lentigolike pigmentation of keratinocytes and skip areas of microscopically benign-appearing changes within the lesion. Consequently, the diagnosis can be difficult histologically as well as clinically. In the early stages, the diagnosis is often missed.

Acral lentiginous melanoma is the least common melanoma, making up about 5 percent or less of all melanomas in Caucasians. Although melanoma is rare in brown- or black-skinned persons, when it does occur, it is mostly of the acral lentiginous type.

PROGNOSIS OF MELANOMA

The best currently available prognostic indicator is the maximum thickness of the melanoma. This is easily measured with the microscope, using a micrometer ocular. This measure is called the Breslow thickness in honor of the physician who demonstrated the usefulness of this simple determination. Table 27–1 gives current generally accepted prognostic ranges.

Another, less used and less useful prognostic indicator is the Clark level, named after its deviser. Depth in Clark levels refers to anatomic units. In Clark level 1, the melanoma is restricted to the epidermis; in level 2, there are a few melanoma cells in the papillary dermis; in level 3, the melanoma cells fill the papillary dermis; in level 4, the melanoma cells invade the reticular dermis; and in level 5, the melanoma cells can be found in subcutaneous fat.

Table 27–1. **FIVE-YEAR MELANOMA SURVIVAL RATES AS RELATED TO TUMOR THICKNESS***

Tumor Thickness (mm)	5-Year Survival (%)
<0.76	96–99
0.76–1.49	85–95
1.50–2.49	75–85
2.50–3.49	60–75
>3.50	40–60

*The ranges reflect figures reported in recent publications. Note these figures deal with 5-year survival. The 5-year disease-free rates are lower.

Several recent studies suggest that tumor volume is the best prognostic index. Unfortunately, estimating tumor volume is a research procedure requiring sophisticated computer devices.

This brief discussion does not attempt to cover the many variables and controversies in melanoma prognosis. There is a vast amount of literature on the influence of variables such as gender, site, clinical type, microscopic regression, inflammation, mitotic activity, and cellular atypia.

CLINICAL DIAGNOSIS

The main problem in diagnosis is distinguishing a benign, growing nevus from a melanoma. It is common for worried parents to bring in their adolescent children because of rapid changes in their moles. Careful examination and explaining to the parents that moles normally grow and enlarge during this period usually suffice. Malignant melanoma is practically unheard of before the age of 16 years, except in congenital nevi. With this in mind, it is almost always possible to reassure parents of a child or teenager regarding the usual melanocytic nevus.

In the adult, distinguishing between a benign melanocytic tumor (i.e., a nevus) and a malignant melanocytic tumor (i.e., a malignant melanoma) is a challenge. Survival of patients with melanoma depends on early diagnosis. If the criteria of a bleeding, nodular black mole are used to diagnose melanoma, it is usually too late to save the patient. The clinical diagnosis of early melanoma is the subject of an excellent review.[1] Melanomas may be suspected early from two findings that are rare in benign nevi:

1. Variegated coloration (Figures C–64, C–67, C–69, C–75, C–77, and C–78). Be suspicious when you see red, white, or blue areas in a brown or black nevus.

2. An irregular border, often with angular induration or notches (Figures C–64, C–67, C–69, and C–73).

Two other objective findings are helpful in differentiating nevi from melanomas. A melanoma tends to be asymmetrical, whereas a nevus tends to be symmetrical. Melanomas are usually larger than nevi; the Skin Cancer Foundation has used a diameter of 6 mm as the cutoff point for diagnosing a benign nevus. In my experience, the size criterion is the least useful in detecting early melanomas. A significant number of persons have nevi larger than 6 mm in diameter, and melanomas smaller than 6 mm in diameter are not rare.

The Skin Cancer Foundation has promoted the widely accepted mnemonic ABCD for the four criteria of asymmetry, border irregularity, color variegation, and diameter enlargement. These criteria should be used together to decide whether there is enough suspicion of melanoma to warrant a biopsy.

The following are subjective signs said to be significant in suspecting a melanoma:

1. Change in color, shape, or size of a mole.
2. Bleeding from a pigmented lesion.
3. Itching in a mole.

By far the most significant of these signs is a change in the appearance of a mole. If an adult reports a significant change in color, shape, thickness, or diameter of a nevus, it warrants a biopsy. Although these lesions are usually benign, I have vivid memories of reassuring patients that a mole appeared perfectly harmless, adding, "let's remove it to be sure," and then getting a pathology report of melanoma. However, when older patients are concerned about a mole "turning dark," they are often talking about a seborrheic keratosis and not a melanocytic nevus.

Bleeding is a late sign in melanoma. A "bleeding mole" is more likely to be a traumatized benign lesion such as a nevus, keratosis, wart, or hemangioma, or a nonmelanoma malignancy such as a basal cell or squamous cell carcinoma. However, every bleeding skin neoplasm deserves an appropriate biopsy, if only for patient reassurance.

The significance of itching in a mole remains in doubt. In the absence of objective findings or a history of change in appearance, it may not be an indication for biopsy.

Not only must nevi be differentiated from melanoma, but seborrheic keratoses and pigmented basal cell carcinoma can perfectly mimic a melanoma (Figures C–79 and C–80). On the other hand, a melanoma, especially the amelanotic variety, may masquerade as a wart or pyogenic granuloma. Do not be fooled by the small, deep hemangioma, which, because of its black color, can mimic a small melanoma (Figure C–83). Firm thumb pressure on a hemangioma for 1 minute usually results in a significant color change resulting from expression of its blood content. If you are still worried, take a tiny punch biopsy. Often not recognized is the pigmented hairy epidermal nevus, or Becker's nevus, which is a pigmented patch that gradually enlarges and usually is first noticed in the patient's teens or early 20s (Figure C–84). Microscopically, the differentiation is obvious, because Becker's nevus does not contain nevus cells.

Good lighting and a low-power magnifier are important in diagnosing skin lesions. The new technique of skin-surface microscopy is sometimes helpful. By using a glass plate and glycerol or mineral oil to render the stratum corneum transparent, the deeper structures are examined in vivo using $10\times$ magnification. Originally, an expensive operating microscope was required; the recent introduction of special hand-held instruments (Dermatoscope, Heine Co.; Epi Scope, Welch Allyn Co.) has made this an office procedure. Skin-surface microscopy is not a technique for the casual user; interpreting what is seen is difficult. I have found it more useful for identifying angiomas and seborrheic keratoses than for distinguishing between a nevus and a melanoma. Whenever there is any question of melanoma, the lesion must be biopsied for appropriate microscopic tissue examination.

HOW AND WHEN TO BIOPSY A SUSPECTED MELANOMA

When you suspect a melanoma, it is best to perform full-thickness excision with a small margin of normal tissue. This provides the pathologist with an adequate specimen for diagnosis and the all-important measurement of depth in case the lesion is indeed a melanoma. It is easy to follow this advice for a small, pigmented lesion of the trunk. What do you do when the lesion is large, especially if it involves the face or other cosmetically sensitive areas? It depends on how strongly you suspect a melanoma, as well as on your surgical expertise.

If the patient calls your attention to a 2-cm, pigmented lesion of the calf that has been present since birth and has gotten thicker and irregular in color in the last few months, you recognize that such changes in a congenital nevus are the equivalent of a flashing red light saying "excise." If you are not comfortable excising the lesion, refer the patient to a surgically inclined dermatologist or a surgeon.

What if the patient rejects your recommendation of a full-thickness excision? Have him get a second opinion from a recognized dermatologist and, if there is concern about scarring, an additional consultation with a plastic surgeon. When it comes to melanoma, share the burden with your colleagues.

With a large or awkwardly located lesion, you may wish to biopsy only a part of the lesion. An incisional biopsy—in contrast to an excisional biopsy, which removes the lesion in toto—is permissible, provided you take a full-thickness specimen (i.e., a punch biopsy) and keep in mind the limitations of this approach. The safety of incisional biopsy has long been debated; some physicians maintain that this approach predisposes the patient to metastasis. However, incisional biopsy appears to be safe and does not worsen the prognosis of a melanoma.

The chief drawback of a punch biopsy is the nonuniform histology of a melanoma. This is especially true of lentigo maligna and acral lentiginous melanoma, which characteristically have areas of benign-appearing histology within the borders of the tumor. In cases in which biopsy is critical, it helps to take multiple, small (2-mm diameter) punch biopsies from darker, more infiltrated sites. The main purpose of a punch biopsy is to be sure the patient does not undergo a significant surgical procedure for a benign lesion. A pigmented seborrheic keratosis can closely mimic a melanoma but can be easily destroyed with liquid nitrogen freezing. However, if the pathologist indicates the presence of a melanocytic lesion, the clinical picture takes precedence over the punch biopsy report in making your decision. If the clinical picture is that of lentigo maligna, acral lentiginous melanoma, or other melanoma, and the pathology is that of a melanocytic lesion, the lesion should be excised even if the biopsy is read as benign.

Never do a shave biopsy of a suspected melanoma. Treatment of a melanoma hinges on its depth. If the shave removal transects the lesion, its depth cannot be measured. Occasionally, only the deep portions of a melanoma show diagnostic features; consequently, the shave biopsy will lead to the incorrect diagnosis of a benign lesion, and the patient will not get the definitive excision that is needed. This is not a condemnation of the shave biopsy, which is an extremely useful procedure in dermatologic diagnosis. However, if melanoma is suspected, a shave biopsy is inappropriate. A possible exception is a purely macular lesion of the trunk or extremities. If you are certain that the lesion is very superficial, some authorities feel a deep shave removal is permissible. This approach is controversial, because lesions that appear to be thin and very superficial may not be.

Mistakes are inevitable. Sometimes benign lesions are overtreated. Much to my embarrassment, I have removed seborrheic keratoses by full-thickness excision believing they were melanomas—an error more commonly made by my surgical colleagues. I have removed my share of histologically benign nevi because of a clinical suspicion of melanoma. At other times, I did not even consider the possibility of melanoma—for example, when I curetted off a bleeding actinic keratosis, or when I biopsied a persistent, pink, scaling plaque that I suspected to be either chronic dermatitis or Bowen's disease. Both turned out to be melanomas.

Such mistakes, although annoying, do no serious damage—the melanoma does get treated. What is disastrous is when a melanoma is treated without a biopsy, or not treated at all. "Let's just burn off that harmless mole that's catching on your bra strap" was what the physician told the patient before electrodesiccating a nevus of her back. Or so she testified later at the malpractice trial, after the recurrence at the treated site was found to be a melanoma that by then had metastasized. It is easy to pass off an early lentiginous melanoma of the foot as a bruise; I have made this error. Clinical judgments must still be made. You cannot send every skin tag, wart, or seborrheic keratosis for tissue examination. No matter how skilled the clinician, an occasional mistake is inevitable. Reduce these inevitable misdiagnoses to a minimum by being suspicious. If you have doubts, biopsy the lesion or get a second opinion.

HISTOPATHOLOGIC DIAGNOSIS OF MELANOMA

The pathologist is the final arbiter of the question: Is it a melanoma? His task is not easy. Unlike basal cell carcinoma, with its distinctive cell type, the diagnosis of melanoma usually depends on analyzing a pattern of change. Especially in early melanomas, the changes may be subtle and difficult to distinguish from those found in atypical or dysplastic nevi. Pathologists recognize this, and often recruit a colleague for a second opinion when diagnosing melanoma.

In my experience, histologic misdiagnosis of melanoma is not a rarity. It is more usual for the diagnosis of melanoma to be missed by a general pathologist than for melanoma to be falsely diagnosed. If you strongly suspect a melanoma on clinical grounds, and the report is that of a nevus, possibly "activated" or "inflamed," it is appropriate to request that it be reviewed, possibly by a trained dermatopathologist. Unfortunately, even full-time, university-based dermatopathologists do not always agree on a diagnosis or are able to give an unequivocal diagnosis.

I am not a histopathologist, but I review slides of all tissue I submit to the hospital-based group of pathologists I use. I do not tell a patient he has a melanoma unless the histology is so typical that I can recognize it, and two pathologists have independently made the diagnosis of melanoma. If these conditions are not met, I request a review by a dermatopathologist. My pathology colleagues readily comply, as we have all learned the importance of sharing the burden of correctly diagnosing melanoma. I tell patients what I have done to ensure that the histopathologic diagnosis of melanoma is correct. It helps the patient deal with this serious diagnosis, improves rapport, and is good medicolegal practice.

TREATMENT OF NEVI

The type of treatment depends on the reasons for having a mole removed. Is the mole unsightly? Is the patient concerned about malignancy? Does the physician suspect melanoma? Is the mole annoying because it protrudes?

Permanent eradication requires all the nevus cells to be destroyed or removed. This can only be achieved by full-thickness skin excision or destruction. Full-thickness skin excision provides an adequate sample for histology as well as ensures removal of the mole. The resulting defect can be closed with sutures or, if small, may be allowed to heal by secondary intention using gelatin foam packing for hemostasis.

Partial or shave removal of a nevus is a useful technique for treating benign nevi that annoy because they protrude (Figures C–61 and C–62). Under local anesthesia, the protruding part of the nevus is removed with a blade or scissors, and the wound is allowed to heal by second intention. It is customary to submit the shaved-off portion for histology. This technique converts a protruding mole into a flat one. Although there is almost always cosmetic improvement, it is rare that the mole becomes invisible. Tell this to your patients. Occasionally, the mole becomes temporarily darker as a result of postsurgical inflammation.

In treating moles, do not use any technique that fails to provide tissue for histology. This eliminates thermal destruction (cautery, electrodesiccation) as well as liquid nitrogen as a therapeutic option. There is another reason for not using liquid nitrogen: It does not work. Nevi are amazingly resistant to liquid nitrogen freezing.

WHEN TO EXCISE FULL THICKNESS

There is one clear-cut indication for full-thickness excision. If you strongly suspect malignancy, full-thickness excision should be performed as initial therapy and to provide the pathologist with an adequate specimen. The prognosis of melanoma—and consequently the type of therapy indicated—correlates closely with the depth of the lesion. The pathologist can only determine the prognosis from a full-thickness skin specimen. If your suspicion of melanoma is strong, infiltrate the anesthetic around the nevus and excise it along with a small margin of normal tissue.

Although there are conflicting opinions about if and when to excise the common, ordinary-sized congenital nevus, full-thickness excision is the treatment of choice. If the patient is a child, wait until he has reached the early teens to ensure cooperation. Full-thickness excision is also a good approach when the patient is annoyed or worried by one or two flat nevi and is not concerned about scarring.

WHEN TO SHAVE-REMOVE A NEVUS

Shave or partial removal of a nevus is an efficient way of dealing with protuberant nevi that are nicked by razors or irritated by garments. Explain that you are simply removing the upper part of the mole and converting it to a flat mole. Nevi that are cosmetically annoying because they are protuberant can also be effectively dealt with by partial shave removal.

Shave surgery is a good way of dealing with a mole that concerns the patient but that you believe to be benign. This technique provides an adequate specimen for the pathologist to issue a reassuring report without the penalty of the significant scarring that usually results from full-thickness excision. Shave removal is recommended only if you believe the lesion is benign; if you share your patient's concern about malignancy, do a full-thickness excision.

WHEN TO PUNCH BIOPSY A NEVUS

A nevus rarely should be punch biopsied. The experienced clinician finds that most nevi are best managed either by full-thickness excision or by shave surgery. When dealing with suspicious lesions in cosmetically sensitive areas, a preliminary punch biopsy may be wise. It is important to select the right portions of the nevus for biopsy. Often, it is best to take multiple small (2-mm) biopsies rather than one medium-sized biopsy. Punch biopsies have the advantage of providing the pathologist with a full-thickness skin specimen, but the drawback of sampling only a small portion of the nevus.

WHEN TO EXCISE ATYPICAL OR DYSPLASTIC NEVI

We lack objective guidelines for treating atypical nevi. In a person having or suspected of having the familial melanoma syndrome, it is obvious that nevi showing significant change should be excised whether or not they meet the clinical criteria of atypical nevi. In those patients without a personal or family history of melanoma, there is currently no generally accepted way of dealing with atypical nevi. Presumably, if there are just a few clinically atypical nevi, it is simplest to excise them and be done with it. When there are multiple atypical nevi without a personal or familial history of melanoma, periodic examination of the patient's entire skin is recommended. At a number of melanoma centers, the entire skin is photographed. The photographs are used as aids in evaluating new or changing pigmented lesions.

WHEN TO DO NOTHING

Often, it is best to do nothing surgically. Parents read the cancer warning signs about a mole enlarging or changing color, become worried, and bring in their offspring for treatment. After careful examination, explain that people continually grow new moles, and this normal process is especially rapid during adolescence. It saves time to have the parent read the patient instruction sheet Moles after you examine the child and pronounce the moles harmless but before the question-and-answer period. Seize this opportunity to educate parents about the dangerous effect of sunburns, and stress that even ordinary sun exposure causes new moles.

Sometimes, it is prudent to modify the "do-not-treat" advice for nevi in children when the parents are very concerned. Snipping off a few nevi that worry the parents and submitting them for histologic examination may provide more reassurance than hours of explanation. Another challenge to the art of benign neglect is the child or young adult, frequently female, who wishes removal of all unsightly moles. These patients are often descended from parents with many nevi, and they wish to be spared a "moley" fate. Frequently, they believe we possess some medical magic that will remove moles without a trace. "Do-not-treat" advice disappoints them and may raise doubts as to your ability. When careful explanation and the printed instruction sheet Moles fail to convince, I refer patients to a conservative plastic surgeon for a second opinion.

Patients should be instructed to return if any mole shows unusual growth patterns. Changes in color pattern, size, and shape are important and should be documented by photographs. Illustrated patient brochures are invaluable; check what is currently available from the Skin Cancer Foundation, the American Cancer Society, and the National Cancer Institute. The Skin Cancer Foundation's (Appendix B) brochure, "The Many Faces of Malignant Melanoma," is a mini-atlas of excellent color photographs that I highly recommend for both patients and physicians.

TREATMENT OF MELANOMA

Adequate surgical excision is the appropriate treatment for melanoma. This should be performed by someone experienced in the treatment and follow-up of melanoma. Guidelines for treatment are being continually revised; therefore, this section will be limited to a few brief generalizations.

What constitutes adequate margins continues to be debated. There is now good data documenting that for melanomas less than 1 mm thick, a 1-cm lateral margin is adequate. For thicker melanomas, margins varying from 2 to 5 cm have been recommended, and current studies are attempting to settle this issue by comparing margin width with cure rates.

So far, no systemic treatment has been effective in prolonging the lives of patients with metastatic melanoma. From the standpoint of patient care at present, an exhaustive search for metastatic disease using techniques such as bone and liver scans and magnetic resonance imaging seems to be a waste of medical resources. However, most physicians treating a patient with melanoma do order a chest x-ray.

There is general agreement that for melanomas less than 1 mm thick, prophylactic lymph node dissection is not warranted. For deeper lesions, published studies are contradictory. Lymph node dissection results in significant morbidity without proven benefit; therefore, I do not recommend prophylactic dissection of asymptomatic lymph nodes. Successful treatment of melanoma depends on excising the tumor before it has metastasized—hence the preoccupation with early diagnosis.

REFERENCE

1. Sober AJ, Fitzpatrick TB, Mihm MC Jr: Primary melanoma of the skin: Recognition and management. *J Am Acad Dermatol* 2:179, 1980

28 *Nickel Allergy*

Patient sheet page P–73

ETIOLOGY

Allergy to nickel is common in women, occurring in about 10 percent of Northern European and American women. Nickel contact dermatitis is usually caused by jewelry, but may also be produced by brassiere hooks, zippers, or the metal in eyeglass frames. In the pre-panty-hose days, thigh dermatitis from nickel-plated garter snaps was common. Persons allergic to nickel may get a rash wherever nickel-containing metal touches their skin. Curiously, nickel-containing coins infrequently cause dermatitis.

All jewelry contains nickel as a hardener; pure 24-karat gold is too soft for jewelry. There is less nickel in 14- or 18-karat gold jewelry than in inexpensive costume jewelry. Most women with weak nickel allergy who cannot tolerate costume jewelry can wear jewelry made of 14- or 18-karat gold. Although stainless steel contains nickel, the nickel is tightly bound within the alloy and doesn't cause dermatitis. Therefore, patients with nickel allergy can wear stainless-steel articles, provided they are not nickel-plated.

Like other allergies, nickel allergy is acquired. Ear piercing sometimes initiates nickel allergy. After nickel allergy appears, it persists for years.

DIAGNOSIS

The history and distribution of the rash usually enable the physician to diagnose nickel contact dermatitis with confidence. When a woman tells you she breaks out from wearing costume jewelry, you can be certain she is allergic to nickel, because nickel allergy is common in women. However, that does not necessarily mean that nickel caused the rash that is troubling her. It is the distribution of the rash (e.g., on the ear lobes, around the neck, on the back, under a ring) in a person with a history of nickel allergy that establishes the diagnosis of allergic contact dermatitis from nickel (Figures C–87 and C–88). Morphology is not helpful, because nickel contact dermatitis resembles other processes, such as atopic eczema, nummular eczema, and seborrheic dermatitis.

The presence of nickel allergy can be confirmed by patch testing.[1] Patch testing is superfluous in a patient with a typical history of breaking out from nickel-containing objects but may be of value in a patient with possible weak nickel allergy. Weak nickel allergy may cause an atypical dermatitis, such as recurrent crusting and oozing of the ear lobes, that is easy to misdiagnose as infection. Another diagnostic problem is recurring dermatitis underneath a ring without a history of dermatitis from other metal contact. Such ring dermatitis is usually not the result of nickel allergy, but represents the cumulative irritant effect of trapped detergents and moisture beneath the ring.

TREATMENT

When nickel allergy causes dermatitis, application of a topical corticosteroid and avoidance of further nickel contact usually clear the rash. Patients with mild nickel allergy frequently tolerate 14- or 18-karat gold jewelry for limited periods of time. The prophylactic use of a topical corticosteroid when wearing jewelry is useful. For women in whom nickel allergy prevents them from wearing wedding rings, a compromise often works; they wear wedding rings only when away from home and apply a topical corticosteroid first.

PREVENTION

Preventing development of allergy to a widely used material is ordinarily impossible; however, nickel allergy presents one special situation: ear piercing. Tissue trauma facilitates sensitization. Nickel sensitization from ear piercing can be prevented by using hypoallergenic nickel-free earrings to maintain patency of the tracts until they heal. Special hypoallergenic stainless-steel ear-piercing kits and earrings are available from firms such as H&A Enterprises, Inc., 143-19 25th Avenue, Whitestone, NY 11357.

DESENSITIZATION

At present, there is no way to desensitize a person allergic to nickel. In some, the intensity of the allergy may spontaneously decrease over the years.

MANAGING THE PATIENT

Emphatically explain to your nickel-allergic patients that the only way to prevent dermatitis is to avoid skin contact with nickel-containing metals. Special stainless-steel hypoallergenic earrings are commercially available. Cloth padding can be inserted between nickel-plated zippers and brassiere hooks to prevent them from touching the skin. Plastic-covered rather than metal eyeglass frames should be worn. The fascinating subject of nickel allergy, as well as a useful spot test for determining which metal objects contain nickel, is reviewed superbly in Fisher's book.[1]

REFERENCE

1. Fisher AA: *Contact Dermatitis,* 3rd edition. Philadelphia: Lea & Febiger, 1986

29 *Perioral Dermatitis (Rosaceaform Dermatitis)*

Patient sheet page P–75

Perioral dermatitis is a common facial rash, usually found in women aged 20 to 50. Despite its unique clinical picture, perioral dermatitis often escapes recognition by physicians. In the classic presentation, small red papules associated with erythema and sometimes scaling patches affect the upper lip, chin, and medial cheeks (Figures C–89 through C–91). A small zone of skin adjacent to the vermilion of the lips is usually spared.

ETIOLOGY

The cause of perioral dermatitis remains unknown. Fluorinated toothpastes, candidiasis, and cosmetics have all been accused of being causative agents, but without convincing evidence. However, it is known that potent topical corticosteroids are a significant aggravating factor, and perhaps the usual cause. This condition was rare before the introduction of potent steroids, and many patients have a history of applying potent topical corticosteroids to the face.

Both patients and physicians may be misled by the apparent beneficial effect of potent topical corticosteroids. Initially, these agents reduce the inflammation of perioral dermatitis, but attempts to discontinue their use result in severe flare-ups. With time, the rash gradually spreads, and there are ever-worsening flare-ups when the medication is discontinued.

Patients with active perioral dermatitis have irritable skin, and sunlight, soap, cosmetics, and moisturizers tend to aggravate the rash. Skin irritability resolves when the perioral dermatitis is brought under control. It is important to stress that cosmetics are not a cause of perioral dermatitis. Also emphasize that perioral dermatitis is not contagious, is not caused by germs or poor hygiene, and is not related to diet.

DIAGNOSIS

The classic presentation—erythematous papules around the mouth—can be diagnosed at a glance. When the distribution and morphology are atypical, acne, rosacea, and seborrheic dermatitis can present problems in differential diagnosis. Adult acne is often localized to the chin or cheeks and can resemble perioral dermatitis, except for the absence of erythema and scaling. Acne papules are perifollicular, whereas those in perioral dermatitis are not. Rosacea tends to affect an older age group, although there is considerable overlap. In rosacea, the nose is usually involved, there is a marked tendency to flushing, and scaling and dermatitis are absent. However, sometimes rosacea is indistinguishable from perioral dermatitis; this accounts for the alternative name for perioral dermatitis—rosaceaform dermatitis. Furthermore, perioral dermatitis and rosacea respond to the same therapeutic agents. When papules are not prominent, perioral dermatitis may resemble seborrheic dermatitis. If this condition is treated with potent topical corticosteroids, the patient will experience ever-worsening facial rash. Perinasal erythema, a fairly common, little-mentioned condition of redness with slight scaling about the nose, often appears to be the disorder preceding perioral dermatitis triggered by topical corticosteroids. Perinasal erythema responds poorly to topical agents but often resolves with systemic antibiotics—much like perioral dermatitis and rosacea.

TREATMENT

SYSTEMIC

Tetracycline is the sovereign remedy for perioral dermatitis. Most patients respond dramatically to a 3-week course of tetracycline, 500 mg twice daily. Thereafter, the tetracycline is tapered by decreasing the dose by 250 mg every 3 to 4 weeks until the patient is no longer taking the medication or finds that a low maintenance dose is required for some months.

At the first visit, go over the patient instruction sheets Perioral Dermatitis (Rosaceaform Dermatitis) and Tetracycline Treatment of Skin Disorders. If there are no contraindications, prescribe a 3-week course of tetracycline, 1 g daily, and ask the patient to return in 3 weeks. Most patients show clear-cut improvement after 3 weeks of treatment. Tell the patient how to taper the tetracycline dose, and give them the patient instruction sheet Long-Term Tetracycline Treatment, which describes the tapering procedure.

Favorable response to treatment is the rule. However, warn patients who have been using a strong corticosteroid that their rash will temporarily get worse. In no case should the corticosteroid be resumed. Flare-ups usually fade in 1 or 2 weeks, but occasionally, many months of systemic antibiotics are necessary before the skin recovers. If tetracycline is not tolerated or if photosensitivity is a problem, minocycline or erythromycin is often effective.

Ask the patient to contact you if the flare-up is severe. Severe flare-ups respond dramatically to a short course of oral prednisone, beginning with 40 mg/day and decreasing the dose gradually over 10 to 14 days.

TOPICAL

Topical therapy is much less effective in controlling perioral dermatitis; patients who cannot or will not take a systemic antibiotic present a considerable therapeutic challenge. The skin of patients with perioral dermatitis is sensitive and tends to be irritated by topicals. In one of the few controlled studies on the topical therapy of perioral dermatitis, metronidazole cream was found to be clearly effective, but less so than systemic tetracycline. However, in the United States, metronidazole is available only as a gel, which is drying and irritating to many patients. Anecdotal experience suggests that topical antibiotics used in acne are of benefit in treating perioral dermatitis. Unfortunately, most of these agents come in irritating hydroalcoholic or gel-type vehicles. However, clindamycin is available as a lotion (Cleocin-T) and meclocycline is available as a 1 percent cream (Meclan). Application of these agents two or three times per day may be tried. However, a prompt and satisfactory clearing of perioral dermatitis usually requires systemic antibiotics.

Some physicians prescribe a low-potency topical corticosteroid such as 1 percent hydrocortisone in addition to systemic or topical antimicrobials to suppress the inflammation of perioral dermatitis. However, there is no evidence that such treatment is beneficial. In view of the irritating effect of potent corticosteroids, it would seem prudent to avoid all topical corticoids when treating perioral dermatitis. The occasional patient who has a severe flare-up on stopping topical corticoids should be treated with oral cortisone, and under no condition should potent topical corticoids be resumed.

Although some textbooks claim that recurrences of perioral dermatitis are rare, and that this characteristic helps to distinguish it from rosacea, this has not been my experience. I have learned to tell patients who respond to their internal antibiotic that the long-term course is unpredictable. Sometimes, low doses of systemic antibiotics are necessary for several months to 1 year.

Recurrences are common, and I encourage patients to resume the antibiotic when they get a clear-cut flare-up. After patients have had this disorder correctly diagnosed and explained to them, they become adept at recognizing their recurrences. Flare-ups are often controlled with low doses of antibiotics. Encourage patients to try 250 or 500 mg of tetracycline initially and proceed to the full 1-g dose only if the lower dose proves ineffective.

Perioral dermatitis is distressing to women, as its papules cannot be hidden with cosmetics. Patients are delighted when the correct diagnosis leads to successful treatment.

Pityriasis Rosea

30

Patient sheet page P–77

ETIOLOGY

Pityriasis rosea is a common, harmless disease of unknown cause. In its typical form, a single scaly patch, the herald patch, precedes the generalized rash.

This generalized rash favors the trunk and spreads to the thighs, upper arms, and neck. Usually, a few spots appear on the face, but they are rarely a cosmetic problem. The generalized eruption lasts for 3 to 6 weeks but occasionally disappears in 1 week or persists as long as 3 months. Mild malaise is common, significant systemic symptoms rare.

While most patients have few skin complaints, 10 to 20 percent are uncomfortably itchy. Severe rashes resemble a florid drug eruption and are rare.

DIAGNOSIS

Pityriasis rosea is commonly misdiagnosed by both patients and physicians as due to a fungus. When only the herald patch is present, microscopy of KOH-cleared skin scrapings may be necessary to exclude tinea corporis. The herald patch may also resemble eczema.

Once the typical generalized rash appears, it is clear that the condition is not tinea corporis, although it sometimes panics patients who believe their "fungus has spread." Secondary syphilis and a drug eruption are the main diagnostic problems. Check the mucous surfaces, palms, and soles, because they are characteristic sites of secondary syphilis that are spared by pityriasis rosea. Pityriasis rosea may resemble any of the papulosquamous disorders, which adds seborrheic dermatitis, tinea versicolor, and psoriasis to the differential diagnosis. Occasionally, the rash "explodes" with myriads of macules that resemble measles or other viral exanthems.

TREATMENT

Most patients need only reassurance that their disease, although dramatic, is harmless and not contagious. This mild skin irritability is minimized by avoidance of soap and use of a lubricant. Skin lubrication is readily accomplished with bath oils.

When itching makes the patient uncomfortable, corticosteroids should be prescribed. Mild-to-moderate symptoms often respond to once-daily application of a high- or ultra-high-potency corticosteroid for 1 to 2 weeks. For severe symptoms, systemic corticosteroids are indicated; a 10- to 14-day tapering course usually produces dramatic improvement. Prednisone is the preferred steroid and should be given as a single morning dose. I use a regimen similar to the one for poison oak and poison ivy and start with 40 to 60 mg the first day, decreasing the dosage by 5 mg/day. Sometimes, a second course of prednisone is necessary to achieve complete resolution of symptoms.

Tell the patient the prednisone is for comfort and is not a cure. Before starting prednisone, inquire about peptic ulcers, diabetes, hypertension, and asthma, although these are only relative contraindications. Because concern about side effects of corticosteroids is common (and well-founded), explain that these concerns generally apply to long-term therapy, not to the 2-week course that you are prescribing.

Ultraviolet light therapy shortens the course of pityriasis rosea. However, the cost and nuisance of multiple ultraviolet light treatments are seldom justified in treating this disease. During warm weather, you may wish to tell patients that moderate sun exposure several times per week will speed healing.

The main treatment of pityriasis rosea is reassurance. Fear of contagion, concern about scarring, and worry about diet are anxieties that a few words and the patient information sheet Pityriasis Rosea should put to rest.

Poison Ivy and Poison Oak (Rhus *Allergy*)

Patient sheets pages P–21, P–79

31

ETIOLOGY

Acute contact dermatitis in North America, from poison ivy in the East and Midwest and poison oak in the West, is exceedingly common. Poison ivy and oak dermatitis is an example of allergic contact dermatitis. Its common occurrence and frequent severity merit a separate patient instruction sheet, Poison Ivy and Poison Oak Dermatitis. The allergens in poison ivy, poison oak, and poison sumac are similar, and the clinical manifestations and treatment are essentially identical. These plants all belong to the genus *Rhus*.

Rhus dermatitis results from skin contact with the plants' oleoresins. The patient may have come into either direct contact with the plant or indirect contact with the oleoresin, which can be carried on the fur of a pet, clothing, or hands, or via particles in smoke. The allergen is not spread by wind or air.

DIAGNOSIS

The diagnosis is generally easy; usually, patients have correctly made their own diagnosis and desire treatment. Irregular patches and streaks of acute contact dermatitis (Figure C–107 through C–109) point to a plant, and in North America, that plant is almost always *Rhus*. A history of a recent outing in areas known to be infested with *Rhus* increases the likelihood that the diagnosis is correct. Other plants, such as *Primula obconica* and Algerian ivy, can cause plant contact dermatitis that is morphologically indistinguishable from *Rhus* dermatitis. Usually, *Rhus* dermatitis is diagnosed when a physician is confronted with a plant contact dermatitis and a history of probable exposure. It helps when the patient knows he is allergic to *Rhus* plants. Patch testing with *Rhus* allergen is not helpful.

Diagnosing *Rhus* dermatitis can be difficult when the contact was indirect—through a pet, clothing, or some other object, even the patient's own skin. Such skin-to-skin transfer is not uncommon in male patients who develop genital dermatitis from transfer of oleoresin from hands to penis while urinating. Indirect plant contact dermatitis does not have the streaky, sharply demarcated patches that suggest plant contact, but consists of diffuse areas of dermatitis. Diagnosing *Rhus* dermatitis caused by indirect contact may require considerable questioning and detective work; sometimes a correct diagnosis can be made only after repeated bouts of dermatitis.

TREATMENT

Treatment of *Rhus* dermatitis consists of suppression with corticosteroids. Corticosteroids provide dramatic relief. Unfortunately, preventing future episodes of contact dermatitis is difficult. Be sure the patient knows the plants' appearance; pictures are useful, but the best approach is to have a friend or neighbor point out the troublemaker. Poison ivy can be a low, creeping plant or a climbing vine; poison oak is a bush that can grow over 6 feet high.

Washing after *Rhus* exposure is a time-honored preventive measure. Unfortunately, it is seldom effective. The allergen is rapidly bound to the skin; in order to prevent dermatitis, it is necessary to wash within 15 minutes of contact. Washing does rapidly destroy the oleoresin, and washing garments or an exposed pet will prevent the indirect spread of oleoresin. Strong soaps and detergents are unnecessary, because the *Rhus* allergen is unstable in the presence of moisture.

Barrier creams as a method of protection from *Rhus* dermatitis have received considerable publicity; however, it is not known whether they are effective. Some of these products will lessen the severity of experimentally produced *Rhus* contact dermatitis. However, the circumstances of these patch test studies have little in common with actual brush exposure. No large-scale field trials to determine whether barrier creams are effective in preventing *Rhus* dermatitis have been performed.

Desensitization as a method of preventing *Rhus* dermatitis remains an unrealized dream. Most preparations designed to desensitize are inactive and without value. Potent *Rhus* extract, given orally or by injection, temporarily decreases sensitivity to *Rhus* plants. When the desensitization treatments are stopped, the sensitivity usually returns to its previous level. Furthermore, such treatment may cause side effects. I have not attempted to desensitize patients to *Rhus* for 25 years; it is simpler to treat acute episodes with a short course of systemic corticosteroids.

SPECIFIC THERAPY

Systemic corticosteroids work quickly and can prevent the weeks of blistering and misery that severe *Rhus* dermatitis causes. Systemic corticosteroids are essential during the acute phase, since topical corticosteroids cannot penetrate the swollen, blistered skin. Use enough corticosteroid to suppress the eruption. Usually, 60 to 100 mg of prednisone per day are adequate; severe cases may initially require daily doses of 200 mg. As the dermatitis improves, the daily amount of corticosteroid is reduced. A 10- to 14-day course of oral steroids usually suffices.

Prednisone is the preferred corticosteroid. In mild-to-moderate *Rhus* dermatitis, prednisone is best taken as a single morning dose. In severe contact dermatitis, when doses of more than 100 mg are required, have the patient divide the daily dose and take one half in the morning and one half in the evening. The prednisone schedule I use for treating moderately severe *Rhus* contact dermatitis is given in Table 31–1. Prescribing 20-mg prednisone tablets, rather than the usual 5-mg tablets, is more convenient for the patient.

Treatment must be individualized, especially for severe cases. When enough corticosteroid is prescribed, the patient should improve daily. Tell the patient to call you if he or she fails to improve each day. The occasional patient who fails to improve day by day is instructed to take extra prednisone for a few days. In the early stages of *Rhus* contact dermatitis, it is impossible to determine whether the attack is going to be relatively mild or severe. When treating patients whose history of repeated severe attacks of *Rhus* contact dermatitis suggests a high degree of allergy, it is wise to initiate treatment with more than the usual amount of corticosteroid.

Table 31–1. **SCHEDULE FOR TREATING MODERATELY SEVERE**
Rhus **DERMATITIS WITH PREDNISONE TABLETS AS A SINGLE**
MORNING DOSE

Day	Prednisone (mg)	Dose (No. of 20-mg Tablets)
1	80	4
2	70	3½
3	60	3
4	50	2½
5	40	2
6	40	2
7	30	1½
8	30	1½
9	20	1
10	20	1
11	10	½
12	10	½
13	0	0

Systemic corticosteroid therapy can be provided in other ways than oral prednisone. Some physicians use injections of ACTH; others inject repository corticosteroids. Injection of long-acting repository steroids such as triamcinolone acetonide should be avoided, because these agents remain in the patient's body much longer than necessary. In addition to oral prednisone, I frequently inject 4 mg of dexamethasone phosphate intramuscularly at the initial visit. This fast-acting, soluble corticosteroid provides the patient with an immediate systemic effect and the psychological boost of having something done for him at once.

The safety of such short courses of systemic corticosteroids has been documented and is attested to by their almost universal use in treating *Rhus* dermatitis in North America. Active peptic ulcers, although not an absolute contraindication, suggest caution and the briefest possible course of corticosteroids. Insomnia, jitteriness, and irritability are fairly common but rarely severe. Diabetics should be warned that corticosteroids may worsen their disease.

The major problem with short courses of systemic corticosteroids is patient concern. Most patients have heard horror stories of persons whose "health was ruined by cortisone." Avoid this potential problem by emphasizing that short courses of corticosteroids are safe (after all, the body makes cortisone); it is prolonged steroid intake over months or years that produces dangerous side effects. Give the patient information sheet Cortisone Taken Internally, which provides detailed advice. For persons who suffer frequent bouts of *Rhus* dermatitis, as many as four courses annually can safely be prescribed. Each time I see the patient, I warn him to take all precautions to avoid future episodes of *Rhus* dermatitis.

It may be advisable to prescribe a supply of prednisone for patients who unavoidably get severe *Rhus* dermatitis occasionally. I do this only for selected patients whose occupations or avocations make repeated exposure unavoidable.

Other systemic drugs, such as antihistamines, sedatives, or tranquilizers, are unnecessary in treating *Rhus* contact dermatitis. Antihistamines do not suppress contact dermatitis, nor are they antipruritic, except for their sedative side effects. When *Rhus* contact dermatitis is adequately controlled by systemic corticosteroids, sedation is unnecessary. There are always exceptions. Occasionally, when there is severe itching and distress, patients are grateful for 2 or 3 days of bedtime hydroxyzine or a similar nonbarbiturate sedative.

TOPICAL THERAPY

During the acute, swollen, vesicular stage, what the patient does not apply to his skin is more important than what he does apply. Topical therapy is of little help at this stage of *Rhus* dermatitis. However, early stages of even severe poison oak contact dermatitis may benefit from twice-daily application of an ultra-high-potency (i.e., class 1) topical corticosteroid. The wrong topical may aggravate the dermatitis, because anesthetic ointments can sensitize, alcohol and astringents may irritate, and calamine and other lotions make a mess without doing much good. Cool water compresses are soothing and help remove debris and crusts. Although water is as good as anything else, Burow's solution, skim milk, saline, or a similar bland liquid can also be used. When the blisters and crusts have cleared up, the compresses should be stopped and topical corticosteroids begun.

Subacute poison oak contact dermatitis is helped by topical corticosteroids. Ultra-high-potency (i.e., class 1) topical corticosteroids such as clobetasol propionate (Temovate), halobetasol propionate (Ultravate), and others (see Chapter 1) may be useful in patients with subacute poison oak contact dermatitis who wish to stop their prednisone because of insomnia or other annoying side effects. Furthermore, topical therapy with such superpotent class 1 corticosteroids helps control mild-to-moderate outbreaks of *Rhus* contact dermatitis, and it may be of some help in the acute phase, when systemic corticosteroid therapy is refused by the patient or is medically contraindicated.

When extensive *Rhus* dermatitis is being treated with systemic prednisone, there is little to be gained by using the expensive superpotent topical corticosteroids. Instead, use inexpensive, generic, 0.1 percent triamcinolone acetonide cream, a moderate- to high-potency corticosteroid, as an adjunct and to subdue any dermatitis remaining after the course of prednisone has been completed.

Patients may bathe as desired but are told not to apply soap to the rash, because soap is an irritant. Dry skin may be annoying in the later stages of the dermatitis; if this occurs, have the patient lubricate the skin as suggested in the patient instruction sheet Dry Skin (Asteatosis, Xerosis).

COMPLICATIONS

Mild corticosteroid side effects are common, especially insomnia and jitteriness. Usually, these respond to reassurance; sometimes a mild tranquilizer at bedtime is helpful. In the rare patient with drastic psychic changes, discontinue the corticosteroid at once. Occasional stomach and abdominal pain may occur; usually, this side effect responds to antacids and rapid tapering of the prednisone.

Diabetes and hypertension are aggravated by systemic corticosteroids. Short courses of these drugs are justified in the treatment of acute *Rhus* contact dermatitis, provided blood pressure is monitored in hypertensive patients and urine and/ or blood sugar levels are checked daily by diabetics.

Corticosteroid side effects bear more relation to the length of treatment than to the amount of drug; it is safer to take 200 mg of prednisone in 1 day than 10 mg daily for 20 days. Too often, one encounters patients who have been itching, blistering, and unable to go to work or school for weeks because of inadequate doses of systemic corticosteroids.

Pyoderma is an unusual complication of *Rhus* contact dermatitis. Secondary infection is an indication for treatment with systemic antibiotics; erythromycin or a semisynthetic penicillin is a good choice.

Postoperative Care

32

Patient sheets pages P–61, P–105, P–107, P–109, P–111

Postoperative care instruction sheets save you time; you will receive fewer telephone calls from anxious patients and be spared answering the same questions many times. The methods of patient education described in this chapter are effective and can be modified for special cases. For example, you may want to keep a sutured wound dry longer than the 2 days advised in the patient sheet.

Skin surgery leaves a wound that either is closed with sutures or remains as an open defect that gradually epithelializes. Postoperative care following open surgery differs from care after closed surgery; they are discussed separately. A third section discusses care after liquid nitrogen destruction.

Do wounds heal better dry than wet? Tradition holds that a dry crust is desirable, as it protects the wound and discourages infection. Recent studies, however, have shown that wounds epithelialize faster if occluded to prevent loss of moisture and drying of the surface. Crusts retard healing by acting as a mechanical barrier to the regenerating epidermis. Moist postoperative care aims to prevent crust formation by using ointments and/or occlusive dressings to keep the wound from drying. Many surgical dressings designed for moist wound healing have been introduced; these are discussed in more detail in Chapter 4. The small, superficial wounds resulting from most types of dermatologic surgery do not justify the expense and special care these dressings entail.

The moist technique is also useful for sutured wounds. Epithelium must fill the gap between the sutured wound edges, and it does so more rapidly if the wound is occluded to prevent desiccation.

OPEN WOUNDS

I use both the dry and the wet approach for caring for open wounds. Use of a chemical styptic such as Monsel's solution or aluminum chloride provides a dry wound with a scab. However, these wounds heal more slowly than those in which a tissue-neutral hemostatic, such as Gelfoam, is used. Most of the time, I use Gelfoam and a moist postoperative regimen. In cases in which bandaging is difficult and in areas of little cosmetic concern—for example, the hairy scalp or inguinal area—I use a styptic. Styptics should be used only on superficial wounds. If deep wounds are left open, use Gelfoam and/or pressure to control bleeding.

The moist postoperative technique should be employed when optimal cosmetic results are important. Superficial wounds without crusts and deep open wounds are best managed by the moist postoperative technique.

DRY TECHNIQUE

Use the instruction sheet Care After Superficial Surgery. The patient is asked to ignore the wound except for painting the crust twice daily with ordinary rubbing alcohol or a hydroalcoholic anti-acne antibiotic solution. Alcohol or antibiotic solution applications decrease bacterial colonization and are something innocuous that patients can put on their wounds—otherwise they are tempted to apply their own "healing" potions.

MOIST TECHNIQUE

Use the instruction sheet Wound Care. Occlusion is achieved with an ointment and a bandage. This method does not provide as perfect occlusion as that achieved by covering the wound with plastic film, but it represents a practical compromise. Some physicians prefer to use an antibiotic ointment to discourage bacterial growth; there is no proof that these preparations are superior to petrolatum. Ideally, the moist technique should be used until the wound has epithelialized. The wound care directions are a compromise between moist and dry healing and allow the patient to leave the wound open after a firm crust has formed, reducing the time a bandage is needed. You may wish to modify the wound care sheet to continue occlusion until healing is complete.

The wound care sheet is used when wounds have been partially closed with sutures. Partial wound closure should be explained to patients so they understand that you left the wound partially open on purpose and not by mistake.

CLOSED SURGERY

Provide the patient instruction sheet Care of the Sutured (Stitched) Wound. Initially, an ointment and bandage are used to prevent desiccation and crust formation, which interfere with epithelialization.

To avoid railroad-track scarring, I remove sutures early and then apply a tape wound support to prevent dehiscence and minimize scar spreading. I currently use flesh-colored "paper" tape (Micropore) applied over spirit gum adhesive. Mastisol is an alternative to spirit gum. Sterile support tapes such as Steri-strip (3M) and Proxi-strip (Ethicon) are available commercially.

This tape support system sticks tenaciously for over 1 week in most wound locations. It will not loosen with water, and patients are glad to be able to bathe as usual. The system is not sterile, but sterility is not necessary at this point. Tape wound supports are not practical in hairy areas. Even on a closely shaved beard, a few days of hair growth loosens tape. On hairy skin, I apply flexible collodion directly to the wound as a support. The collodion is shed in a few days. Although not as good as tape support, it is better than nothing.

When gut is used for wound closure (see Chapter 4), provide the patient instruction sheet Care of Wounds Closed With Dissolving Stitches. This sheet explains that the sutures will be shed spontaneously and need not be removed.

LIQUID NITROGEN INSTRUCTIONS

The patient instruction sheet Liquid Nitrogen Treatment differs from the other postoperative instructions in that it discusses liquid nitrogen treatment and follow-up care. Patients may be unfamiliar with liquid nitrogen treatment. I explain that the pain lasts only a short time and that the growth is intact after freezing and will be shed later.

When freezing lesions deeply, stress that marked blistering can occur and is part of the treatment, not a complication. Patients are sometimes frightened by pronounced eyelid swelling following liquid nitrogen treatment about the eyelids. Alert patients to the possibility of marked swelling when lesions about the eyelids are treated. Reassure them that the swelling will disappear spontaneously over a few days.

Liquid nitrogen treatment of lesions on the dorsa of the hands may lead to huge, tense blisters (Figure C–58) that interfere with use of the hands and may rupture when the patient puts the hands in his pockets. In treating large keratoses of the hands, I usually ask the patient to return in 1 or 2 days so I can drain any large blisters by puncturing one edge with a large needle or the tip of a No. 11 blade. For reliable patients, I provide a large, sterile, 22-gauge needle so they may drain any annoying blisters. The top of the blister is not removed; only the fluid is drained.

Liquid nitrogen treatment frees the patient from worry about follow-up care. The wound almost invariably heals nicely whatever the patient does. The liquid nitrogen patient instruction sheet does not mention infection as a possible complication, because infection is rare following the superficial liquid nitrogen freezing used in treating benign lesions.

The last paragraph of the patient instruction sheet asks the patient to return if liquid nitrogen treatment does not eradicate his lesion. I reinforce this instruction when talking with the patient, because liquid nitrogen is used on lesions clinically diagnosed as benign, but sometimes we err. Diagnostic error is a particular problem in freezing actinic keratoses, because a skin cancer may mimic a benign keratosis. Biopsy any keratosis that fails to respond to liquid nitrogen treatment. These concerns about recurring lesions do not apply to recurrence of typical warts, which is, unhappily, a frequent event.

33 *Pruritus Ani (Rectal Itch)*

Patient sheets pages P–19, P–81*

ETIOLOGY

Pruritus ani is common in North America; because of their embarrassment, patients often admit they have it only after direct questioning. As a result of popular advertising for hemorrhoid preparations, patients frequently misdiagnose their anal itching as hemorrhoids. Hemorrhoids themselves do not itch; sometimes, if numerous, hemorrhoids may cause retention of fecal material with resulting anal itching.

DIAGNOSIS

In most patients, pruritus ani has no obvious cause. Although some texts state that diseases of the anal canal cause pruritus ani, cases that result from anal disease are distinctly unusual. Of the specific causes of pruritus ani, psoriasis is the most common. Dermatitis of the perianal skin occurs frequently in psoriasis, characteristically with extension into the gluteal cleft. All patients complaining of pruritus ani should be thoroughly examined for psoriasis. Psoriatic involvement of other skin areas may be minimal, and only some pitting of the fingernails or a scaly plaque on the scalp, elbows, or knees will lead to the correct diagnosis. Not infrequently, pruritus ani appears to be a forme fruste of psoriasis.

Fungal infection is a less frequent cause of pruritus ani. It may occur in men in association with tinea cruris and its sharply demarcated scaly patches of the inner thighs. Fungal infections usually extend well onto the skin of the buttocks, whereas idiopathic pruritus ani is limited to the immediate perianal skin. Candidiasis, with its macerated skin, superficial erosions, and satellite lesions, may sometimes be superimposed on idiopathic pruritus ani.

In the majority of patients with idiopathic pruritus ani, two factors play an etiologic role: (1) the irritant effects of the stool; and (2) the relative irritability of the perianal skin. Stools are irritating to skin; witness the inflammation produced in babies or incontinent adults when fecal matter is not promptly cleaned from perianal skin. Most persons, however, although having experienced transient irritation from stools, do not complain of pruritus ani. Patients with pruritus ani have unusually sensitive, easily irritated perianal skin. Many patients with pruritus ani show additional signs of skin dysfunction—for example, hand dermatitis, otitis externa, or seborrheic dermatitis of the scalp.

*Refer to the *Universal Medication Summary Sheet*, page xxi.

TREATMENT

SPECIFIC

In the few cases when a specific cause for pruritus ani can be found, treatment is directed at the cause. Dermatophyte infestations respond well to one of the broad-spectrum, relatively nonirritating antifungal creams such as ciclopirox (Loprox), econazole (Spectazole), or naftifine (Naftin). Psoriasis of the anal area and gluteal cleft responds to 1 to 2 percent topical hydrocortisone applied sparingly two or three times daily. In most patients with pruritus ani, therapy must be aimed at soothing the perianal skin and reducing irritation.

MINIMIZING IRRITATION

Reducing the irritant effects of stools with careful anal hygiene is the most important step in treating idiopathic pruritus ani. Cleansing after bowel movements must be meticulous and gentle and is best accomplished with water. European authors often advise using a bidet—a measure which is not practical in North America. Some patients, especially those with much perianal hair, find it necessary to shower for adequate post-bowel-movement cleansing. Dry toilet paper must be avoided. A reasonable compromise is to use moist tissue or toilet paper gently until all traces of stool are gone, then blot the area gently with dry toilet paper. Moistened, foil-wrapped tissues designed for anal cleansing are commercially available. Although these products are useful for the traveler, they are more expensive than water-moistened toilet paper, and occasionally their alcohol content irritates the skin. A spray of water from a rubber-bulb syringe may prove useful for patients in whom hemorrhoids, excessive hair, or tender skin renders moist toilet paper an ineffective method for proper anal cleansing.

Diarrhea, fecal leakage, and mucoid discharge all aggravate pruritus ani by exposing the perianal skin to irritant bowel contents. Sometimes, diarrhea is caused by an antibiotic. Chronic diarrhea is an indication for help from a consultant. Fecal leakage is occasionally the result of anal canal disease, such as fissures or cryptitis. Pruritus ani is rarely relieved by elimination of anal-canal disease or other proctologic procedures.

In some persons, certain foods, especially coffee and spicy dishes, induce gastrointestinal hyperactivity, with increased bowel movements and mucoid anal discharge. Eliminating the foods responsible for the bowel irritability may be dramatically effective in resolving pruritus ani. Not much can be done to relieve pruritus ani in patients with slight sphincter incontinence and frequent flatus. One approach is to keep a pledget of cotton outside the anus, held in place by the buttocks, to absorb anything expelled per anum. Commercial nonwoven fabric patches cut especially for this purpose (Tucks) are available.

The patient instruction sheet Pruritus Ani (Rectal Itch) stresses the role of gentle, careful anal hygiene. Scrubbing with soap and water is an almost universal response to itching. Soap is irritating; it should never be used on the perianal skin, because water alone provides adequate cleansing. The instructions prohibit self-treatment with proprietary anti-itch remedies, which can irritate the skin.

TOPICALS

Topical corticosteroids, when properly used, are effective in treating pruritus ani. Only hydrocortisone-containing topicals should be employed; more potent corticosteroids interfere with cell replication and may cause skin thinning with disastrous consequences. If possible, try to control the pruritus with 1 percent hydrocortisone cream. Higher hydrocortisone concentrations such as 2.5 percent, although more effective, carry the risk of skin thinning (see Chapter 1). Patients should apply the hydrocortisone topical sparingly with a fingertip after bowel movements, at bedtime, and possibly once or twice more daily. As the dermatitis improves, the topical corticosteroid can be tapered. The relapse rate after successful treatment of pruritus ani is high; recurrences usually yield to a repetition of the original regimen.

WARNING. Topical medicaments frequently irritate perianal skin. Even topical corticosteroids may irritate and aggravate pruritus ani. Be wary of irritation, and avoid potential sensitizers such as topical anesthetics.

SYSTEMIC THERAPY

When there is severe perianal dermatitis, especially with a superimposed allergic contact dermatitis from a topical medicament, a brief course of systemic corticosteroids is indicated. Usually prednisone taken for 7 to 14 days as a gradually decreasing daily morning dose suffices. Sometimes, pruritus ani requires longer periods of a systemic corticosteroid for control. This is a problem mainly when previous therapy with potent corticosteroids has resulted in a thin, extremely irritable perianal skin not responsive to topical hydrocortisone. When confronted with this dilemma, I usually initiate a 3- to 6-week course of alternate-day prednisone. Tell your patient that the systemic corticosteroid therapy is a temporary measure to provide some relief while his skin recovers sufficiently for control by topical medication.

Some physicians view pruritus ani as a psychosomatic illness and are fond of prescribing sedatives for it. The pruritus ani is allegedly part of a compulsive, perfectionistic personality. Although some pruritus ani patients are preoccupied with anal hygiene, the majority have objective evidence of other skin abnormalities, and a psychosomatic explanation does them injustice. From the standpoint of therapy, the question of psychosomatic causation of pruritus ani is moot. A patient's personality will not change with counseling and sedatives. With proper dermatologic care, most patients obtain relief.

Psoriasis

Patient sheets pages P–19, P–83, P–85*

34

ETIOLOGY

Psoriasis is difficult for both the patient and the physician. Textbooks invariably and appropriately describe psoriasis as a chronic dermatitis. Despite intensive research, little more is known than that psoriasis involves excessively rapid turnover of epidermal cells. It is generally considered an inherited disorder. Recently, this view has been challenged by studies suggesting that psoriasis occurs in two patterns: (1) as an inherited disorder that usually begins before age 30 years; and (2) as sporadic cases in which the patient's relatives do not have psoriasis.

DIAGNOSIS

Diagnosis of the classic presentation—sharply demarcated, scaling plaques of the scalp, elbows, and knees—is easy, but psoriasis can appear in ways that baffle even the most experienced clinician. Psoriasis may present difficulties when it affects only the palms (Figure C–103), soles, or fingernails (Figure C–105). Psoriasis may begin insidiously and initially resemble such disorders as seborrheic dermatitis, nummular eczema, dry-skin dermatitis, atopic eczema, or hand dermatitis (Figures C–103 through C–106). Most dermatologists have learned to view with suspicion stubborn seborrheic dermatitis of the scalp; years later, it often develops into classic psoriasis.

TREATMENT

Psoriasis affects between 1.5 and 3 percent of the Caucasian population and thus represents an important therapeutic challenge. Patients with newly developed psoriasis often become disenchanted with their treatment and switch physicians in the hope of finding a cure. Although there is no cure, treatment usually offers significant temporary relief and sometimes clears the rash. Because psoriasis is a disorder requiring long-term treatment, therapy should be simple and inexpensive. The effective, currently available treatment modalities for psoriasis are listed in Table 34–1. More than 95 percent of psoriatics require only topical therapy. Systemic treatment should be reserved for patients whose severe psoriasis fails to respond to topicals.

The patient information sheet Psoriasis mainly contains background information and emphasizes that the aim of treatment is control rather than cure. Because

---

*Refer to the *Universal Medication Summary Sheet*, page xxi.

Table 34–1. **TREATMENT MODALITIES FOR PSORIASIS**

Topical therapy	Ultraviolet light
Corticosteroids	Alone
Calcipotriol	With topical potentiation
Tar	With systemic potentiation by psoralens (PUVA therapy)
Anthralin	Systemic
Intralesional injections of corticosteroids	X-ray
Sunlight	

the treatment of psoriasis varies with severity and location of disease, routine printed treatment instructions are not feasible. Treatment is often complicated; therefore, it is wise to write out specific treatment instructions for each patient.

TOPICAL THERAPY

The topicals used for psoriasis are corticosteroids, tars, calcipotriol, and anthralin, in addition to a few miscellaneous agents of limited usefulness, such as salicylic acid and phenol.

Corticosteroids are the most popular topicals; they neither stain nor stink. The major disadvantages of these agents are that the control they achieve is usually transient, and daily applications are generally needed. Skin atrophy occurs readily in skin-fold areas, even with moderate-potency corticosteroids. The super-potent (i.e., class 1) corticosteroids cause atrophy at any skin site and should not be used on skin-fold areas. Although intermittent pulse therapy with one or two *weekly* applications of a super-potent corticosteroid has been advocated for treatment of plaque-type psoriasis on glabrous skin, even this may cause atrophy.

Tars are of modest benefit in treating psoriasis. In the United States, chiefly coal tars are used in treating psoriasis; wood tars are preferred by some. All tars stain and have a characteristic odor. Coal tar is a potent photosensitizer. Both coal and wood tars occasionally produce allergic sensitization and a resulting contact dermatitis.

Numerous proprietary coal-tar preparations are available in lotions, creams, gels, or tar-oil bath additives. Traditionally, coal tar was compounded in petrolatum—an effective but messy preparation. Proprietary tar preparations are less messy and less expensive than tar ointments compounded to order. Every dermatologist has his or her favorites.* Coal-tar solution is a solubilized fraction of coal tar that can be diluted to 25 percent in alcohol as a scalp tincture or added at 5 to 10 percent to a corticosteroid cream.

Calcipotriol, a noncalcemic vitamin D derivative, is an exciting development in the topical treatment of psoriasis. For plaque-type psoriasis, calcipotriol is as effective as betamethasone valerate ointment or short-contact anthralin therapy. Consequently, there is a treatment for plaque-type psoriasis without the risk of steroid atrophy or the messiness and staining of anthralin. Calcipotriol is somewhat irritating and occasionally causes facial dermatitis even though it is not used on the face. There is no effect on serum calcium when less than 100 g of ointment per week is used. In late 1993, calcipotriol was available only in Europe; however, FDA approval for U.S. use is expected.

Anthralin is an effective but difficult-to-use topical, because it irritates the skin. It stains clothing permanently and skin temporarily. Corticosteroids increase the irritating effect of anthralin; these agents should not be used together. Despite

---

*Some over-the-counter preparations are Alphosyl and Doak-Tar (lotions and creams), Psorigel and Estar (gels), and Balnetar, T-Derm and Doak-Oil (tar-oil combinations). The tar-oil combinations, although sometimes marketed as bath additives, are useful when painted directly on the skin.

these drawbacks, anthralin is a valuable preparation. When used judiciously, it can work wonders in treating extensive body psoriasis. When applied for only 10 to 30 minutes as short-contact therapy, the problem of stained clothing is eliminated. Unlike tar, anthralin does not smell. In short-contact therapy with anthralin, the only aesthetic objection is temporary skin staining. This staining, as well as skin irritation, is reduced by applying a topical containing triethanolamine after washing off the anthralin. As of fall 1993, triethenolamine is available in the United States as an over-the-counter spray, CuraStain.

Correct use of anthralin is difficult because, to be effective, it must be used at the threshold of irritation. Precise application to the psoriatic site is critical; a patient information sheet Anthralin Treatment of Psoriasis is provided. Although only a minority of patients with psoriasis will be able to use anthralin successfully, success in that minority makes it well worth the effort.

Anthralin may be used in two ways: as the traditional overnight application and as the newer, short-contact therapy. I now use only the short-contact treatment. Anthralin is available in the United States in a cream base as Dritho-Creme, and in a petrolatum vehicle as Anthra-Derm ointment in concentrations of 0.1, 0.25, 0.5, and 1 percent. Most patients prefer the cream vehicle (Dritho-Creme), as it is easier to wash off.

For short-contact therapy, the patient starts with 0.25 percent anthralin. When the patient tolerates the 0.25 percent preparation, the time of application is gradually increased. When the application time exceeds 30 minutes, have the patient switch to the 0.5 percent concentration, and reduce the application time sharply until the degree of response to that concentration is determined; then the application time should be increased gradually. When the 0.5 percent preparation is tolerated for 30 or 40 minutes, switch to the 1 percent concentration. Studies using short-contact anthralin treatment have shown the benefit of increasing the concentration stepwise to 2, 4, and 6 percent, compounded in petrolatum by a skilled pharmacist.

Precise application of a small amount of anthralin to the exact confines of the lesion is critical to the success of treatment. Demonstrate this to the patient, using any nonstaining cream if you prescribe Dritho-Creme, or nonstaining ointment if you prescribe Anthra-Derm.

I have patients return in 1 week, because despite oral and written instructions and a careful demonstration, almost all of them use too much ointment and cause irritation of the surrounding skin. This irritation is the reason why anthralin is not used as widely as it deserves to be. Point out that the irritation is due to spreading of the ointment from the lesion, which will not occur if it is applied sparingly and precisely. Marked irritation is an indication for decreasing the application time, whereas a lack of effect suggests the need for longer application times or higher concentrations.

Another checkup is scheduled in 2 to 3 weeks, because it generally takes 3 to 4 weeks to determine whether anthralin treatment will be of benefit. If there is improvement, treatment is continued vigorously until the psoriasis clears or the best possible result has been obtained. When clearing or reasonable control is achieved, the patient must determine by trial how frequently he needs to use anthralin treatment to control the psoriasis.

If you prescribe anthralin: (1) be cautious, because it is irritating; (2) do not use corticosteroids at the same time; and (3) warn the patient that it can stain clothing permanently.

In psoriasis, the response to topical medications shows striking regional variations. Medications useful in the groin and armpits will have no effect on scalp psoriasis, whereas topicals designed for scalp psoriasis are usually too irritating to be used in skin-fold areas. This variation in response accounts for the complexity of topical therapy.

Scalp

1. The patient should shampoo daily, if possible. This is to remove the continuous accumulation of scale. The type of shampoo the patient uses makes little difference; medicated shampoos are of limited benefit.

2. A coal-tar preparation should be applied sparingly to the psoriatic areas 3 to 12 hours before each shampoo. By applying it sparingly and precisely, the patient can minimize the smell and staining. Tar-oil bath additives can be painted sparingly with a cotton-tipped applicator on psoriatic patches, preferably by someone other than the patient. Tar gels are good alternatives that patients can easily apply themselves.

3. Topical corticosteroids—solutions, lotions, or gels—work well on scalp margins but are of less benefit on the hairy scalp. Creams and ointments are hard to apply to the scalp and should be avoided. Hydrocortisone has little impact on psoriasis of the scalp; a high-potency corticosteroid should be used.

4. Anthralin used as short-contact therapy is effective. Applying triethanolamine spray, available over the counter as CuraStain, after washing out the anthralin minimizes hair and scalp staining.

5. Ketoconazole cream or one of the broad-spectrum antifungal lotions or creams applied 2 to 10 hours before shampooing is sometimes beneficial.

Ears and Scalp Edges

High-potency corticosteroid creams, gels, and ointments usually nicely suppress psoriasis of the ears and scalp edges. Surprisingly often, patients prefer ointments. If used sparingly at bedtime, ointments are cosmetically acceptable. Psoriasis of the ear canals can be stubborn; a concentrated corticosteroid ointment applied thinly once or twice daily with fingertip or cotton-tipped applicator usually suppresses this condition. In some persons, ear psoriasis is prone to repeated infections, which are often treated as "chronically infected otitis externa" by nondermatologists. Vigorous treatment of ear-canal psoriasis with topical corticosteroids generally prevents such episodes.

Combining a topical nonsensitizing antibiotic such as tetracycline or erythromycin with a potent corticosteroid will often control exudative psoriasis of the ears when a corticosteroid alone fails. Unfortunately, such combinations are no longer available commercially in the United States. Although pharmacists can mix an antibiotic ointment with a corticosteroid ointment, it is simpler for the patient to apply a thin layer of antibiotic ointment once or twice during the day, and a corticosteroid ointment at bedtime. Another approach is to apply one of the new broad-spectrum antifungal creams (e.g., ketoconazole, econazole, naftifine) in the morning and a corticosteroid ointment at bedtime.*

Face

When psoriasis involves the face, it is generally mild. A cream containing 1 to 2.5 percent hydrocortisone applied sparingly twice daily usually controls this condition. If this treatment does not suffice, add 2 percent sulfur and 2 percent salicylic acid to the hydrocortisone topical. Sometimes, alternating applications of ketoconazole cream with hydrocortisone will control psoriasis of the face when hydrocortisone alone fails. Avoid potent corticosteroids on the face; they may cause rosaceaform eruptions as well as atrophy with telangiectasia.

---

*Topical ketaconazole, as well as some of the newer broad-spectrum topical antifungals, has a significant beneficial effect on seborrheic dermatitis and, to a lesser extent, on psoriasis. These agents have antibacterial, antifungal, and anticandidal activity and also appear to possess an intrinsic anti-inflammatory action.

Psoriasis of the armpits, groin, and perianal skin must be treated differently from lesions elsewhere. These skin folds are sensitive to traditional remedies such as anthralin and tars, which often irritate, and to the potent corticosteroids, which may cause skin thinning and atrophy. Perianal involvement in psoriasis is common. The most frequent cause of pruritus ani is mild, often unrecognized psoriasis. Gentle skin care is essential in perianal psoriasis. Provide the patient instruction sheet Pruritus Ani (Rectal Itch). Start the patient on 1 percent hydrocortisone cream applied very thinly two or three times per day and instruct him to use it less often when there is improvement.

Psoriasis of the inguinal folds and armpits should be treated similarly to psoriasis of the gluteal cleft: by avoiding irritants and using hydrocortisone topically. Patients should be instructed to avoid soap in these areas. Deodorants are irritating to many patients with armpit psoriasis. Suggest either a drying powder as a deodorant, or prescribe a topical antibiotic lotion or cream of the type used in treatment of acne. My current favorite is clindamycin lotion. Avoid the hydroalcoholic antibiotic formulations, which tend to irritate the skin.

If 1 percent hydrocortisone does not work, try alternating the hydrocortisone topical with ketoconazole cream or another broad-spectrum fungicide. If necessary, increase the concentration of hydrocortisone to 2.5 percent. This will control the majority of rashes. Patients using 2.5 percent hydrocortisone topicals should taper them as soon as they are better.

Do not use strong corticosteroids in the armpits, groin, or perianal area. While often dramatically effective over the short term, they tend to cause thinning and atrophy, with resulting irritable, hypersensitive skin. The patient uses the strong steroid more and more, the skin gets thinner and thinner, and the rash gets steadily worse. It often takes months to reverse the atrophy produced by just a few weeks of strong corticosteroids. Even 2.5 percent hydrocortisone occasionally causes skin thinning in skin-fold areas.

Body, Arms, and Legs

1. Potent corticosteroids are the simplest therapy for psoriasis of these areas, and they suffice in many patients. However, when there is extensive psoriasis, the physician must consider both the cost of these preparations and the degree of systemic absorption. Corticosteroids used in psoriasis tend to produce a temporary effect; relapse usually occurs within days of discontinuing them. The effect of corticosteroids can be greatly accentuated by occluding them with plastic film for 3 to 8 hours each day as described in Chapter 1.

2. Calcipotriol may well become the treatment of choice.

3. Coal tar is a traditional remedy for body psoriasis. Although it stains and has an odor, it is often effective. For mild-to-moderate body psoriasis, try combining coal tar applied at bedtime with a potent corticosteroid applied sparingly in the morning. The patient may wish to use old pajamas and sheets and remove any remaining tar with a morning shower.

4. The use of anthralin ointment has been described previously.

Hands

Psoriasis of the hands (Figure C–103) is best treated with topical corticosteroids according to the location and severity of the dermatitis. Details are given in Chapter 15. Most often, treatment with moderate-potency corticosteroids and plastic occlusion will be necessary. These agents can cause skin thinning; use them carefully. Psoriasis of the hands may be a difficult therapeutic challenge. Localized areas respond dramatically to intralesional injections of triamcinolone acetonide suspension as described later in this chapter.

Feet

Psoriasis of the feet tends to involve the soles, often with formation of deep-set vesicles and pustules. Potent corticosteroids applied at bedtime and covered overnight with plastic are the most effective therapy of psoriasis of the soles. Plastic occlusion of the feet is best accomplished by using a small plastic bag (the type available in grocery stores for food storage) cut down and held in place with a sock overnight. As an alternative, use Saran Wrap or similar pliable plastic food wrap held in place with a sock. Cautions regarding skin thinning with this treatment apply to the soles as well as the hands. As the patient improves, he should use the treatment less often. Friction markedly aggravates psoriasis; patients with psoriasis of the feet should be encouraged to wear shoes and socks and avoid going barefoot, especially on rough surfaces. For limited areas, intralesional triamcinolone injections are very effective.

INTRALESIONAL THERAPY

Intralesional injection of repository corticosteroids is a practical approach to limited areas of psoriasis, especially for the patient who has cosmetically annoying psoriasis of the elbows and knees (Figures C–100 and C–101). For psoriasis, use triamcinolone acetonide suspension 10 mg/ml (Kenalog-10) injected at a depth of 3 to 7 mm as described in Chapter 1.

SUNLIGHT

Most psoriasis is improved by sunlight. Sunburn should be avoided as it—like any other skin injury—may aggravate psoriasis. If coal tar is used, caution patients that tar is a potent photosensitizer. I encourage those patients who benefit from sunlight to take sunbaths two or three times per week when possible. The face should be protected with a sunscreen; the benefits of sun must be weighed against its skin-damaging effects. Be aware that there is a small subset of psoriatics whose disease is aggravated by sunlight.

ULTRAVIOLET LIGHT

Short-wave "sunburn" ultraviolet light, termed ultraviolet B (UV-B), has significant benefit in treating psoriasis. Traditional hot quartz mercury lamps, as well as fluorescent sun bulbs, emit UV-B. The effectiveness of UV-B is potentiated by coal tar. Systematic use of coal tar and ultraviolet light, termed the Goeckermann treatment, is an effective although rather involved method of treating extensive psoriasis.

Long-wave ultraviolet light, ultraviolet A (UV-A), is of little value by itself. However, when psoralens are used as photoactivators with UV-A, it is a powerful tool in the treatment of psoriasis. Treatment with oral psoralens and UV-A light (PUVA) is a very effective treatment for severe, extensive psoriasis. Both special light sources and special expertise are required.

STABLE VERSUS UNSTABLE PSORIASIS

The traditional therapy of psoriasis applies to stable psoriasis—scaly, hyperkeratotic patches present for months or years. At times, psoriasis becomes unstable and spreads rapidly. When this happens, traditional treatments must be stopped. Unstable, spreading, irritable psoriasis is made worse by the tar or anthralin remedies often necessary to subdue chronic psoriasis.

Treat unstable psoriasis with utmost caution and gentleness. Lubrication and topical corticosteroids in nonirritating vehicles are the best treatment, possibly augmented by mild tars or low-dose ultraviolet light. With time, unstable psoriasis usually becomes stable and then responds to traditional antipsoriasis remedies.

Unstable psoriasis is markedly irritable and prone to aggravation by inappropriate therapy. Strong remedies not only worsen unstable psoriasis and cause additional lesions, but may lead to exfoliative dermatitis. Warn the patient that his or her skin is sensitive; anything that irritates must be avoided and the condition is likely to get worse before getting better. Resist the temptation to use potent antipsoriatic remedies in the face of rapidly spreading psoriasis.

What causes psoriasis to become unstable and spread? Streptococcal pharyngitis is a well-documented triggering factor, especially in young patients. The resulting droplike showers of new psoriatic lesions (i.e., guttate psoriasis) usually respond nicely to mild treatment over a period of months. Other types of physical stress (e.g., infections, injuries, surgery) may cause psoriasis to become destabilized. A severe sunburn, irritating topical therapy, unrelated contact dermatitis (e.g., poison ivy, poison oak), or similar skin insult may activate psoriasis. Often, the cause of psoriatic instability is unknown. Whatever the cause, it is important to recognize psoriatic instability and suitably modify treatment.

SYSTEMIC TREATMENT

Antimetabolites

Antimetabolites have been used with success in psoriasis. These cellular poisons reduce the excessive turnover of psoriatic epidermal cells. All antimetabolites have significant side effects and require careful monitoring. Methotrexate is the drug best studied and most commonly used. Antimetabolites are best left to the experts; anyone attempting their use should carefully review the recent literature.

Corticosteroids

Systemic corticosteroids are rarely indicated in the treatment of psoriasis. Psoriatic erythroderma may be one exception. Although systemic corticosteroids are temporarily dramatically effective in controlling psoriasis, the disease flares up severely when side effects require their withdrawal. Few things are more difficult than weaning a psoriatic patient from long-term corticosteroids.

Psoralens

The use of PUVA or photochemotherapy has been discussed previously in this chapter.

Etretinate

Etretinate (Tegison), a vitamin A derivative, has adverse effects similar to those of another systemic retinoid, isotretinoin. Both etretinate and isotretinoin are potent teratogens, frequently cause elevation of triglycerides, may cause hyperostosis, and have ophthalmic effects. Etretinate causes elevation of liver-function enzymes in approximately 25 percent of patients, and serious hepatic toxicity is an occasional complication. Although isotretinoin is rapidly removed from the body and women may safely become pregnant 2 months after discontinuing it, etretinate lingers in the body for years. It is not known when, if ever, it is safe to become pregnant after a course of etretinate. Etretinate is best avoided in women of childbearing potential.

The toxicity of retinoids is related to the length of exposure; in treating acne with isotretinoin, a 4- to 5-month course usually results in a remission lasting years. Unfortunately, etretinate does not produce long-lasting remissions of psoriasis, although it is possible to reduce the total dose of etretinate by combining it with PUVA (RE-PUVA) therapy. Etretinate is probably best left to tertiary treatment centers experienced in managing severe psoriasis.

Other Systemic Drugs

A variety of drugs, including nonsteroidal anti-inflammatory agents and drugs that suppress immune responses, are undergoing therapeutic trials in the treatment of severe psoriasis. Toxic effects, including carcinogenesis, have forced abandonment of some of these agents. Because these drugs have significant adverse effects, their use should be considered experimental and restricted to research centers.

X-RAY THERAPY

Superficial x-ray and grenz-ray therapy is often effective in suppressing psoriasis. Many dermatologists have used these treatments successfully to provide temporary clearing of stubborn, localized psoriasis. As a therapeutic tool in psoriasis, x-ray therapy is of limited value. Psoriasis is a chronic, usually lifelong disease, and the total amount of x-ray exposure that may be given is limited. Given patient and physician concerns about the safety of radiation, and considering the medicolegal climate, I consider x-ray therapy of psoriasis to be of historical interest only.

MANAGING THE PATIENT

Psoriasis presents a challenge in psychological management as much as in clinical therapy. Psoriasis is not psychosomatic; part of the psychological management of psoriasis is to stress that psoriasis is not caused by nerves or emotions but is a genetically determined defect of skin growth. It is bad enough to have psoriasis; the patient should not have to feel guilty about being responsible for it. However, this is not to deny that emotional stress may aggravate psoriasis, just as it does many other somatic disorders.

The emotional impact of psoriasis is often overwhelming. Advertisements referring to the "heartbreak of psoriasis" do not exaggerate its effects on some patients. The true physician prescribes more than topical medicaments; he helps and supports patients' efforts to cope with this disorder. The patient must understand the course of psoriasis and the limitations of treatment. Explain that treatment is long-term and that there is no magical cure. It helps to point out that this is also true for diabetes, hypertension, and arthritis.

It is equally important to reassure patients with stable, chronic psoriasis of a few areas (e.g., scalp, elbows, perianal area) that in all likelihood, their psoriasis will remain a localized nuisance. Only a small percentage of psoriatics have severe, "life-ruining" eruptions.

Approach treatment with enthusiasm and provide specific instructions so that the patient realizes you have a therapeutic program in mind and are not groping in the dark. Avoid the "You might try this ointment" approach. Remind discouraged patients that psoriasis often improves spontaneously and may clear for many years.

Rosacea

Patient sheets pages P–89, P–113

35

ETIOLOGY

Rosacea is a skin dysfunction characterized by papulopustules and areas of erythema. Its resemblance to acne is emphasized by the antiquated term for this disorder, acne rosacea. Its cause is unknown. Older textbooks often discuss imagined relations to emotions, diets, and/or gastrointestinal disorders. Eye disorders, chiefly conjunctivitis and rarely keratitis, occasionally accompany rosacea.

DIAGNOSIS

Diagnosis is easy in the typical case with both papulopustules and areas of erythema. Unlike acne vulgaris, the nose is usually prominently affected (Figure C–99). Sometimes, when papulopustules are sparse, seborrheic dermatitis, discoid lupus erythematosus, and eczema enter into the differential diagnosis. The chronic application of high-potency corticosteroids to the skin of the face can produce a dermatitis closely resembling rosacea, which has been termed rosacealike dermatitis from steroids, steroid rosacea, and corticosteroid facies (Figures C–97 and C–98). Atypical forms of rosacea are common and often are not recognized.

TREATMENT

In the past, only systemic antibiotics were consistently successful in suppressing rosacea. Today, there is metronidazole, an effective topical treatment of rosacea. Metronidazole is available in gel form in the Unites States (Metrogel). Most cases of mild-to-moderate rosacea can be adequately controlled with topical metronidazole. If control is satisfactory, it may be continued indefinitely. Severe cases usually require systemic antibiotics. Antibiotics are also indicated when there are eye symptoms, even though the skin involvement may be mild. In paired comparison trials, systemic tetracycline, 1 g/day, has been shown to be superior to twice-daily applications of metronidazole.

TOPICAL TREATMENT

Metronidazole gel applied twice daily is a proven, effective treatment for rosacea. Improvement usually begins after 3 to 4 weeks, but optimal clearing may require 2 to 3 months of treatment. Metronidazole gel is drying and may cause skin irritation. The manufacturer has suggested counteracting this side effect by using a bland lubricant between Metrogel applications. Even though the skin is inflamed, do not prescribe a topical corticosteroid; it will aggravate rosacea.

There are topical alternatives to metronidazole. Sulfur 10 percent in a cream base applied at bedtime has been shown to be moderately effective in treating rosacea. However, patients do not like the smell or feel of this preparation, and it may irritate the skin.

SYSTEMIC TREATMENT

For patients with severe rosacea or with eye involvement, systemic antibiotics are indicated. I generally start with tetracycline 500 mg twice daily on an empty stomach. Rosacea generally responds to this regimen in 3 to 4 weeks (Figures C–92 through C–96). When satisfactory control occurs, patients gradually reduce their tetracycline dose by 250 mg each month, using the patient instruction sheet Long-Term Tetracycline Treatment. Such gradual reduction determines whether the patient can discontinue the oral antibiotic or needs a low maintenance dose for control. For the occasional patient who fails to respond to a 4-week course of 1 g tetracycline daily, I prefer to increase the tetracycline dose to 1.5 or 2 g/day before switching to alternative antibiotics—either erythromycin 1 g/day or minocycline 100 to 150 mg/day.

Rosacea aggravated by topical corticosteroids responds much more slowly to antibiotic treatment than ordinary rosacea. It is often necessary to continue systemic antibiotics for 3 to 6 months before an adequate response is obtained. In these patients, do not switch to a different antibiotic if you fail to get a response in 1 month; continue the one you have been using, perhaps at a higher dose, for at least 3 months. The problems involved in treating steroid-aggravated rosacea or rosaceaform dermatitis are described in more detail in Chapter 29.

It is the rare case of roscea that cannot be suppressed with systemic antibiotics. In these patients, systemic isotretinoin may be effective. However, this is not a drug for casual use.

Is it worthwhile to add topical metronidazole to a systemic antibiotic? I am not aware of any study that has addressed this question. I often treat patients with severe rosacea with both oral tetracycline and topical metronidazole. As they improve, the tetracycline is gradually phased out to determine whether topical metronidazole alone will control the condition. This is my personal approach; it has not been validated by controlled studies.

FLUSHING

Both oral antibiotics and topical metronidazole suppress the papular component of rosacea much better than the erythema. Patients with rosacea tend to flush easily, and the flushing probably aggravates rosacea. Hot beverages, hot foods, alcohol, and spicy foods tend to cause flushing; it is traditional to advise patients to avoid such stimuli. Reassure your patients that it is not the caffeine in coffee or tea that causes flushing; it is the heat of the beverage. Lukewarm or iced tea or coffee will not cause flushing.

LONG-TERM CONTROL

Emphasize to your patients that once rosacea develops, it is a long-term, usually lifelong problem. Although it may clear for several months or years, it tends to recur. For patients with occasional bouts of rosacea alternating with long disease-free periods, intermittent treatment is a logical choice. For those patients whose rosacea promptly relapses when treatment is discontinued, continuous, long-term treatment is best. In long-term patients, topical metronidazole used once daily may be effective. If tetracycline is used, as little as 250 mg/day may suffice.

36 *Scabies*

Patient sheet page P–91

ETIOLOGY

Scabies, a fascinating disorder, results from infestation with the mite *Sarcoptes scabiei.*

DIAGNOSIS

Diagnosis depends on the physician's index of suspicion and experience. Typical cases can be diagnosed at a glance by the experienced; however, scabies can present in unusual fashions that fool even experts. Suspect scabies when dealing with any intensely itching eruption that spares the face. The brief review by Orkin and Maibach is excellent.[1]

The diagnosis of scabies can be proven by demonstrating the mite, a challenging task. Although a patient with scabies may have hundreds of itching papules, he often has fewer than one dozen mites. The generalized eruption is a hypersensitivity response. The chances of finding a typical burrow and extracting a mite are best on the hands and wrists, especially in the webs between fingers (Figure C–110). Sometimes, the ankles yield burrows; in male patients, the penis should be carefully examined. The burrow is a short line that resembles a superficial scratch, except that it is curved or wavy (Figure C–111). The tiny brownish dot at one end is the mite (Figure C–112). A magnifying glass or binocular loupe is essential in the search.

When a suspected burrow is located, you can confirm the mite's presence microscopically in either of two ways:

1. If you see a tiny black dot at one end of a burrow, this is probably the mite; insert a small hypodermic needle (25- or 26-gauge) or the tip of a pointed scalpel blade into the skin. The mite will stick to it and can be transferred to glycerol, water, or immersion oil on a slide, covered with a coverslip, and examined under low power. A needle is the best method of extracting the mite, but this technique requires experience.

2. An alternative approach is to slice off the whole burrow with a sterile scalpel blade held parallel to the skin. You will draw some blood if you do this properly. Put the slice on a slide, cover it with glycerol or mineral or immersion oil, add a coverslip, and examine it under a microscope. The presence of the mite, ova, or feces—small, brownish, rounded objects—proves the diagnosis. When you cannot find any burrows, try vigorously scraping an area of multiple papules or excoriations in the finger webs or wrists and examining the scrapings after clearing with one of the above media.

Even the most expert physician will sometimes fail to prove the diagnosis. If there are strong clinical suspicions of scabies, a therapeutic trial is indicated even if the mite cannot be demonstrated. A therapeutic trial should be just that: A one- or possibly two-time application of a scabicide.

CONTAGION

Scabies is cured by killing the mite. The patient will stay cured only if the possibility of reinfection is eliminated. Close contacts must be treated. There are many misconceptions about the contagiousness of scabies; transmission requires close personal contact. In our society, transmission between adults is usually the result of sexual activity. Child-to-child and child-to-adult transfer occurs readily without sex. Scabies is practically never spread by clothing or bedding. There is no need to call in exterminators or process bedding or clothing in any special manner. Scabies is no longer contagious 24 hours after effective treatment.

How wide to spread the treatment net in an effort to eradicate all potential sources of the mite remains controversial. Some physicians treat only those contacts they have personally examined and found to harbor scabies. I believe this approach is impractical, not only because it may be virtually impossible to get all contacts in for a medical examination but also because early scabies may be overlooked even by a skilled examiner. I believe it best to treat all sexual contacts and all family members of a patient with proven scabies. Proven usually means that the mite has been demonstrated, although when two or more members of a family or sexual partners have a clinical picture typical of scabies, there is little likelihood of the condition being anything else.

TREATMENT

The treatment of choice is 5 percent permethrin cream (Elimite). This agent is essentially nontoxic to humans and therefore preferable to the previous standard treatment of 1 percent lindane (Kwell). Also, comparison trials have shown permethrin to be a more effective scabicide than lindane. The only drawback to permethrin is its cost.

Prolonged scabicide-to-skin contact is critical to the success of treatment. Although the package insert recommends 8 to 14 hours of contact, I prefer 24 hours. At bedtime, the patient applies the scabicide to the entire skin, except the face and scalp. Emphasize that every bit of skin below the face, including the neck, genitalia, perianal area, and toes, must be covered with a thin coat of permethrin cream. Infants must also have it applied to the face and scalp. The permethrin cream is washed off in the shower or bath the next night; emphasize that no bathing or showering is permitted for 24 hours after application.

Special attention must be given to treatment of the hands, because they are a favorite site for the mite. For the first 8 hours, the patient is to reapply the cream to the hands if they are washed. Patients are instructed to wash their hands before eating and reapply the cream to hands and wrists after breakfast, lunch, and snacks.

Permethrin cream is packaged in 60-g tubes. Although 30 g of cream suffice for one thin application to the entire skin of an adult, patients usually apply it more generously; one 60-g tube will be needed for each adult. Prescribe enough permethrin so that all sexual contacts and family members can be treated simultaneously.

Successful treatment requires precise patient compliance. Review the patient instruction sheet Scabies, and emphasize the following points:

1. All sexual contacts and family members must be treated simultaneously.

2. The cream must be applied to every part of the skin below the face.

3. The cream must be reapplied to the hands and wrists if the hands are washed before eating or after using the toilet.

4. The patient may not shower or bathe for 24 hours.

5. The itching will stop gradually. The severe itch of scabies is caused by allergy to the mite and generally clears in 2 to 3 weeks. Unless this is explained, patients will assume that the continued itching is caused by persistence of the infestation and will repeatedly apply the scabicide on their own. This may cause an irritant dermatitis with ever-worsening itch.

With proper application, permethrin cream is almost always curative in one treatment. Treatment failures are usually the result of failure to treat a sexual contact or family member at the same time. No one is immune to scabies; unless all close personal contacts are treated at the same time, reinfestation may occur. When it is likely that all potential contacts cannot be treated at the same time (e.g., the patient has multiple sexual partners; family members live in different households) I usually advise a second application of permethrin cream 1 week later.

In my practice, accompanying dermatitis is so common that most adult patients are also given a 10- to 14-day tapering course of prednisone by mouth. When there are signs of secondary infection with oozing and crusts, a 5- to 7-day course of an oral antibiotic such as erythromycin is indicated in addition.

I routinely tell patients with dermatitis to avoid soap and to use bath oils or other lubricants if their skin is dry. Generally, patients are asked to return in 10 to 14 days, because postscabetic dermatitis is quite common. Postscabetic dermatitis usually yields to a 2- to 3-week tapering course of prednisone combined with topical corticosteroids and avoidance of soap. Occasionally, longer courses of systemic corticosteroids are necessary. When this is the case, try to shift the patient to every-other-day prednisone taken as a single dose in the morning. The follow-up examination reassures the patient that any continuing itching is not due to scabies. This lessens the temptation for patients to reuse their scabicide whenever they itch—which some do despite strict warnings to the contrary.

COMPLICATIONS

Postscabetic dermatitis is the main complication of scabies and occasionally persists for months with persistent itching nodules. Men may develop indurated, severely itching scrotal and inguinal nodules. When it is impossible to distinguish postscabetic dermatitis from a treatment failure, a second course of antiscabetic therapy is permitted. Unfortunately, patients frequently use potent antiscabetic agents daily for weeks and even months with the mistaken notion that their persistent itching represents persistent scabies. Therefore, do not make prescriptions for scabicides refillable.

REFERENCE

1. Orkin M, Maibach HI: This scabies pandemic.
   N Engl J Med 289:496, 1978.

Seborrheic Keratoses

Patient sheets pages P–61, P–93, P–107

37

ETIOLOGY

Seborrheic keratoses are benign, genetically determined growths that usually first appear in adulthood. They gradually increase in number. Elderly patients may have a great many keratoses covering the trunk (Figure C–65). They are not caused by sun damage. Their former name of seborrheic verruca is appropriate to these wartlike lesions.

DIAGNOSIS

Differential diagnosis includes viral warts, nevi, actinic keratoses, basal cell carcinoma, squamous cell carcinoma, and, when the keratoses are highly pigmented, malignant melanoma.

TREATMENT

There are two indications for treatment: (1) the diagnosis is in question; or (2) the patient wants the growths removed. Seborrheic keratoses may itch, are often unsightly, or may be otherwise annoying to the patient.

The superficial nature of seborrheic keratoses makes removal easy by either curettage or liquid nitrogen freezing. If there is a question of diagnosis, curette them to provide a specimen for histology. Otherwise, the choice between liquid nitrogen and curettage depends on the availability of liquid nitrogen and the physician's preference.

Although cosmetic results with liquid nitrogen are slightly superior to those obtained by curettage, on the face, both methods produce excellent results, often without any scars (Figures C–113 through C–115). In treating seborrheic keratoses of the trunk and extremities, both curettage and liquid nitrogen frequently leave slight scars. Liquid nitrogen may produce temporary hyperpigmentation. The slight scarring that either method may cause is much preferable to the appearance of the original growths.

Liquid nitrogen treatment is discussed in Chapter 4. Judging the depth of adequate liquid nitrogen freezing can be difficult. I tend to be conservative and freeze seborrheic keratoses lightly. The patient is asked to return for a no-charge checkup visit in 4 to 5 weeks and is told that any residual keratoses will be frozen a second time without additional charge. Remember that you can always freeze a second time, but the scar from heavy-handed use of liquid nitrogen can never be undone.

Removal by curettage is simple (Figures C–113 through C–115). After giving local anesthesia, stretch the skin with the fingers of one hand and, using a 5- or 6-mm-diameter curette, scrape off the keratoses to a clean base with short, firm strokes. If optimum cosmetic results are critical, use pressure or a tissue-neutral homostatic, such as gelatin foam, to control bleeding. Otherwise, styptics such as Monsel's solution or aluminum chloride can be used. Do not electrodesiccate keratoses, as this procedure needlessly worsens scarring. Details of curettage treatment and postoperative care are discussed in Chapter 32.

Skin Aging and Skin Care

Patient sheets pages P–95, P–99

38

SOLAR DAMAGE

CAUSE

In our youth-oriented society, skin aging is a frequent concern. Much of what is commonly referred to as skin aging—fine wrinkles, irregular pigmentation, and patchy roughness—is not the result of age but a consequence of sun damage. Fair-skinned persons are especially prone to such effects; darker-skinned persons suffer less sun damage because of the protection provided by their pigment. It is common to underestimate the age of middle-aged blacks, because their youthful-appearing skin represents an absence of actinic damage. Not all skin aging is caused by sun damage, however; age is responsible for the deep wrinkles of the elderly.

The deleterious effects of sun damage are not fully appreciated. We have forgotten the wisdom of our great-grandmothers, who, with wide-brimmed hats, gloves, long sleeves, and parasols, carefully avoided the sun. Not only does sunlight age skin, but it is also responsible for basal cell carcinomas (which hardly ever occur in blacks) and most squamous cell carcinomas. Sunlight plays a role in the etiology of malignant melanoma. It is suspected that the increasing incidence of malignant melanoma—a worldwide phenomenon—is related to the "sun worship" that is so widely practiced.

As in other forms of radiation injury, there is a latent interval between sun exposure and the appearance of skin damage. Youthful sunbathing is a time bomb that may not go off for decades. Sun damage is cumulative and largely irreversible. A common misconception is that sun damage is caused by sunburn and that moderate sun exposure is safe. This is not true; moderate sun exposure and careful tanning will avoid sunburn but not actinic damage. Actinic damage is permanent. Although the skin cannot be rejuvenated, dermabrasion and deep chemical peels can improve the skin's appearance and texture.

PREVENTION

The idea of preventing disease has become fashionable; diseases caused by the sun can be prevented. Solar damage is produced by the sunlight's invisible ultraviolet rays. Clothing provides the best protection from these rays; sunscreens should be used on unprotected parts of the body. The most effective sunscreens contain pigment and mechanically block sunlight. The paintlike pigments make them unsightly and messy. Nevertheless, they are effective and practical when appearance is not at a premium; note the widespread use of zinc oxide to protect nose and lips at the beach. Commercial preparations of this type (A-Fil ointment, RVPaque oint-

169

ment) are sometimes given a flesh-colored tint to make them cosmetically more acceptable.

A number of fairly cosmetically acceptable "chemical-free" sunscreen lotions are available. These rely on zinc and/or titanium oxides for their modest sun protection, usually in the SPF 15 range. Trade names and formulations change; therefore, it is a good idea to occasionally review the druggist's shelf of sunscreens. A thick, heavily colored makeup base is also an efficient sun protective.

Most sun protectives are "clean," transparent preparations that act by chemically absorbing ultraviolet rays. The better ones—those with a high SPF—are very effective in blocking the shorter, ultraviolet B sunburning rays. They are of little value as blockers of the longer-wave ultraviolet A rays, which are the usual cause of photosensitivity reactions. The ultraviolet-absorbing chemicals often irritate, especially about the eyes, and occasionally, they sensitize the skin. I have patients test their tolerance for a sunscreen by applying it to the same small area of skin for 4 to 7 days. Some formulations, labeled "waterproof," resist washing and provide significant protection during swimming if applied 1 hour or so before water exposure. Detailed instructions are given in the patient instruction sheet Sunlight and Your Skin.

The sun protective factor, or SPF, on sunscreen labels is a quantitative measure of the product's efficacy. It is the ratio of the amount of light needed to produce erythema in the presence of the sunscreen to the amount of light producing erythema with no sunscreen. The higher the number, the better the protection. Patients should use products with an SPF of 25, or higher.

There are innumerable effective over-the-counter sun protectives. I will not try to list the many and changing brand names. The patient instruction sheet Sunlight and Your Skin has blank spaces for names to be inserted; you may also wish to provide samples.

Lips should be protected from the sun with an ultraviolet-absorbing lip pomade such as Shade Stick 30, or a heavily pigmented lipstick. Ordinary lubricating lip pomades do not give adequate protection.

Body lotions, baby oil, and tanning creams are frequently used by sunbathers who believe these preparations afford significant sun protection. They do not. Tanning lotions are simply weak sun protectors designed to screen out some of the ultraviolet light to minimize the risk of a sunburn.

Aim at moderation. The message is to minimize sun exposure, not avoid it. Occasionally, one encounters patients who have become so frightened of sun exposure that they have renounced all outdoor activities. Such overreaction is rare; it is more common for patients to continue their avid sun worship in spite of our warnings.

"SAFE" TANNING

Patients frequently ask, "Will I tan when using a sun blocker?" "Unfortunately, yes," is the answer. Even the most efficient, clean sun protectives allow a significant amount of solar radiation to reach the skin. Tell patients they should try to prevent tanning, because it is impossible to tan without damaging the skin.

Not only must patients be educated to protect themselves from solar radiation, they must be warned that artificial ultraviolet radiation also damages the skin. Ultraviolet light systems used in tanning parlors and the ultraviolet lamps present in many gyms and health spas are dangerous to the skin. Ultraviolet A is used rather than ultraviolet B in these artificial light sources, and it is claimed that this ultraviolet radiation is safe. Ultraviolet A has a longer wavelength and less sunburning tendency—for a given tanning effect—than does ultraviolet B. Although ultraviolet A permits tanning without sunburning, it causes chronic cellular injury.

Ultraviolet A radiation has produced skin cancers in animals. Tanning parlors and other sources of ultraviolet radiation—either A or B—should be shunned.

Instant tanning creams or lotions provide a safe, temporary way of darkening the skin. These products contain dihydroxyacetone, which combines with skin proteins to form a brownish pigment. The color change requires a few days of application for satisfactory darkening. Unless applications are continued, the artificial tan fades rapidly, because the pigmented compound is in the outermost skin layer and is rapidly lost by desquamation.

COSMETIC TREATMENTS

Patients often ask how they can prevent—or reverse—skin aging, wrinkles, and other signs that betray their age. The public is bombarded with advertisements that claim various products or procedures will rejuvenate the skin and smooth away wrinkles. Newspapers and magazines feature articles on the latest "breakthroughs" to achieve radiantly healthy skin, including exercise and diet. Dermatologists, plastic surgeons, and other health professionals increasingly extol the virtues of collagen injections, facelifts, liposuction, and special cosmetics. It is no wonder patients turn to their physicians for guidance.

Adequately answering such questions is a lengthy process, and physicians usually give such "trivia" short shrift. However, a patient's skin is not trivial to him. Most people have similar concerns; therefore, the patient information sheet Skin Aging and Treatments is a timesaver and a patient pleaser. Furthermore, we can give categorical answers to most questions on skin aging.

TRETINOIN

Tretinoin (Retin A) has been in use for almost two decades as a topical agent in the treatment of acne. In recent years, it has been promoted as a skin rejuvenant that reduces fine wrinkling and mitigates uneven pigmentation. In using tretinoin, some patients observe a gradual improvement in skin tone with diminution of wrinkles, as well as a more uniform skin color. Lentigenes often become less noticeable. The process is gradual and requires months of applications to achieve a perceptible effect. Any beneficial effect of Retin-A is modest and far less dramatic than what has been implied in advertisements and some of the "research" articles underwritten by the manufacturer. In my experience, fewer than one out of three users find the cosmetic benefits great enough to continue long-term tretinoin applications.

The effect of tretinoin is temporary; when applications are discontinued, the skin usually returns to its previous state. Long-term application of tretinoin appears to be safe. Tretinoin makes the skin sensitive to sunlight and mechanical trauma. Beauty salon operators warn against wax removal of facial hair in those using tretinoin.

Tretinoin is an irritant; consequently, some patients are unable to use it because of intolerable redness, scaling, and discomfort. Initiate treatment gradually with the most dilute formulation; then gradually increase the frequency of application and the concentration. Tretinoin is available in cream, gel, and liquid formulations; which preparation is best for treating aging skin has not been determined. My technique, which is admittedly arbitrary, is to start with applications of 0.025 percent cream every other night. The patient is instructed to apply the tretinoin nightly after 2 weeks, and twice daily after an additional 2 weeks, provided each level of use is tolerated. The patient's progress is checked after two to three months; depending on the response, I may increase the tretinoin cream concentration to 0.05 percent, and later 0.1 percent.

COLLAGEN, FIBREL, AND FAT INJECTIONS

Collagen injections are expensive and of moderate duration, yet they are popular with those who desire immediate smoothing of wrinkles. The greatest drawback to collagen injections is their temporary nature. The collagen is gradually absorbed, and its effects last only about 1 year, often less. Another disadvantage is allergy. Despite negative skin tests, occasionally patients develop unsightly papules and plaques at the injection sites; these persist until the collagen is absorbed. Because collagen is derived from cattle, concerns and unanswered questions remain about possible long-term effects of injections of a foreign protein.

Fibrel is the trade name for a mixture of gelatin, aminocaproic acid, and the patient's own plasma. This mixture must be freshly prepared for each treatment. The injection technique is more complicated than that used with collagen. Because Fibrel injections are painful, a local anesthetic is advisable. I have not seen good photographic documentation of Fibrel's benefit. Fibrel is not widely used.

Injection of the patient's own fat into the upper subcutis eliminates one objection to collagen; allergy is unlikely to develop. So far, this technique has not proven itself, because the injected fat cells are usually absorbed in a matter of months.

Collagen, Fibrel, and fat injections are best left to specialists with experience in these techniques.

CREAMS

A highly respected dermatologist, Alexander Fisher, has suggested that antiwrinkle creams should bear the warning "This product may be detrimental to your purse." He adds: "It's highly unlikely that patients will consult a dermatologist about these magic cosmetics that promise so much. After all, what do dermatologists know about magic?"

Still, there are advantages in educating people that wrinkles cannot be prevented or smoothed away by creams, that face washing need not be a complicated ritual, and that cosmetics can improve their appearance only temporarily. They may be able to save money, simplify their hygienic routine, and avoid feelings of guilt over their failure to preserve their skin.

EXERCISES

Facial exercises may actually worsen wrinkles, not prevent them. Wrinkles, after all, are the result of facial movement; witness their absence in persons whose facial muscles are paralyzed by stroke or neurologic disorder.

SURGERY

The two most common procedures consist of mechanical destruction of superficial layers of the skin by dermabrasion or chemical peeling with phenol or trichloroacetic acid. In properly selected patients, both dermabrasion and deep chemical peels are capable of dramatic results. Because both procedures may produce complications, including scarring, leave them to competent, experienced specialists.

Tetracyclines in the Therapy of Skin Disorders

39

Patient sheets pages P–113, P–127

Tetracycline is so widely used in dermatology that it merits two patient instruction sheets: One when initiating treatment, the other describing its long-term use. Tetracycline is the drug of choice for treating rosacea and perioral dermatitis; it is the most commonly employed systemic agent in treating acne. About 90 percent of patients with rosacea or perioral dermatitis do well with tetracycline suppression (Figures C–89, C–90, C–92 through C–96, and C–99). With acne, the process is less certain; probably fewer than two-thirds of acne cases respond satisfactorily to the usual doses of tetracycline. Rosacea and acne are long-term disorders that may require years of antibiotic suppression.

Many patients are apprehensive about treating a skin disorder with an internal antibiotic. The patient sheet Tetracycline Treatment of Skin Disorders aims to inform your patients of tetracycline's safety, its interactions, and its occasional, and usually minor, side effects. When I believe tetracycline treatment is warranted, I find it invaluable to have the patient read and digest this information sheet before discussing the treatment. It answers most questions, allays most fears, and instructs them in the correct way of taking their medicine. Those patients who respond to tetracycline will need to learn how to use it over the long term and adjust their dose to control their disorder with as little medicine as possible. Such long-term instruction is the goal of the second patient information sheet dealing with tetracycline, Long-Term Tetracycline Treatment.

Minocycline and doxycycline are two tetracycline derivatives widely used in treating skin disorders. Their dosages and side effects differ from those of tetracycline, and each will be discussed briefly in separate sections. Many dermatologists believe that these two newer tetracyclines, especially minocycline, are superior to tetracycline in the treatment of acne. Both minocycline and doxycycline are excellent alternatives for patients with rosacea or perioral dermatitis who fail to respond to or do not tolerate tetracycline. Minocycline has the advantage of not being a photosensitizer. It may be taken with food, but not with dairy products. It can cause dizziness and is expensive; however, less costly generic forms are available. Doxycycline may be taken with food and dairy products and is reasonably priced. Doxycycline is a significant photosensitizer and is not suitable for patients who receive intense sun exposure.

CAUTIONS

ORAL CONTRACEPTIVE FAILURE

Tetracyclines, erythromycin, penicillin, and other commonly used antibiotics may be associated with occasional oral contraceptive failure. This possibility arose from the observation that rifampin and phenytoin can interfere with the effectiveness of oral contraceptives. Rifampin and certain anticonvulsants induce liver enzymes that accelerate the metabolism of sex hormones. The resulting reduced blood sex hormone levels may lead to oral contraceptive failure. However, the tetracyclines, erythromycin, and penicillin do not induce these enzymes and do not reduce blood levels of sex hormones. There is no evidence that tetracycline interacts with oral contraceptives. Oral contraceptives fail in 0.2 to 1 percent of women taking them each year, and it is likely that any failure associated with tetracycline ingestion is a chance event.

Because it is impossible to prove that such an interaction cannot occur, it is important to describe this possible association to women who rely on oral contraceptives to prevent pregnancy. My personal approach is to discuss the possible association, and after explaining that I do not consider it a significant risk, leave the decision up to the patient. This temporal association of antibiotic ingestion and oral contraceptive failure occurs not only with long-term tetracycline treatment, but also with short-term use of penicillin, erythromycin, or other common antibiotics prescribed for such acute infections as sinusitis, dental abscesses, and boils.

TOOTH ENAMEL DEFECTS

Any tetracycline may cause tooth enamel defects if ingested when enamel is being formed during early childhood. Tetracyclines should not be used in patients younger than 8 years of age. Fortunately, acne is rare before puberty.

THE PATIENT STARTING TETRACYCLINE

Tetracycline should be taken on an empty stomach, because food, especially dairy products, binds it in the gastrointestinal tract and interferes with absorption. Taking tetracycline split into two daily doses is as effective as and simpler than the older, four-times per day regimen. A simple system will help your patients remember to take their antibiotic regularly. Tell the patient to count out the entire day's antibiotic ration when entering the bathroom on arising. Stress that this should be done even before using the toilet. The patient should take one half of the daily tetracycline ration at once with a full glass of water and put the other half in a small glass bottle or dish in a prominent place in the bathroom (assuming there are no small children about). The container with the medication serves as a reminder for the patient to take it in the evening. Ask the patient to check the dish at bedtime; if it is not empty he obviously forgot it earlier. When a patient is taking 500 mg or less of tetracycline daily, the entire dose is taken at one time on arising. This simple routine virtually eliminates forgotten doses—not an uncommon problem with patients on long-term oral therapy.

Acute side effects of tetracycline therapy—the not uncommon mild gastroenteritis or yeast vaginitis—are discussed in Chapter 5. The vexing question of tetracycline's interaction with birth control pills is also discussed in Chapter 5 and in the introductory patient information sheet Tetracycline Treatment of Skin Disorders, which also warns about drug interactions with lithium and phenytoin, as well as the binding of tetracycline in the intestinal tract by dairy products, iron, and calcium. Pregnant women should not take tetracycline. Tetracycline does not appear to be teratogenic; however, it is incorporated into the fetal bones and teeth, and this is not desirable.

Photosensitivity is a troubling side effect of tetracycline in sunnier climes. Photosensitivity is dose-related and is rarely a problem when the daily dosage of tetracycline is 500 mg or less. With 1 g/day, most fair-skinned persons will observe easier sunburning when exposed to summer sunshine. Individuals taking 2 g of tetracycline per day usually experience easy sunburning. Reversible photo-onycholysis (i.e., separation of the nails from their bases as a result of sun exposure) is an occasional side effect, mainly in young women taking 1 g or more of tetracycline daily. For some reason, photo-onycholysis occurs more commonly in women than in men. Tetracycline photosensitivity in North American patients is a problem principally during summer; however, be sure to alert skiers and patients taking a mid-winter vacation on a sunny island. The patient information sheet Tetracycline Treatment of Skin Disorders warns about sun sensitivity and advises the use of sun-protective measures. You may wish to give patients on higher doses of tetracycline or who are heavily exposed to the sun the patient instruction sheet Sunlight and Your Skin.

When acne and rosacea patients respond to tetracycline, long-term control usually requires long-term ingestion of tetracycline. The long-term use of systemic antibiotics to treat what are essentially cosmetically handicapping skin disorders seems to contradict traditional medical teaching. All physicians have been told to use antibiotics sparingly, and only for definitely diagnosed bacterial infections, yet nearly all dermatologists—and many other physicians as well—prescribe enormous amounts of tetracycline in treating acne, rosacea, and perioral dermatitis. Patients frequently voice concern about the long-term effect of tetracycline.

Fortunately, there is good evidence that long-term tetracycline therapy is remarkably safe. Several careful studies, as well as extensive clinical experience, have shown that patients on long-term tetracycline therapy are just as healthy as those who are not. There is no need to monitor tetracycline therapy with blood counts and urinalyses.

MINOCYCLINE

The usual starting dose of minocycline is 100 mg/day, taken either as 50 mg twice daily or, more simply and cheaply, as a single 100-mg dose. Fairly often, the dose must be increased to 150 or 200 mg/day to achieve a satisfactory response. Dizziness is an occasional, dose-related side effect. Dizziness is infrequent in patients on a daily dose of 100 mg or less, but it is a good idea to warn all patients of its possibility. Very rarely, prolonged use of minocycline colors the skin gray or blue-black; this effect is reversible. Rarely, minocycline may cause tooth discoloration in *adults*.

Minocycline causes less gastrointestinal irritation than tetracycline or doxycycline. For those with very sensitive stomachs, start with 50 mg daily taken with food. If this dose is tolerated, gradually increase the dose by 50-mg increments, always with food but not with dairy products.

DOXYCYCLINE

Doxycyline may be taken with food and is much less expensive than minocycline. Its main drawback is that it is a significant photosensitizer. The photosensitization is dose-related. Doxycyline causes more gastrointestinal irritation than minocycline, but most people tolerate it. It should be taken with food, and dairy products do not interfere with its absorption. The usual anti-acne dose is 100 mg/day. Some patients require 100 mg twice daily for control.

LONG-TERM CONTROL

The patient instruction sheet Long-Term Tetracycline Treatment stresses its safety. Be sure to mention this to patients. It will not only help to reassure them but also open the way for them to voice their concerns and fears. Not infrequently, patients have heard that it is dangerous to take antibiotics for a long time. Occasionally a patient worries about addiction. Stress that tetracycline has no mood-altering effects.

In long-term tetracycline therapy, the aim is to take the minimum dose required to suppress the eruption effectively. Because this minimum effective dose can vary widely, it needs to be determined for each person. After it has been determined that full doses of tetracycline are effective, the next step is to reduce the dose gradually to the point of a mild flare-up to determine the smallest amount required.

The patient instruction sheet Long-Term Tetracycline Treatment provides a schedule with dates and number of tablets to be filled in by the physician. Because there is a significant lag between taking tetracycline and the appearance of its effect, decreases in tetracycline dose should be gradual. Generally, 6 weeks should be allowed at one dose level before further reduction is attempted. Stress that patients should follow their schedules and reduce their tetracycline only gradually.

With some guidance, most patients adjust their tetracycline dosages successfully. Patients are told that they may adjust their dosages upward to the previous original amounts if pimples occur with lower doses. This is especially important to those patients whose acne is improved with summer sunshine but flares up during fall and winter. Occasionally, a patient varies the dosage from day to day, depending on how many pimples he finds in the morning. This practice should be stopped, and the reason why it is pointless explained. When patients understand that there is a lag of 1 to 3 weeks between the ingestion of tetracycline and the appearance of its effect, they recognize the uselessness of day-to-day adjustments.

How frequently should you ask patients on long-term tetracycline therapy to return? In general, acne patients require closer follow-up than patients with rosacea. Rosacea tends to run a more stable course than acne, and it affects adults, who are more reliable than adolescents about taking long-term medications. It would seem wise to see acne patients on long-term tetracycline therapy every 3 months for the first half year, and then, if their skin eruptions are reasonably well controlled on relatively small (i.e., less than 1 g) doses of tetracycline daily, see them every 6 months to 1 year thereafter. Patients should be told that if their acne is not adequately controlled, they should return promptly. There is no point in taking any medicine if it is ineffective.

Tinea Cruris (Jock Itch)

40

Patient sheet page P–115

ETIOLOGY

Tinea cruris is an infection of the skin of the groin with fungi, notably *Trichophyton mentagrophytes, Trichophyton rubrum,* and *Epidermophyton floccosum.* Tinea cruris is frequent in men and rare in women. Jock itch is a lay term referring to any itchy groin rash.

DIAGNOSIS

Tinea cruris usually shows sharply demarcated, scaling patches (the old term was eczema marginatum) extending from the inguinal folds onto the thighs and often the buttocks (Figure C–102). A fine collarette of scales or tiny papules is often present. Finding typical hyphae on microscopy of KOH-cleared skin scrapings taken from the edge of the lesion proves the diagnosis. Candidiasis, nonspecific intertrigo, seborrheic dermatitis, and psoriasis are the chief differential diagnostic problems.

It used to be important to distinguish candidiasis from tinea cruris, because the treatments of these disorders differed. Fortunately, there are now effective topical fungicides that act against both tinea cruris and candidiasis. Older fungicides (e.g., tolnaftate, undecylenic acid preparations) are ineffective against yeasts, and anti-*Candida* agents such as nystatin (Mycostatin, Nilstat) and amphotericin (Fungizone) are not effective against the dermatophytes that cause tinea cruris. It is not uncommon to encounter patients who have been unsuccessfully treating their tinea cruris with a nystatin preparation prescribed by a physician who mistakenly thought that nystatin was an antifungal agent.

Candidiasis usually shows satellite lesions beyond the border of the main rash, and superficial vesicles that may have ruptured, leaving small, round, denuded areas. Seborrheic dermatitis of the groin and inguinal psoriasis can perfectly mimic tinea cruris. It is not rare to have tinea cruris coexist with groin psoriasis; confirmation of the diagnosis by microscopy of skin scrapings is essential.

A frequent complication of tinea cruris is superimposed dermatitis from excessive scrubbing with soap and water or application of irritating remedies. The dermatitis can mislead the physician by obscuring the underlying tinea cruris. The inguinal folds are particularly prone to irritation from topical medicaments. This often leads to a remarkable similarity in appearance among groin rashes of different etiologies.

TREATMENT

GENERAL PRINCIPLES

Tinea cruris usually responds promptly to the newer topical broad-spectrum fungicides. Unfortunately, recurrences are common, especially when the infecting organism is *T. rubrum*. Dermatophytes thrive in a moist, warm environment; flare-ups and recurrences of tinea cruris are likely during hot weather, after prolonged wearing of a bathing suit, and with heavy sweating. Patients with persistent or recurrent tinea cruris should be advised to wear loose cotton underwear and use a bland dusting powder in the groin. Prophylactic use of miconazole powder sometimes works wonders; this over-the-counter fungicide (Micatin) is well tolerated in the groin.

When dermatitis coexists with tinea cruris, the two disorders must be treated simultaneously. The combined use of a corticosteroid topical and antifungal topical is wise. Depending on severity, you may combine a brief course of oral prednisone with topical antifungals or prescribe griseofulvin or another systemic antifungal by mouth and a topical corticosteroid. Prescribe only gentle measures. Topicals that itch, burn, or aggravate the eruption should be stopped.

Groin skin is easily irritated. Instruct patients not to apply home remedies. Soap should not be used on the groin; cleansing with plain water suffices. Soap may be used on normal skin when showering, because transient contact with dilute soapy water does no harm.

SPECIFIC TREATMENT

Topical

Tinea cruris usually responds dramatically to one of the newer broad-spectrum topical fungicides such as econazole (Spectazole), naftifine (Naftin), or ciclopirox (Loprox). These three agents are slightly more effective than miconazole (Micatin) or clotrimazole (Lotrimin, Mycelex). However, it appears that topical terbinafine (Lamisil) will prove superior to all previous agents in its persistence of antifungal action. These broad-spectrum fungicides are effective against yeasts (*Candida*) as well as dermatophytes.

The skin of the inguinal fold is sensitive; even the newer broad-spectrum fungicides, which are moderately irritating, should be used sparingly. In the groin, the cream formulations are better tolerated than liquids or gels. Clioquinol (Vioform) is a less effective fungicide and has the drawback of staining clothes; I consider it obsolete. Also obsolete is tolnaftate (Tinactin), because it fails to suppress yeasts. The highly irritating undecylenic acid preparations (Desenex) are of historical interest only.

Although simple, uncomplicated tinea cruris usually responds to topical fungicides, this is not the case when there is accompanying dermatitis. When tinea cruris and dermatitis coexist, treat the patient by alternating applications of 1 percent or 2.5 percent hydrocortisone cream with one of the newer broad-spectrum fungicides. Have the patient apply each agent twice a day at different times. As improvement occurs, direct him to first phase out the hydrocortisone cream. Any corticosteroid stronger than 2.5 percent hydrocortisone should be employed reluctantly, and only for a few days.

When there is severe dermatitis, avoid topical fungicides. Because the inflammatory process causes shedding of the fungi, fungicides are usually unnecessary in this stage and are likely to irritate the already inflamed skin. After the acute dermatitis has been controlled, fungicides—either alone or in conjunction with hydrocortisone—are often beneficial.

Systemic

Certain systemic antifungals are very effective in clearing tinea cruris. They should be reserved for severe cases not responding to topical therapy or when tinea cruris coexists with another skin disorder, such as psoriasis. Griseofulvin is a traditional agent; however, it appears that the newer antifungals fluconazole, itraconazole, and terbinafine are even more effective. Generally, only 10 to 14 days of treatment with these agents is required to produce clearing. Although they are reasonably safe for short courses, griseofulvin and the newer systemic antifungals produce significant drug interactions and side effects. Ketoconazole is best avoided; it may cause severe liver failure, although rarely, when given for longer than 1 week.

41 *Tinea Pedis (Athlete's Foot)*

Patient sheet page P–117

ETIOLOGY

Athlete's foot is the lay term for tinea pedis, the infection produced by fungi called dermatophytes. This is usually a chronic, lifelong infection; asymptomatic intervals, often prolonged, are common.

DIAGNOSIS

Although careful examination suggests the diagnosis, finding fungal elements on microscopic examination of KOH-cleared skin fragments is necessary for confirmation. Patients refer to almost any foot rash as "athlete's foot"; often they have psoriasis, eczema, shoe contact dermatitis, or hyperhidrosis. Tinea pedis is readily suspected when there is interdigital maceration, scaling, and fissuring, but it may be overlooked when the patient presents with blisters of the sole or the side of the foot (Figure C–121). In chronic *Trichophyton rubrum* infections, there is often a reddened, thick, scaling sole that may be dismissed as dry skin by patient and physician (Figure C–123).

Because so many conditions can mimic tinea pedis, even the experts rely on microscopy to confirm the diagnosis. Although you may be clinically certain of the diagnosis, it is reassuring to have objective confirmation. Appendix A provides step-by-step directions for this useful technique. Demonstrating the fungus microscopically only proves the patient has tinea pedis; it does not establish that all the skin signs are caused by tinea pedis. Tinea pedis occasionally coexists with psoriasis or other skin disorders, providing a diagnostic and therapeutic challenge (Figure C–104).

TREATMENT

TOPICAL

Imidazole derivatives and related topical antifungal agents have greatly simplified and improved the topical therapy of tinea pedis. These agents are not only more potent but also less irritating than the older undecylenic acid preparations. Furthermore, these agents are active against yeasts, and most have significant antibacterial activity. Secondary bacterial infection is a common complication of tinea pedis, and superinfection with yeasts also occurs. Consequently the new fungicides have rendered undecylenic acid preparations, as well as tolnaftate, obsolete in the treatment of tinea pedis.

It is important to distinguish between chronic tinea pedis with low-grade fissuring and scaling of the interdigital webs and acute flare-ups with edema, pain, and blistering. Chronic low-grade interdigital tinea pedis is controllable with any of the newer antifungals (e.g., econazole, naftifine, ciclopirox, sulconazole, terbinafine). These agents are effective when applied just once daily, thus simplifying the traditional advice of applying the medicament two or three times per day. In a small-scale trial, once-weekly applications of terbinafine cream controlled tinea pedis. Because tinea pedis is almost always a chronic condition, control with relatively infrequent applications is a tremendous boon.

The thick, chronic, scaling lesions of *T. rubrum* infections interfere with the penetration of topical antifungals. Gel vehicles improve penetration. Another approach is to alternate applications of a peeling agent, such as Keralyt gel, with the antifungal. Use peeling agents only for the hyperkeratotic, dry type of tinea pedis; they are not suitable for treating interdigital webs. Unfortunately, current topical therapy of hyperkeratotic tinea pedis is poor, and systemic antifungals are usually needed to achieve clearing.

Acutely inflamed, swollen, tender tinea pedis requires different therapy. The acute, oozing intertriginous eruption of the toes represents superinfection with bacteria and requires a systemic antibacterial agent. The systemic antibiotic (e.g., penicillin, erythromycin, minocycline) should be combined with bland soaks and a topical antimicrobial. The hydroalcoholic topical antimicrobials used to treat acne—especially clindamycin solution—are excellent, because they do not macerate.

An alternative topical would be one of the newer antifungals that have significant antibacterial activity (e.g., econazole, ciclopirox). After the acute phase is controlled, follow-up treatment consists of once- or twice-daily applications of one of the new, potent antifungals.

Acute blistering of the soles in athlete's foot is usually the result of active fungal infection; sometimes hypersensitivity also plays a role. Systemic antifungal therapy is frequently helpful, along with bland soaks and possibly a topical antibiotic. On occasion, a 2- to 4-day course of a systemic corticosteroid is dramatically effective—but only if you are certain that bacterial infection is not present. After the acute, blistering phase has subsided, treat as in chronic tinea pedis with topical imidazoles or similar agents.

The fungi that cause athlete's foot thrive on warmth and moisture; this accounts for flare-ups during hot weather and as a result of wearing occlusive shoes. Patients should dry their feet carefully after bathing and wear well-ventilated shoes. An antifungal powder applied to the feet in the morning is often helpful. These points are detailed in the patient instruction sheet Tinea Pedis (Athlete's Foot).

SYSTEMIC

Although most cases of tinea pedis can be controlled with topical antifungals, occasional cases require systemic treatment. As mentioned previously, the hyperkeratotic, dry type of tinea pedis responds poorly to topical agents. An occasional person will have repeated attacks of vesicular tinea pedis affecting the plantar surface. When symptomatic, both situations are indications for systemic antifungals.

Currently, the five systemic antifungals effective against dermatophytes are griseofulvin, ketoconazole, fluconazole, itraconazole, and terbinafine. All are available in the United States except terbinafine, for which FDA approval is expected shortly.

Griseofulvin has been used for more than 30 years, and the majority of patients with tinea pedis respond to it. Resistant dermatophyte strains have been reported but apparently are rare. Griseofulvin has a good overall safety profile, but it produces severe headaches as a significantly frequent side effect. Occasionally, gastrointestinal side effects are so annoying that patients stop taking the drug.

Ketoconazole is a potent anti-androgen and may rarely produce severe liver disease when given for longer than 10 days. I do not use it to treat tinea pedis.

Fluconazole in a dose of 100 mg/day is very effective against tinea pedis. Of interest are recent reports that 150 mg of fluconazole once weekly is highly effective in treating a variety of dermatophyte infections. Unfortunately, fluconazole is very expensive. Liver disease may occur with fluconazole, but apparently it is safer in this regard than ketoconazole.

Both itraconazole and terbinafine are highly effective antifungals. Paired comparison trials have shown them to be superior to griseofulvin in the treatment of recalcitrant tinea pedis. These drugs may become the systemic treatment of choice for dermatophyte infections. Hopefully, there soon will be data on optimal dosing and relative risk-to-benefit ratios for these and other newer antifungals. The situation regarding new systemic antifungals is currently undergoing such rapid change that any textbook advice probably will be out of date by the time it is printed.

CONTAGION

Epidemiologic studies on coal miners sharing common shower facilities and on public swimming pools have shown that athlete's foot is moderately contagious. Unfortunately, there is not much that can be done about it. Patients with athlete's foot do shed the fungus and thus expose family members. It is impossible to permanently sterilize showers, bathtubs, and other surfaces. Reassure patients that special precautions are not only futile but pointless, because family members cannot avoid exposure to the fungus outside the home.

Tinea Versicolor

Patient sheet page P–121

42

ETIOLOGY

Tinea versicolor is a superficial fungal infection caused by *Malassezia furfur,* which is identical to the microorganism *Pityrosporon orbiculare* found on normal skin. Tinea versicolor is caused by overgrowth of an inhabitant of normal skin. It is not contagious.

Patients usually seek treatment because their lesions are cosmetically annoying; rarely, there is slight itching. Tinea versicolor is more common in the tropics and often flares up in hot weather.

DIAGNOSIS

Tinea versicolor is characterized by variable coloring and mild scaling. On untanned skin, tinea versicolor is a pink-to-coppery tan. On tanned skin, the tinea versicolor patches are lighter than normal skin, because tanning does not occur in the rash areas (Figures C–126 through C–128). Occasionally, tinea versicolor is misdiagnosed as vitiligo. Close examination, however, shows fine scaling which is absent in vitiligo, and usually, tinea versicolor produces only partial pigment loss. Seborrheic dermatitis, pityriasis rosea, and sometimes tinea corporis are the chief differential diagnoses.

Microscopy of KOH-cleared scrapings, a useful diagnostic tool, shows short, curved hyphae and clusters of round yeast cells. Examination of the skin under ultraviolet black light (i.e., Wood's light) may be helpful, because active lesions in tinea versicolor may have a yellowish fluorescence. This is often absent, however, and black-light examination is less useful as a diagnostic aid than to demonstrate the extent of the process, which is usually more widespread than ordinary light reveals.

TREATMENT

Many remedies clear this disorder, but clearing is usually temporary, because the disease is not the result of infection by an exogenous agent but is caused by overgrowth of a normal skin inhabitant. Eventually, tinea versicolor recurs. Not only is there no cure, it is not definitively known which of the many recommended treatments is best.

It is difficult to know when to stop treatment if depigmentation is prominent.

Treatment does not repigment the skin; after tinea versicolor has cleared, the skin will repigment normally. Prescribe a course of treatment, and wait 1 or 2 months for the color contrast to fade. If the color contrast persists or scaling continues, repeat the treatment.

The patient instruction sheet Tinea Versicolor reflects the uncertainty as to the best treatment; it presents a menu of options. Selenium sulfide suspension used in treatment of dandruff (Selsun, Exsel) has long been popular and is often effective. It can be used either as a single, thorough, overnight application that is removed by showering the next morning, or as daily 10-minute applications before showering for 1 week. Whichever approach is used, have the patient wait for 1 month after treatment; if tinea versicolor has not cleared, have him repeat the treatment monthly until a satisfactory result is obtained. Selenium sulfide is cheap and usually effective. However, if tinea versicolor does not clear in 2 months of using one treatment, it is time to try another.

An antidandruff shampoo containing zinc pyrithione can be used similarly to selenium sulfide suspension before the daily shower. It should be applied for 10 minutes before the shower, then thoroughly rubbed in; the treatment should be repeated daily for 2 weeks. These preparations are available over the counter.

A clean and inexpensive treatment that is often effective is twice-daily applications of 50 percent propylene glycol in water for 2 weeks.

The newer broad-spectrum antifungal agents such as miconazole (Micatin), clotrimazole (Lotrimin, Mycelex), ciclopirox (Loprox), and econazole (Spectazole) are effective in treating tinea versicolor, but they are expensive and no more effective than the less expensive medications discussed previously. Sodium thiosulfate, a traditional remedy, stinks and requires numerous applications; I prefer to use other agents.

The systemic antifungal antibiotic ketoconazole will clear tinea versicolor. The schedule I use is 400 mg taken daily with a carbonated beverage on two successive days for a total dose of 800 mg. This 2-day course seems as effective as 1- and 2-week courses, which have also been recommended.

The patient instruction sheet Tinea Versicolor describes the 2-day course. Because extensive tinea versicolor invariably recurs, I usually prescribe enough ketoconazole for three courses of 2 days each and caution the patient to allow at least 3 months between courses. Although ketoconazole may rarely cause liver toxicity, the reported cases have all involved courses longer than 10 days. The 2-day ketoconazole treatment appears to be very safe.

The newer systemic antifungals fluconazole, itraconazole, and terbinafine are effective in treating tinea versicolor. In one study, a single 400-mg dose of fluconazole cleared 74 percent of cases of extensive tinea versicolor; however, fluconazole is expensive. Another study demonstrated that 5 days of itraconazole, 200 mg/day, produced clearing in over 90 percent of patients. Which systemic antifungal has the best benefit-to-risk profile remains to be determined. It is likely that brief systemic treatment will largely replace the often tedious and messy topical therapy of tinea versicolor.

Tinea versicolor routinely recurs. Tell patients to repeat the treatment *when*— not *if*—tinea versicolor recurs.

Warts

Patient sheets pages P–61, P–107, P–121, P–123, P–125

43

DIAGNOSIS

Diagnosis of warts is usually easy; most patients make the correct diagnosis themselves. One exception is plantar warts, which may closely resemble corns. Often, it is necessary to pare down a plantar callus before the characteristic speckled appearance of the plantar wart is evident. Flat warts, especially on the face, may be misdiagnosed as a rash or pimples (Figure C–129). Lesions of molluscum contagiosum may resemble warts until, on closer inspection, molluscum contagiosum's smooth papule with umbilication is recognized (Figure C–86). Warts always have a rough surface. At times, warts may be indistinguishable from seborrheic keratoses. Flat warts can closely resemble benign keratoses or epidermal nevi; when grouped, they are sometimes mistaken for a rash. Genital warts may resemble bowenoid papulosis, genital papules that are histologically malignant but usually clinically benign. Bowenoid papulosis appears to be caused by certain strains of wart virus.

GENERAL PRINCIPLES OF TREATMENT

Warts appear to have a bad reputation among primary physicians, because patients are frequently referred to dermatologists for "expert" therapy. Yet the unpredictable nature of warts "ruins dermatologists' reputations," as one dermatologist has put it.

Because there are no systemic antiwart viral agents, unsatisfactory best describes the destructive methods employed in treatment. Warts often fail to disappear with treatment, or they recur after apparent cure. Fortunately, warts may disappear by themselves, especially in children. This tendency of warts to disappear spontaneously makes it difficult to evaluate treatments. There is no way to prevent warts, and both patient and physician may become discouraged by an apparently endless succession of new warts.

The goal of treatment is to destroy the wart while sparing normal skin. Many people have scars from overenthusiastic wart destruction, often by electrodesiccation. Scars on the face or legs are unsightly; on the soles they may be painful. Warts do not produce scars; scars are the result of treatment.

The traditional view that warts are a banal nuisance is not correct when it comes to genital warts in women. Certain strains of wart virus can induce carcinoma in situ of the cervix and even frank cervical cancer. Consequently, it is important not only to eradicate genital warts in women, but also to destroy warts of the penis, the usual source of infection in women. Men with penile warts should be instructed to use latex condoms so as not to infect their sexual partners. There is good evidence that women with genital warts should be routinely screened for cervical dysplasia.

The benign nature of warts requires that treatment be limited to methods that have proven safe. This excludes, with rare exceptions, x-ray therapy. Deliberately sensitizing patients to a potent allergen such as dinitrochlorobenzene, followed by application of the sensitizer to warts to produce a brisk dermatitis, is still an experimental procedure. Be skeptical of new wart treatments; few are effective, and some are dangerous.

The absence of a truly effective wart treatment makes it important that the patient understand that warts are unpredictable. The patient information sheet Warts is suitable for all patients with warts. Once adequately informed, patients hopefully will blame treatment failures or the development of new warts on the capricious wart virus rather than on the therapy.

A great variety of thermal and chemical irritants have been proclaimed effective in treating warts. Repeated irritation of the wart is the common factor in these remedies. It is speculated that repeated irritation alters the body's response to warts, probably by some immune process, and causes wart necrosis. No one agent is superior in this respect, because the actions of these irritants are nonspecific.

Most dermatologists have simple wart treatment routines. Different types of warts require different routines. The treatment must be tailored to the wart's structure and location. From the standpoint of treatment, warts can be grouped into several types: (1) verruca vulgaris, the common wart; (2) plantar warts, warts of the sole; (3) flat warts; (4) acuminate or moist warts on the mucocutaneous junctions of the anogenital area; and (5) periungual warts.

Specific step-by-step directions for treating each type of wart are given in the next section of this chapter. Look upon these detailed directions as a collection of wart treatment "recipes"; review and follow them just as a cook carefully follows a new recipe. The instructions are designed so that the occasional wart therapist can proceed with confidence. As repetition brings familiarity, you will find yourself referring to them less and less frequently.

Before scanning the specifics of wart treatment, please carefully read the remainder of this section on general principles. An understanding of why certain methods are advisable—and why others are not—will help you avoid unpleasant results and unhappy patients.

Sometimes a wart persists no matter what therapy is provided. If tissue histology confirms the diagnosis of wart (carcinoma can masquerade as warts), advise the patient to live with the wart. Suggesting that the wart may disappear spontaneously helps the patient tolerate it.

I struggled unsuccessfully with a persistent wart on the third toe of a 62-year-old woman. The wart resisted chemical destruction, repeated liquid nitrogen treatments, and two curette removals. Histology confirmed the diagnosis. I suggested that the patient live with her wart and pare it down when it became protuberant. Unwilling to accept this, she sought treatment from another dermatologist, who included a course of x-ray therapy along with many other unsuccessful remedies. Subsequent excision and grafting by a plastic surgeon failed to eradicate the tenacious growth. Later, while hospitalized for a cholecystectomy, the woman persuaded an orthopedic surgeon to amputate her toe. This got rid of the wart, of course, but left her with persistent pain at the amputation site. Fortunately, such horror stories are rare.

SPECIFIC METHODS

This section provides detailed instructions for treating the five types of warts. The methods included are practical and safe. Some warts are best treated at home by chemical destruction. To be successful, these self-treatment approaches require careful instruction of patients. This instruction is made easier by using the patient instruction sheets Chemical Destruction of Warts and Plantar Warts.

VERRUCA VULGARIS (COMMON WART)

Surgery

Surgical treatment of the common wart is rapidly and easily accomplished by scoop removal, using scissors and curette, and has a better than 90 percent cure rate. This simple surgical method usually results in a small, sometimes invisible scar. Because even a tiny scar on the sole can be troublesome, surgery should be avoided in treating plantar warts. In cosmetically significant areas such as the face, elbows, and knees, liquid nitrogen treatment is preferable, although gentle scissors and curette removal usually provides cosmetically acceptable results if only pressure or gelatin foam packing is used for hemostasis.

Surgical treatment of warts by scoop removal or blunt dissection is described in detail in Chapter 4. After local anesthesia, the epidermis is incised circumferentially around the wart with the tip of a small, curved scissors. Using a large curette or a blunt dissector, a cleavage plane is established around the wart, and the wart is shelled out. Bleeding is controlled by pressure or packing with gelatin foam. Electrodesiccation should be avoided in treating ordinary warts, for it unnecessarily increases scarring (Figure C–132). Surgical wart removal means scissors and curette removal—never full-scale excision and suture. Because warts are neoplasms limited to the epidermis, full-thickness skin excision is unnecessary.

Liquid Nitrogen Treatment

From a cosmetic viewpoint, liquid nitrogen is an excellent treatment for warts. It is the treatment of choice for warts of the face and cosmetically sensitive areas of the hands, arms, and legs, especially in women. On the fingers and palms, where warts tend to be deeper, liquid nitrogen treatment often fails; I use surgical removal. Provided the freezing is superficial, scarring does not occur. The technique of liquid nitrogen therapy is discussed in Chapter 4.

Repeated liquid nitrogen treatment, sometimes combined with a home chemical-destruction approach, is one way of managing multiple warts. When treating warts repeatedly with liquid nitrogen, you do not have to freeze deeply; repeated superficial freezings have been shown to be effective.

Cantharidin

Application of the blistering agent cantharidin (Cantharone) to warts has a discouragingly high failure rate. Sometimes, it makes the wart larger and doughnut-shaped. Since cantharidin is painless, I sometimes use it in treating multiple warts in children despite its drawbacks.

Cantharidin is a powerful blistering agent and should be used with caution. The details of treatment with cantharidin are described in Chapter 26, because cantharidin is an ideal treatment for molluscum contagiosum lesions.

Chemical Destruction

Chemical destruction is my preferred treatment for numerous warts. Although surgical removal is excellent for one or a few common warts, it is not practical when there are more than five. Chemical destruction is painless; therefore I use it with small or anxious children even though they have only one or two warts that could be surgically removed in a fraction of the time needed to explain the chemical destruction treatment.

A self-treatment method using chemical destruction is the best therapy for the patient with numerous ordinary warts, because it allows treatment of emerging warts as well as established ones. Please note that I did not claim chemical destruction is a "good" answer to the treatment of numerous warts; it is merely one of the best of the inadequate available treatments. Chemical self-treatment of warts is slow and requires perseverance and encouragement.

Chemical wart destruction requires the repeated application of a moderately strong caustic such as salicylic acid, formalin, or lactic acid. There are numerous, well-advertised, over-the-counter salicylic acid–containing wart removers. Until recently, there were a number of prescription wart paints containing higher concentrations of salicylic acid. However, the FDA has ordered these to be removed from the market. One useful formulation is 40 percent salicylic acid ointment.

These caustics are used in a similar way and require the following:

1. Precise application to the wart with a toothpick or applicator. The caustic is applied most conveniently at bedtime. When a commercial wart-removing liquid is used, instruct the patient to allow 5 minutes for thorough drying before covering with tape.

2. An occlusive covering for about 8 hours for adequate penetration of the destructive agent. Occlusion is best accomplished by covering with waterproof tape. The nonocclusive "paper" tapes are not suitable. The moisture-retaining and macerating effects of waterproof tape are desirable; there is no harm in the patient getting the tape wet. If removal of the tape injures the surrounding skin, have the patient apply nail-polish remover between tape and skin when removing the tape. In patients with myriads of warts, occlusion with plastic film (e.g., plastic gloves on hands, Saran Wrap elsewhere) is a practical measure.

3. Mechanical removal of dead wart tissue using a pumice stone, the tip of a metal nail file, curved scissors, or a similar instrument. This should be done after bathing, when the necrotic tissue will be soft. The mechanical removal step is crucial to effective treatment. Unfortunately, all too often it tends to be neglected. I frequently have to nag patients into performing adequate necrotic tissue removal.

4. Some flexibility in treatment. If destruction is inadequate, the patient should gradually increase the period of occlusion. If there is too much irritation, let the patient stop treatment for 1 or 2 days.

5. Patient compliance. Chemical wart destruction is self-treatment carried out at the physician's instruction. Patients must understand both the details of treatment and the need to continue it faithfully every day. While there is no substitute for demonstrating the technique and explaining the need to continue treatment faithfully, a patient instruction sheet is also essential. I ask patients to read the instruction sheet Chemical Destruction of Warts once per day for 3 days to fix it in their minds.

6. Flexibility of follow-up. If a patient has numerous warts, have him return 2 to 3 weeks after starting treatment to check on progress. Patients often do not perform the treatment properly. Usually, as mentioned previously, they are too timid about removing the dead wart tissue. For patients who are using chemical destruction on only one or two warts (usually, these are small children), I use a more casual follow-up procedure, telling them to return only if no progress has been made in 1 month or if the wart is still present after 3 months of conscientious self-treatment.

The chemical destruction of warts can be combined with other modalities. In treating patients with multiple warts, I often combine light liquid nitrogen freezing with chemical destruction. The light freezing at the initial visit is not aimed to cure, but simply to start the destructive process and give the patient a psychological boost. I generally repeat light liquid nitrogen freezing at follow-up visits. In this situation, I do not know of a good substitute for liquid nitrogen. The stronger escharotics such as trichloroacetic acid, phenol, and the very destructive monochloroacetic acid are unpredictable and difficult to control. They often produce little effect and sometimes cause nasty scars. If liquid nitrogen is unavailable, pare down warts with a No. 15 blade at follow-up visits.

Bleomycin

Intralesional injection of bleomycin is a treatment of last resort for stubborn warts. Bleomycin is a potent teratogen and should be used only if there is no possibility of pregnancy. It is expensive, and its solutions have limited stability. Unfortunately, Raynaud's phenomenon has occasionally occurred in fingers treated with intralesional bleomycin for warts, and may rarely occur on toes. I restrict my use of bleomycin to painful plantar warts that have resisted chemical destruction.

PLANTAR WARTS

Plantar warts have a well-deserved reputation as a persistent, painful nuisance. Treatment often fails or is prolonged. The aim of therapy is to eradicate the wart without any scarring, because a plantar scar can be painful. Scars following electrodesiccation of plantar warts sometimes become painful only after a latent period of years.

Many dermatologists claim scarring can be avoided if electrodesiccation is carefully performed. They are wrong. I have seen too many patients with painful electrodesiccation scars caused by dermatologists who have personally assured me that when they electrodesiccate plantar warts, scarring never occurs. Sometimes, patients consult another physician months or years after electrodesiccation of a plantar wart, complaining of a wart recurrence when the actual problem is a painful, hypertrophic scar (Figures C–130 and C–131). Never electrodesiccate a plantar wart.

Even careful surgical scoop removal may cause scarring. Sometimes, when a solitary plantar wart defies chemical destruction, careful surgical removal may be justified. If you undertake surgical removal, observe the same precautions recommended in surgically treating warts on cosmetically significant areas; be gentle with your instruments and control bleeding with pressure and/or gelatin foam packing. Do not electrodesiccate, and do not use styptics such as Monsel's solution.

It is easy to state categorically what not to do in treating plantar warts. Advising how to treat them is more difficult. Most perceptive clinicians use some type of chemical destruction.

There are innumerable formulas for chemical destruction of plantar warts. They all have about the same cure rate; therefore I use the gentler approaches that cause little or no pain. For one or a few plantar warts, I use one of the commercial salicylic acid paints or 40 percent salicylic acid ointment. The patient applies the medicine at bedtime and covers it with tape overnight. Removal of dead wart tissue is essential.

Plantar warts are often painful. Suitable padding will relieve the pain by taking pressure off the wart. Commercially available corn pads are usually too small; I prefer a foam pad with one adhesive-coated surface (Dr. Scholl's Foot and Shoe Padding). A piece of foam is cut large enough to cover either the entire heel or forepart of the foot, and a hole (or, if the wart is at the edge of the foot, a notch) corresponding to the position of the wart is cut into the foam. After sticking the pad on his or her foot, the patient stands for a few moments to promote adherence to the skin and then rolls a sock or stocking carefully over the pad. The technique of making and applying the protective pad and the method to be used in treating the wart should be demonstrated to the patient in the office. The patient instruction sheet Plantar Warts is also essential.

When there are numerous plantar warts, or in the presence of the extensive "mosaic" plantar wart, application of a chemical destructive to each wart is not practical. For multiple or very large plantar warts, dilute formalin soaks are useful. The patient is instructed to mix 1 tablespoon of commercial formalin, which contains 37 percent formaldehyde, with one pint of cool water. The warty area of the sole is soaked in the diluted formalin for 10 to 15 minutes every night. The patient must systematically scrape off dead wart tissue after bathing. If there is soreness or itching, the treatment should be stopped, because irritation or sensitization occasionally occurs.

FLAT WARTS

Flat warts are superficial; gentle treatment measures are indicated, especially because they often affect cosmetically sensitive areas (Figure C–129). For a few warts, very light liquid nitrogen freezing is useful. Cautious chemical destruction using a salicylic acid paint is often effective. This paint should first be used without occlusion. If the flat wart is not in a cosmetically sensitive area, very gentle curettage can be tried.

With multiple flat warts, especially on the face, gentle peeling chemicals are widely used. For this purpose, use one of the peeling acne preparations containing sulfur, salicylic acid, or resorcinol; an alternative is a retinoic acid acne topical (Retin-A). These preparations are designed to be used on the face and therefore will do no harm. Flat warts sometimes respond to topical 5-fluorouracil (Efudex, Fluoroplex) when the peeling anti-acne preparations have failed. The results with this technique are not spectacular; warts usually take a long time to disappear and sometimes resist the treatment completely. Counsel the patient and practice patience. Stress that the treatment is gradual, and if possible, allow 2 or 3 months between visits. Do not let the patient's frustration stampede you into using harsh measures that produce scars.

ACUMINATE WARTS

Acuminate warts, also known as moist or venereal warts, affect primarily the anogenital region. The term venereal is often used and is appropriate, because many of these warts are related to sexual activity. Moist describes both their location and their surface covering, which is softer and more permeable than the keratinous layer of warts that occur elsewhere. This permeability explains the effectiveness of podophyllin (podophyllum resin) treatment.

Keep in mind that not all papular or verrucous lesions of the anogenital region are warts. The condyloma of secondary syphilis can mislead the physician; a serologic test will settle the diagnosis. Malignancies—especially Bowen's disease—can closely resemble anogenital warts. Biopsy any atypical or persistent warty anogenital lesion.

Treatment Controversies

The treatment of anogenital warts is replete with controversies. Warts often resist therapy, and old warts recur as new ones appear. Who has not treated a patient with genital warts month after month, heaving a sigh of relief when all visible warts were gone, only to have the patient return months or years later with a new crop of warts. One reason treatment methods do so poorly is because the wart virus often resides in normal-appearing skin some distance from the wart.

A major controversy in the management of anogenital warts is the use of acetic acid soaks to detect otherwise invisible warts. If 4 percent acetic acid (i.e., vinegar strength) is applied for some minutes to the skin of a patient with genital warts, small whitish papules often appear. Some, but by no means all, of these papules can be shown to be warts that would otherwise be invisible. These acetowhite areas, the presumptive subclinical warts, are then removed surgically or destroyed by using liquid nitrogen, electrosurgery, or laser therapy. Although this rigorous approach is logical, it has not been shown that it provides a better cure rate than simply removing only the grossly visible warts. Because the wart virus may reside in clinically normal skin, it is reasonable to question the need for the tedious business of finding and destroying acetowhite lesions.

Although there is no really effective treatment for acuminate warts, the most popular is podophyllin and a significant advance is the new purified active principle, podofilox. Podofilox is available as a 0.5 percent topical solution (Condylox) designed for patient application. Condylox, unlike podophyllin, is effective on glabrous (dry) skin, whereas podophyllin is not. Controlled studies have demonstrated the effectiveness and safety of podofilox. Its great advantage is that home use by the patient eliminates the multiple office visits required for podophyllin treatment. Podophyllin and podofilox should not be used in pregnant women.

Cryotherapy is also popular and effective in treating warts in all areas of the body. Surgical removal, electrosurgical destruction, and laser surgery have their champions. Topical 5-fluorouracil has its advocates, especially for hard-to-treat vaginal and urethral warts. Kling[1] thoroughly reviews the literature dealing with these treatment options. A flurry of recent papers on interferon injection of genital warts indicates that this expensive and repetitive treatment is usually unsuccessful in eradicating warts.

A Practical Treatment Approach

For moist warts on mucous surfaces, either application of podophyllin by the physician, as detailed later in this chapter, or self-treatment with podofilox solution (Condylox) is recommended. For warts on dry (glabrous) skin, such as the shaft of the penis, liquid nitrogen destruction or self-treatment with Condylox should be used. If liquid nitrogen is unavailable or fails, light electrodesiccation or superficial excision with a delicate scissors is a reasonable alternative.

CAUTIONS. Podophyllin and podofilox solutions are teratogens and should not be used in pregnant patients. Only small amounts of podophyllin should be used, because toxic absorption has been documented when large warts are liberally painted with podophyllin. When freezing warts with liquid nitrogen, discard the applicator after each use.

Podofilox solution (Condylox) is applied by the patient twice daily for 3 consecutive days. It is essential to explain this treatment in detail and then demonstrate the technique of application and which lesions are to be treated. Treatment instructions are packaged with each bottle of Condylox, and the manufacturer can provide an excellent illustrated patient instruction sheet. These instructions nicely supplement an actual demonstration on how and where to apply Condylox. Alert your patients that Condylox is expensive.

There are many techniques for using podophyllin. I paint acuminate warts with 20 percent podophyllin tincture (alcoholic solution) on a cotton-tipped applicator. Most cotton-tipped applicators are too bulky; remove about 90 percent of the cotton, and tightly twirl the remainder around the stick. After dipping this slimmed-down applicator into the podophyllin tincture, allow it to dry in the air for 1 minute to thicken the mixture so that it will not run onto normal tissue. Apply a small amount of podophyllin precisely to the wart, and allow at least 3 minutes for thorough drying.

Warn the patient to expect mild to moderate discomfort. Sitz baths in luke-warm water are advised if soreness develops. I also give the patient a sample tube of some nonmedicated lubricant (not a potent corticosteroid) to apply to any sore warts. Although some physicians advise patients to wash the medicine off 6 or 8 hours after application, I have found this measure to be superfluous. There is also little use in applying petrolatum (Vaseline) to the surrounding normal skin prior to podophyllin applications.

If warts respond poorly to 20 percent podophyllin tincture, I switch to a 20 percent salicylic acid–20 percent podophyllin tincture, which must be compounded by a pharmacist. This preparation causes stinging at the time of application and results in whitish discoloration of the treated wart. If warts resist this stronger medication (rare in perianal warts, but not uncommon in genital warts), try liquid nitrogen, superficial scissors excision, or light electrodesiccation.

PERIUNGUAL WARTS

Warts around the nails, or periungual warts, are especially frustrating to the wart therapist. Periungual warts of the posterior nail fold must be treated gently to avoid damage to the nail-forming matrix; otherwise, a permanently deformed nail may result. When periungual warts grow under the nail to become subungual warts, the nail plate becomes a shield against treatment.

I do not know of any satisfactory treatment for periungual warts. The nonder-matologist will do himself a favor by referring these patients to a specialist. If the patient has only one or two periungual warts, I prefer surgical scoop removal, provided the warts are not in the posterior nail fold. Frequently a bit of nail must be cut away to detect and remove subungual wart extensions. About 40 percent of periungual warts treated this way recur, partly because it is difficult to find a precise cleavage plane between the wart and the pulpy fingertip tissue. The blister-ing agent cantharidin is sometimes effective in clearing periungual warts. Multiple treatments are usually needed.

For multiple periungual warts, or those of the posterior nail fold, chemical destruction and/or repeated superficial liquid nitrogen freezing are my treatment choices. These therapies do not produce scars and are often successful, although the many months that may be required for treatment will annoy both the patient and the physician. The patient must not only vigorously scrape away dead wart tissue but also steadily cut the nail away to expose subungual wart extensions to the destructive chemicals.

REFERENCE

1. Kling AR: Genital warts—therapy. *Semin Dermatol* 11:247, 1992

Appendices

Microscopic Examination for Fungus

Microscopic examination of skin scrapings for fungi is essential in dermatologic diagnosis. I do it daily. Fungal eruptions may closely resemble dermatitis. Most dermatologic diagnoses are made on clinical grounds; microscopy of skin scrapings provides objective information. A positive test clinches the diagnosis of fungal infection; a careful negative test makes it unlikely.

Many nondermatologists overdiagnose fungal infection. On the other hand, we all see cases of "stubborn dermatitis" in which the correct diagnosis of fungal infection is made only after the suspicious—or desperate—physician microscopically examines skin scrapings. Microscopy of potassium hydroxide–cleared skin scrapings—called a KOH exam—takes only a few minutes and is simple in principle. Doing it right takes expertise one can acquire only by practice. KOH exams should be performed by a physician or well-trained assistant.

TECHNIQUE

Using a sterile scalpel blade (No. 15 is convenient) moistened with tap water, scrape the edge of the lesion. Having the blade—or the skin—wet with water prevents scales from flying about. Transfer the scales to a slide that holds a small drop of water to prevent tissue loss. If there are blisters—not uncommon in tinea pedis—unroof them with the blade and a pointed forceps and put the blister roof on the slide.

After collecting the tissue, add 1 or 2 drops of 20 percent KOH, put on a coverslip, and warm the slide gently for 15 to 30 seconds to hasten clearing. A wooden kitchen match provides a simple source of heat. The addition of 40 percent dimethylsulfoxide to the KOH solution accelerates clearing.

Examine the specimen using the low-power (10×) objective with *condenser racked down* and the condenser diaphragm partly closed to provide minimum illumination (Figure C–124). The 3- to 5-power scanning objective is not adequate. Lowering the condenser and closing the diaphragm are essential to accentuate the contrast between fungal elements (hyphae) and cellular borders.

While searching the slide, raise and lower the focus. Changing the focus will help you spot hyphae—thin, often branching strands of uniform diameter that lighten when you raise the focus and darken when you lower it. When you've located a suspect element, switch to the high-dry (43×) objective to confirm your finding. This requires raising the condenser and opening its diaphragm (Figure C–125).

In candidiasis there are frequently thin pseudomycelia. It may be difficult to distinguish them from the hyphae in a dermatophyte infection. You can tell if you are looking at *Candida*, however, by the presence of groups of small, round yeast cells that glisten as you adjust the focus. On examination under the high-dry objective, these bodies are uniform in size—unlike oil droplets. Some are budding.

ERRORS

Intercellular lines are the chief cause of error in the microscopy of skin scrapings. They show as thin *single* lines, whereas hyphae are strands with two borders. Hyphae have a smooth continuity, and intercellular lines a sort of zigzag appearance. The distinction is readily made by adjusting up and down with the fine focus while using the high-dry (43×) objective.

Clothing fibers are another artifact. Fibers are irregular in width and often look frayed; hyphae are smooth and spaghetti-like.

DANGER

KOH is caustic to microscopes and tissues. Keep it in a bottle distinctively different from any treatment-room medication bottles. It should be marked **Danger, Poison** and stored out of children's reach. If excess KOH spills over the edge of the slide, carefully wipe it off before placing the slide on the microscope stage.

SPECIAL SITUATIONS

In tinea capitis, skin scrapings are usually negative; one must examine the hair to find the fungi. Look for broken-off hairs; often the broken, infected hairs have a grayish coating. With pointed tweezers, pluck a broken-off hair and examine it microscopically after thorough clearing with KOH. An infected hair will have masses of small refractile bodies—the spores—in or around the hair shaft. The high-dry (43×) objective is needed to delineate the spores. Spores are distinguished from oil droplets and other debris by their uniform small size.

In inflammatory ringworm, especially ringworm acquired from animals (zoophilic fungi), skin scrapings are frequently negative. Search for broken-off hairs, pluck them, and examine them under the microscope.

Inflammation is one mechanism by which skin rids itself of fungi. It's more difficult to demonstrate fungi in an inflamed lesion than in one showing only some scaling and slight erythema, particularly in inflammatory ringworm.

SIGNIFICANCE OF POSITIVE AND NEGATIVE TEST FINDINGS

A reliably performed positive KOH exam establishes the diagnosis of fungal infection. Unfortunately, a negative test doesn't exclude the possibility of fungus disease. Although one can usually demonstrate fungi in noninflamed tinea pedis or tinea cruris, repeated scrapings may be necessary. Furthermore, in the presence of inflammation, even repeated KOH exams are often negative. A negative KOH exam from an inflamed lesion means little. Repeat the microscopic examination in a few weeks, when the inflammation has subsided.

Sources of Products

Acuderm Inc.
5370 NW Terrace
Fort Lauderdale, FL 33309
Telephone 1–800–327–0015
Office and surgical products, especially disposables.

Allerderm Laboratories, Inc.
P.O. Box 2070
Petaluma, CA 94953
Telephone 1–800–365–6868
Protective gloves, patch test materials, and other products useful in management of dermatitis and contact dermatitis.

Arista Surgical Supply Co., Inc.
67 Lexington Ave.
New York, NY 10010
Telephone 1–800–223–1984
Surgical instruments and supplies. *Catalog.*

Bernsco Surgical Supply, Inc.
6653 NE Windermere Road
Seattle, WA 98115
Telephone 1–800–231–8409
Surgical instruments and supplies for dermatologic surgery. *Catalog.*

Delasco Dermatologic Lab and Supply
608 13th Ave.
Council Bluffs, IA 51501
Telephone 1–800–831–6273
An exceedingly useful source for surgical supplies, magnifiers, lights, KOH solution, stains, and many other special items dear to the dermatologist's heart. *Catalog.*

George Tiemann and Company
25 Plant Ave.
Hauppauge, NY 11788
Telephone 1–800–TIEMANN
Extremely wide selection of dermatologic instruments. *Catalog.*

Hermal Pharmaceutical Labs
163 Delaware Ave.
Delmar, NY 12054
Telephone 1–800–HERMAL–1
Patch test materials and kits.

Robbins Instruments, Inc.
2 North Passaic Ave.
Chatham, NJ 07928
Telephone 201–635–8972
Specialized instruments for cutaneous surgery. *Catalog.*

Skin Cancer Foundation
245 Fifth Ave., Suite 2402
New York, NY 10016
Telephone 212–725–5176
Excellent illustrated patient information sheets and brochures on sun protection, skin cancer, nevi, melanoma, and so forth.

Storz Instrument Co.
3365 Tree Court Industrial Blvd.
St. Louis, MO 63122
Telephone 1–800–325–9500
A premier supplier of surgical instruments. Many plastic surgical and ophthalmologic instruments are useful for the dermatologist. *Catalog.*

Illustrations in Color

Where possible, the photographs on the following pages have been grouped to provide visual "mini" case histories. The following is a guide to these "capsule" case histories.

C-1: Erosions in diaper area from topical corticoids.
C-2 and C-3: Hyperkeratosis of heels treated with topical corticoids.
C-4: Subcutaneous atrophy following repository corticoid injection.
C-5 and C-6: Skin thinning from topical corticoids.
C-7 and C-8: Acne abscess.
C-9: Excoriated acne.
C-10 and C-11: Stretching the skin to detect basal cell carcinoma.
C-12 to C-16: Tangential excision of thin basal cell carcinoma.
C-17 and C-18: Extensive basal cell carcinoma.
C-19 to C-21: Treatment of keratoses with topical 5-fluorouracil.
C-22 to C-24: Basal cell carcinoma mimicking dermatitis.
C-25 to C-31: One-step definitive surgery of inflamed cysts.
C-32 to C-34: Excision of giant scalp cysts.
C-35 and C-36: Treatment of hand dermatitis.
C-37 to C-41: Biopsy and liquid nitrogen freezing of dermatofibroma.
C-42: Nevus resembling dermatofibroma.
C-43 to C-45: Treatment of dermatofibroma.
C-46 to C-48: Impetigo.
C-49 and C-50: Herpes simplex.
C-51: Pitted keratolysis.
C-52 to C-54: Treatment of keloid with intralesional corticoid.
C-55 to C-59: Liquid nitrogen destruction of actinic keratoses.
C-60: Intralesional corticoid injection of localized dermatitis.
C-61 and C-62: Shave removal of a nevus.
C-63 and C-64: Malignant melanoma arising from a congenital nevus.
C-65 and C-66: Nodular melanoma and seborrheic keratoses.
C-67 to C-69: Examples of superficial spreading melanomas.
C-70 to C-72: Acral lentiginous melanoma.
C-73: Malignant melanoma arising from a lentigo maligna.
C-74 and C-75: Melanoma arising in compound nevus.
C-76 to C-78: Lentigo maligna.
C-79 and C-80: Pigmented seborrheic keratoses resembling melanoma.
C-81: Multiple atypical nevi.
C-82: Blue nevus.
C-83: Hemangioma resembling a nevus or melanoma.
C-84: Becker's nevus.
C-85 and C-86: Molluscum contagiosum.

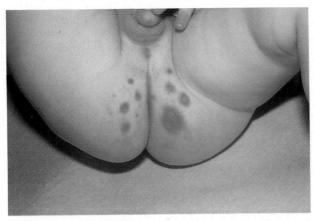

Figure C–1. Erosive diaper dermatitis secondary to the use of triamcinolone acetonide cream to treat mild diaper rash.

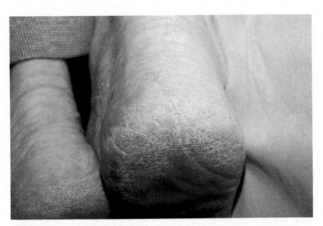

Figure C–2. Painful hyperkeratosis of the heels in a 74-year-old woman—a fairly common problem.

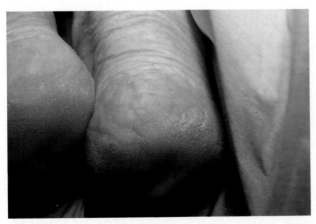

Figure C–3. Smoothing of hyperkeratotic heels after 1 month of twice-daily sparing applications of an ultra-high-potency corticosteroid ointment. The medication's skin-thinning property was put to therapeutic use.

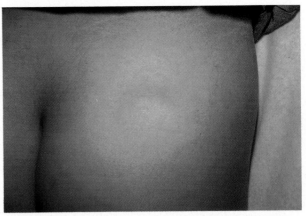

Figure C–4. Subcutaneous atrophy 9 months after injection of repository methylprednisolone for systemic treatment of eczema in a 7-year-old girl. The atrophy completely resolved in another 6 months, as it usually does; when it does not, it has led to malpractice suits. Do not use the shoulder or arm as a site for injecting repository corticosteroids for systemic effect; should atrophy occur in this location, it will be much more noticeable.

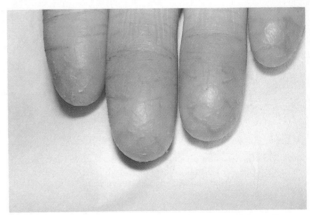

Figure C–5. Tender, fissuring fingertips in an 18-year-old man after treatment of hand psoriasis with a high-potency corticosteroid and occasional overnight occlusion. Note the absence of skin ridges. This condition may be misdiagnosed as dermatitis, rather than being recognized for what it is; an adverse effect of highly potent topical corticoids.

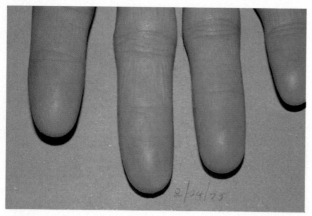

Figure C–6. The same hand 4 months after the patient was switched to 2.5 percent hydrocortisone ointment used with occlusion. The psoriasis is controlled, and skin ridges have returned.

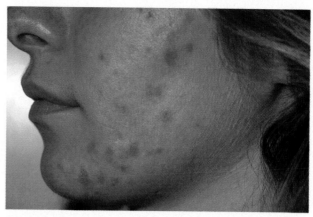

Figure C–9. Severely excoriated acne in a young woman. The lesions are mainly the result of her picking. Behavior modification is just as important as medication in suppressing such patients' acne.

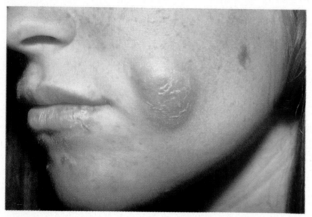

Figure C–7. Large acne abscess in a 19-year-old woman, which was injected with triamcinolone acetonide suspension, 2 mg/ml. To suppress new lesions, oral tetracycline was prescribed. The abscess was injected a second time 3 weeks later.

Figure C–10. Ill-defined depression on the forehead of a fair-skinned man.

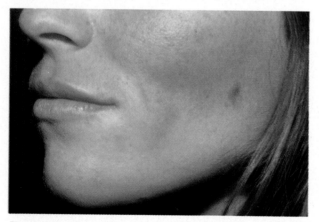

Figure C–8. Five weeks later, resolution is nearly complete without scarring. Incision and drainage, which leave a scar, are best reserved as a last resort for acne abscesses that don't respond to intralesional repository corticosteroids.

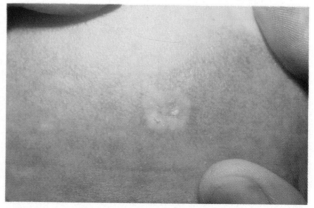

Figure C–11. Close-up view of the same lesion, after the skin has been stretched to help delineate the margins, reveals this lesion to be an infiltrating basal cell carcinoma. Stretching the skin is a useful technique in examining skin tumors.

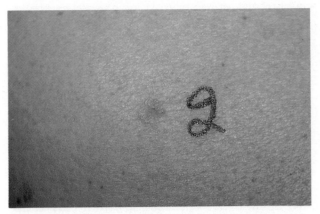

Figure C–12. A 5-mm, superficial basal cell carcinoma of the upper back. The sharply demarcated, infiltrated border suggests the diagnosis.

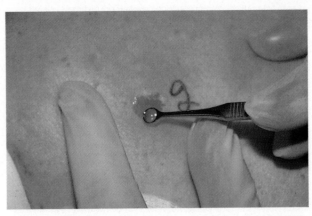

Figure C–15. The edges of the excision are lightly beveled with a curette. Hemostasis is achieved by packing with gelatin foam, a tissue neutral hemostatic.

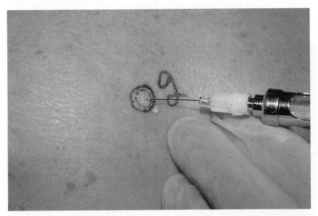

Figure C–13. The margin of the tumor has been outlined with green ink, and a black circle 1.5 mm beyond this indicates the limits for excision. Local anesthetic is injected very superficially to raise up the lesion.

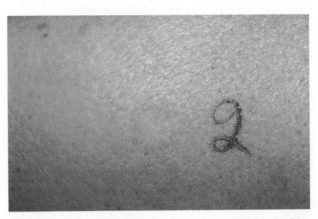

Figure C–16. The wound has healed to leave a slightly atrophic, hypopigmented, flat scar.

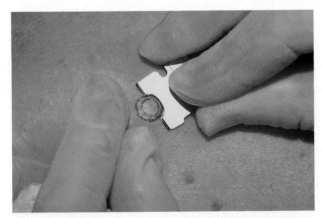

Figure C–14. Using a straight razor blade cut in half, the lesion is precisely sliced off along the black line. Note the left hand stretches the skin.

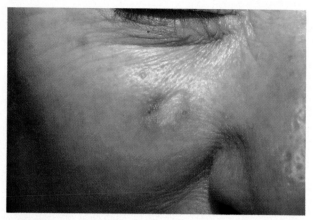

Figure C–17. Biopsy of a nondescript scaling area surrounding an atrophic plaque revealed infiltrating basal cell carcinoma. The histology and the indistinct clinical margins were indications for referral for Mohs micrographic surgery.

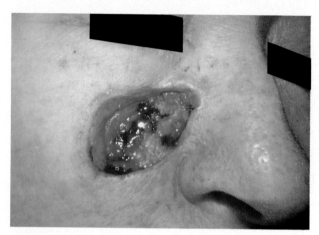

Figure C–18. The extent of the defect after all strands of infiltrating basal cell carcinoma have been traced out and removed. The lesion extended widely into clinically normal skin. Fortunately, this is uncommon, but it illustrates how tricky and dangerous basal cell carcinomas occasionally can be.

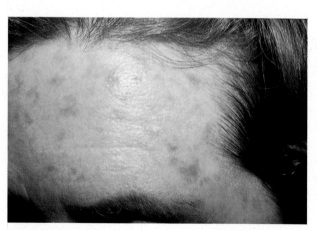

Figure C–19. Multiple actinic keratoses on the forehead of a 52-year-old woman.

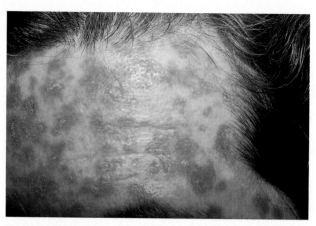

Figure C–20. Erosions after 17 days of twice-daily applications of 5 percent fluorouracil cream. Treatment was continued for 4 more days.

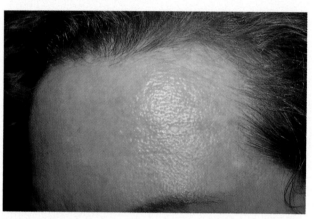

Figure C–21. Seventeen months later, the patient's forehead remains clear.

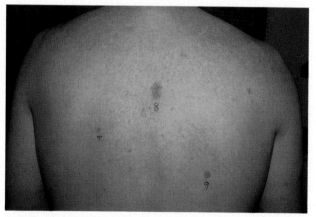

Figure C–22. Multiple superficial basal cell carcinomas on the back of a 33-year-old man. The back is a typical location for this type of tumor.

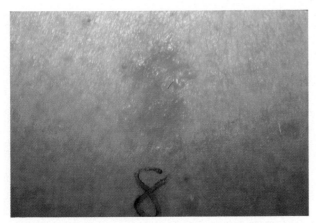

Figure C–23. Close-up view of the largest lesion reveals the infiltrated, pearly border that indicates a neoplastic rather than an inflammatory process.

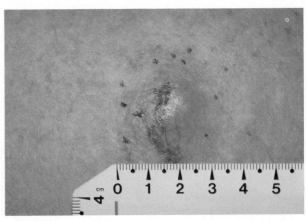

Figure C–26. Close-up view following infiltration of lidocaine around the entire cyst. The cyst borders had been marked with dots of green ink, and the proposed margin of incision is marked with a line.

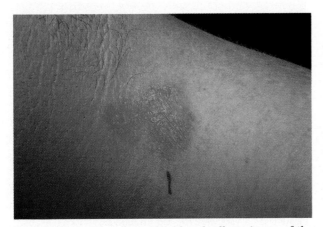

Figure C–24. A 30-mm, superficial basal cell carcinoma of the neck in the same patient. The uncanny resemblance to a dermatitis had led two physicians to diagnose these spots as a rash.

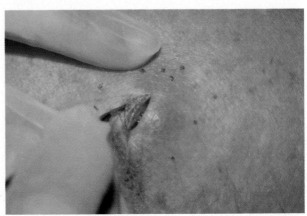

Figure C–27. A thin ellipse of overlying skin is excised with a No. 11 blade.

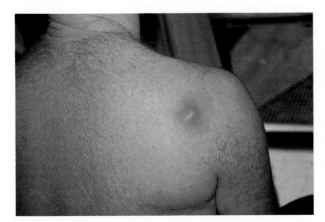

Figure C–25. Inflamed cyst on the shoulder of a 47-year-old man.

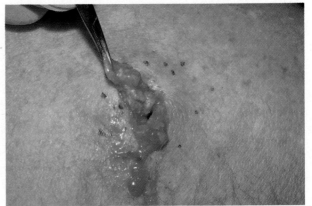

Figure C–28. The cyst wall and necrotic material are tugged out of the wound with a hemostat. A chalazion curette was also used to scoop out the cyst contents.

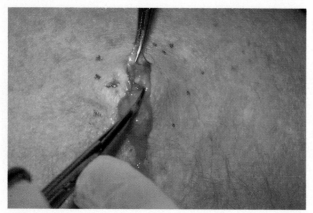

Figure C-29. Cyst wall remnants are removed and dissected away from fat with a hemostat and scissors.

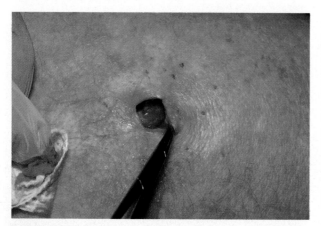

Figure C-30. The cavity is carefully inspected to ensure that all cyst remnants have been removed. A bulky dressing is applied, and the wound is allowed to heal by secondary intention.

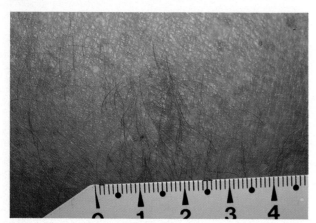

Figure C-31. Four months later, a barely noticeable scar marks the site of the cyst removal.

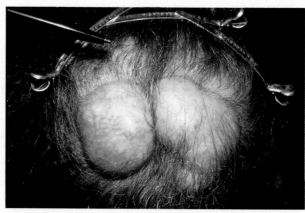

Figure C-32. Two large cysts on the scalp of a 70-year-old woman (pen shows relative size). Clips keep hair out of the surgical field; the scalp was not shaved.

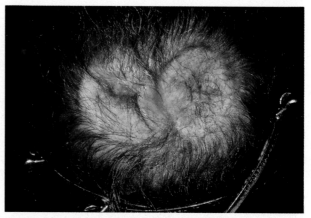

Figure C-33. Cysts were excised through small incisions, using the technique described in the text. Each incision was closed with four interrupted sutures of 5-0 plain gut.

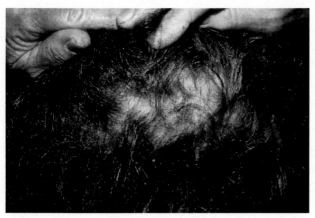

Figure C–34. Same patient's scalp 1.5 years later. The redundant cyst wall tissue has shrunk to the scalp contours, and the surgical sites are not discernible.

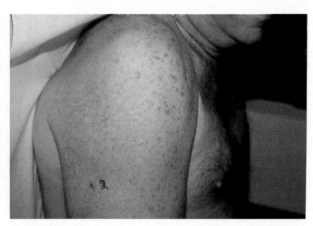

Figure C–37. An 8-mm, enlarging papule of the right upper arm in a 51-year-old man.

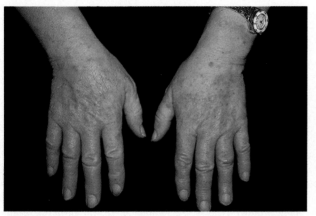

Figure C–35. Housewife's hand dermatitis in a 60-year-old woman who had been doing housework without wearing protective gloves. She had tried a number of over-the-counter remedies.

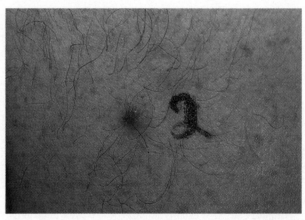

Figure C–38. Although clinically this suggests a dermatofibroma, other possibilities include nevus and melanoma. After a 1.5-mm punch biopsy, the lesion was frozen with liquid nitrogen. Biopsy confirmed the clinical diagnosis of dermatofibroma.

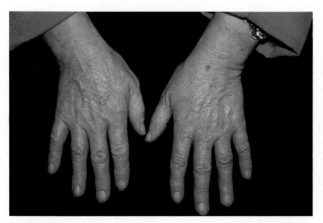

Figure C–36. Improvement following 2 weeks of frequent use of a medicated hand lubricant containing hydrocortisone, wearing protective gloves for housework, and stopping her over-the-counter remedies. Most patients with nonspecific hand dermatitis respond nicely to a regimen of hand protection, lubrication, and a mild topical corticosteroid.

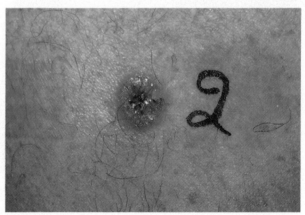

Figure C–39. Healing blister at 5 days. Deep freezing is required for treatment of a dermatofibroma.

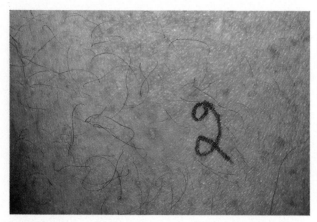

Figure C–40. Four weeks later, the lesion is flat. The punch biopsy site is visible.

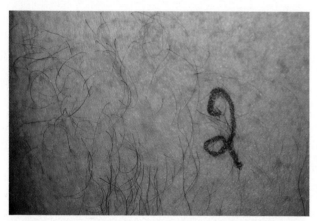

Figure C–41. The treated site 4 years later. Thorough freezing with liquid nitrogen usually produces permanent flattening of these lesions.

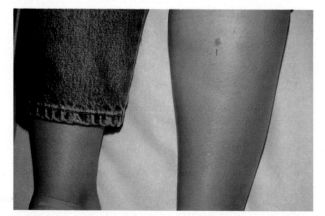

Figure C–42. A 6-mm lesion on the calf of a 20-year-old woman. The calf is a typical site for a dermatofibroma; however, punch biopsy proved it to be a spindle-cell nevus. This is why I prefer to biopsy dermatofibromas just before freezing them with liquid nitrogen.

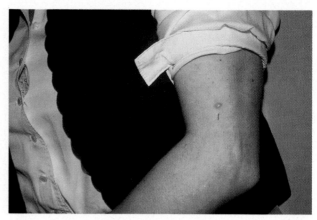

Figure C–43. A 7-mm firm papule that had been present longer than 1 year on the upper arm of a 43-year-old woman.

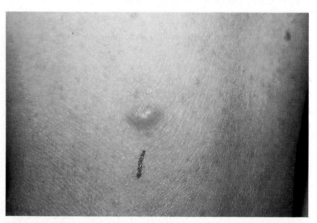

Figure C–44. Close-up view of the same papule shows a smooth, dome-shaped, reddish lesion suggestive of a dermatofibroma. Full-thickness excision in this area often causes an unsightly scar. The patient was treated with deep liquid nitrogen freezing after a 2-mm punch biopsy.

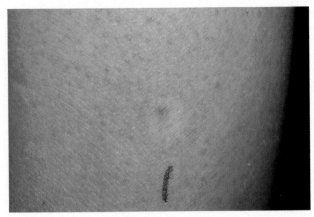

Figure C–45. A flat, hypopigmented, hardly noticeable spot is the result of this fast, simple treatment, which combines the reassurance of a histologic diagnosis with generally satisfactory cosmetic results. Regrowth is rare; this photograph was taken 8 years after treatment.

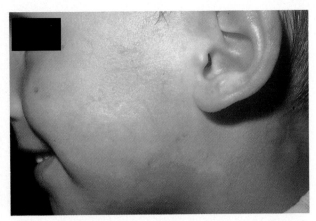

Figure C–48. Three days of oral dicloxacillin produced almost complete clearing. Impetigo is a superficial process that responds rapidly to antibiotics that are effective against both staphylococci and streptococci.

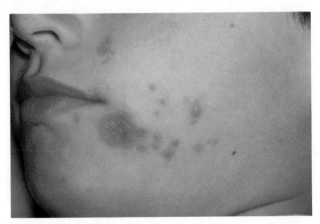

Figure C–46. Impetigo of the face in a child. An unusual number of intact blisters are evident. These blisters are superficial and will soon rupture, leaving crusted patches, often with telltale borders. Localized impetigo such as this responds well to frequent applications of mupirocin ointment.

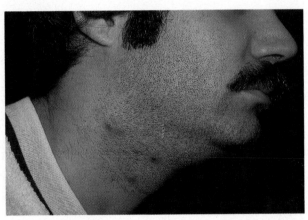

Figure C–49. Lesion on a young man's neck at first glance appeared to be pyoderma of the beard area—a common problem.

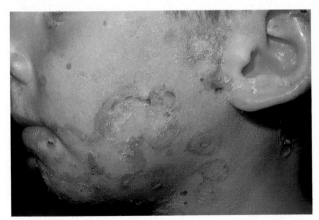

Figure C–47. Florid impetigo, as in this 5-year-old boy, is an indication for systemic antibiotics.

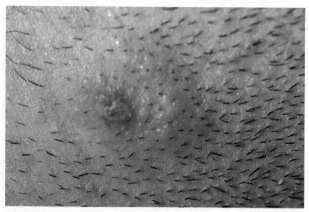

Figure C-50. Close-up view of the same lesion shows the typical picture of herpes simplex with grouped blisters on an erythematous, edematous base. The patient's girlfriend had facial herpes simplex.

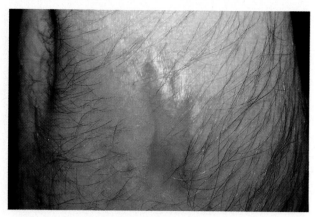

Figure C-53. Moderate flattening 2 months after intralesional injection of 1 ml of triamcinolone acetonide, 10 mg/ml, given in six injections.

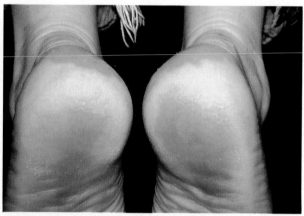

Figure C-51. Pitted keratolysis secondary to hyperhidrosis of the feet. White, macerated tissue and punched-out, superficial erosions are typical of this condition.

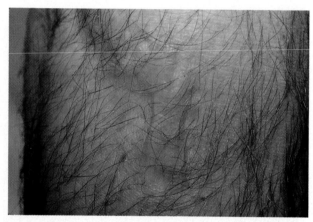

Figure C-54. One year after a second injection of triamcinolone acetonide suspension—an unusually good result from only two treatments.

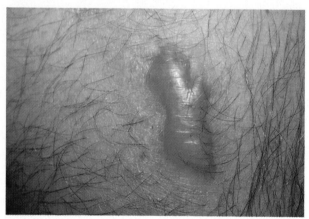

Figure C-52. A 30- by 12-mm keloid of the forearm present for more than 1 year in a 26-year-old man. It followed a burn.

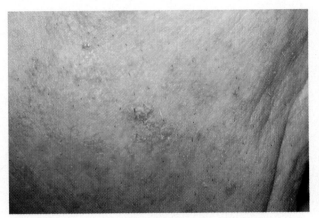

Figure C–55. An 11-mm actinic keratosis on the cheek of a 74-year-old man.

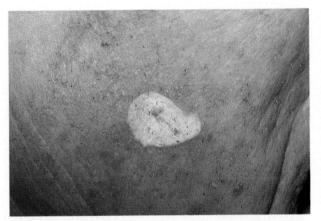

Figure C–56. The freezing front should extend just beyond the border of the lesion. Liquid nitrogen freezing highlights the margin between normal skin and the keratosis.

Figure C–57. Lasting clearing of the lesion 2 years later. Slight atrophy and hypopigmentation are usual after treatment of actinic keratoses.

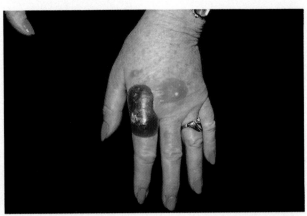

Figure C–58. Liquid nitrogen treatment of actinic keratoses on the loose skin of the dorsa of the hands tends to produce huge, sometimes hemorrhagic blisters.

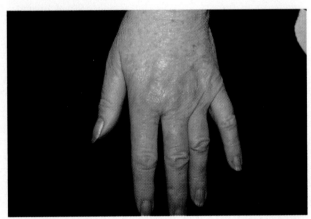

Figure C–59. Fortunately, healing is usually uneventful, without scarring. Draining the blisters with a sterile needle is painless and appreciated by the patient.

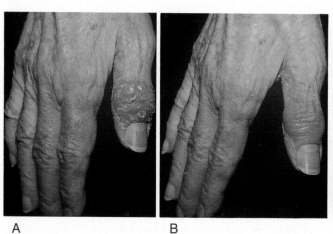

A   B

Figure C–60. *(A)* Psoriasiform dermatitis of the thumb present for 1 year that had failed to respond to self-treatment. A diagnosis of Bowen's disease (intraepidermal squamous cell carcinoma) or other malignancy was considered, but dermatitis seemed most likely because the patient had dermatitis elsewhere. *(B)* Six days after injection of 0.7 ml of triamcinolone acetonide suspension, 10 mg/ml, into the plaque through multiple injections. The patient was told to apply only petrolatum. Intralesional repository corticosteroids are an ideal treatment for localized, chronic, infiltrated dermatoses. If this patient had not responded to the intralesional steroid, I would have biopsied the lesion to rule out a malignancy.

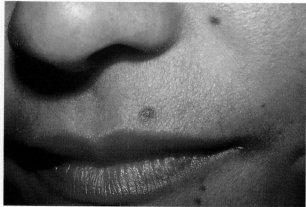

Figure C–62. After shave removal, the nevus is flat and less noticeable. Shave removal provided a specimen for microscopy, which confirmed the clinical diagnosis of a benign compound nevus.

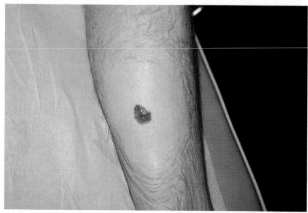

Figure C–63. Malignant melanoma of the leg arising in a congenital nevus in a 32-year-old man.

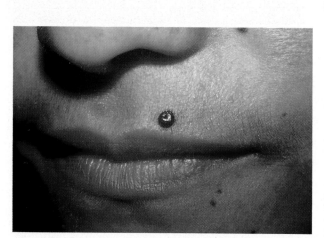

Figure C–61. Prominent, dark, benign-appearing nevus that worried the patient, a 21-year-old woman.

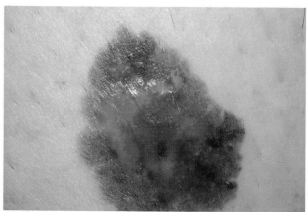

Figure C–64. Close-up view shows all the hallmarks of a melanoma: asymmetry, irregular border, and marked color variation, including reddish and purple shades.

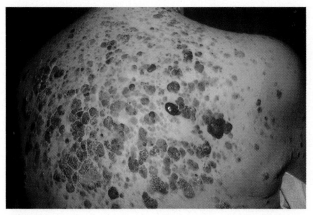

Figure C–65. An 18-mm malignant melanoma on the back of a 75-year-old woman with multiple seborrheic keratoses. The many benign keratoses camouflaged the early stages of the melanoma.

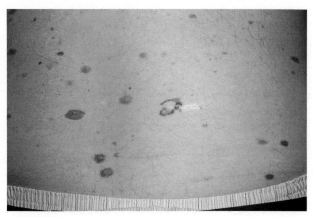

Figure C–68. A 22-mm superficial spreading malignant melanoma adjacent to an old scar on the lower back of a 62-year-old man. Other large, unusual-appearing nevi are also present.

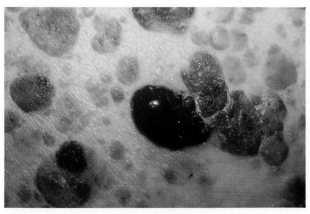

Figure C–66. Close-up view of the same melanoma. Excisional biopsy showed it to be 6.1 mm deep. The poor prognosis of deep melanomas was borne out by the patient's death from this malignancy 15 months later.

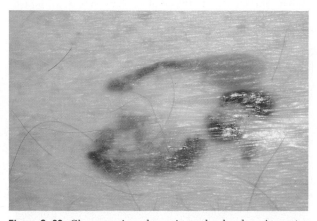

Figure C–69. Close-up view shows irregular border pigmentation, variation in color, and asymmetry. The central whitish area is the result of spontaneous regression of portions of the melanoma. The white area next to the melanoma is an old scar.

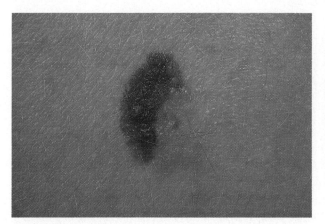

Figure C–67. Superficial spreading melanoma—the pigmented area at left—arising from a long-standing fleshy nevus of the back. The variation in color, irregular outline with notching in the lower portion, and recent color change made the lesion suspect and led to excisional biopsy.

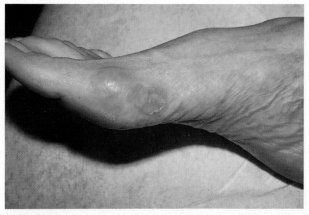

Figure C–70. This nondescript but persistent 16-mm scaling patch on the side of the foot is a superficial spreading melanoma.

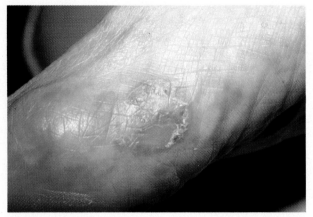

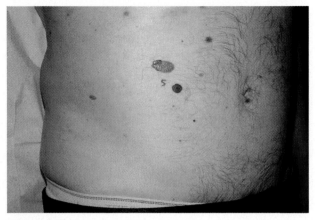

Figure C–71. Even a close-up view does not suggest the diagnosis. After negative KOH microscopy ruled out fungus infection, I prescribed a topical corticosteroid believing this was either dermatitis or Bowen's disease. After 3 weeks of this regimen failed to clear the lesion, I took two small punch biopsies. Wide excision and grafting by a plastic surgeon was followed by uneventful healing.

Figure C–74. Melanoma in situ arising in a long-standing compound nevus in a 64-year-old man.

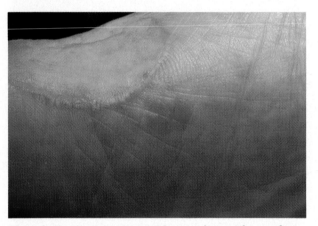

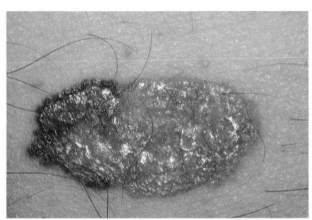

Figure C–72. However, 3 years later, a brownish macule appeared at one border. Biopsy demonstrated superficial spreading melanoma, which led to further surgery and grafting.

Figure C–75. Close-up view shows irregular pigmentation as well as border irregularity, which are clinically suspicious of a melanoma.

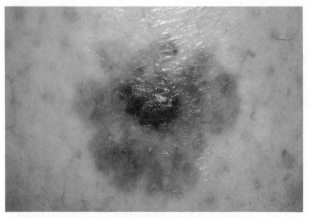

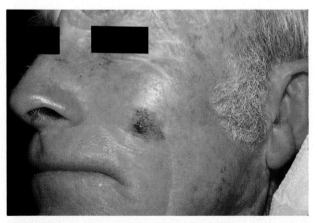

Figure C–73. Nodular malignant melanoma arising from a lentigo maligna. Note the irregular, notched border of the brownish lentigo maligna.

Figure C–76. Typical lentigo maligna (melanoma in situ) in a 73-year-old man.

Figure C–77. Close-up view shows an irregular, darkly pigmented network superimposed on the uniform, light-brown surface of a lentigo.

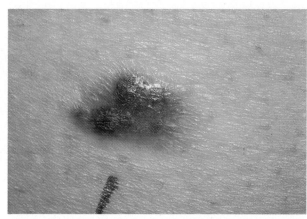

Figure C–80. The irregular pigmentation, irregular border, and asymmetry led to its excision as a probable melanoma. However, the dermatopathologist's diagnosis was inflamed seborrheic keratosis.

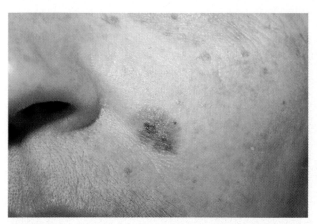

Figure C–78. Early lentigo maligna (melanoma in situ) in a 65-year-old woman. Distinguishing this malignancy from the common solar lentigo can be difficult. The two dark areas are a clue; solar lentigines usually have uniform pigmentation.

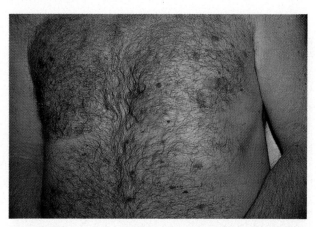

Figure C–81. Assessing changes when there are multiple atypical nevi can be a formidable task, as illustrated by this case in a 63-year-old man, whose copious body hair adds an additional impediment. His wife noted a change in a lesion on his left chest, below and medial to the nipple. She circled it with a red marker, an excellent technique. It turned out to be a hemangioma.

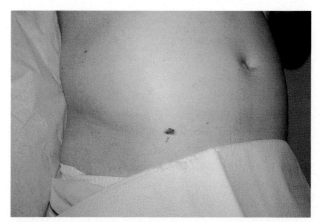

Figure C–79. Ominous-appearing, 13-mm lesion on the abdominal skin of a 64-year-old man.

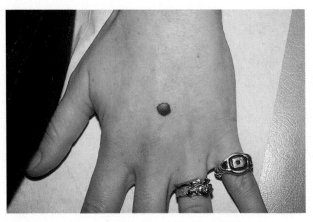

Figure C–82. Blue nevus on hand of a 26-year-old woman. Although the growth is benign, its ominously dark color is the result of pigment deep in the dermis. Clinically, a blue nevus may be indistinguishable from a nodular melanoma.

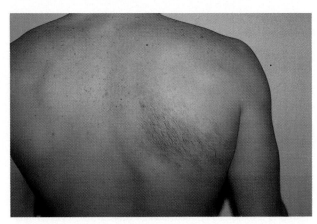

Figure C–84. The pigmented, hairy patch on the right mid-back of this 24-year-old man is known as Becker's nevus. This benign lesion is not composed of nevus cells; it results from hyperpigmentation accompanied by hair follicle hyperplasia. Rarely, there may be associated abnormalities of deeper connective tissue or muscle.

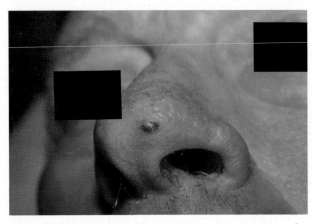

Figure C–83. Hemangiomas may resemble blue nevi or melanomas with their dark, bluish black color. Prolonged digital pressure sometimes—but not always—results in diagnostic blanching. At times, a superficial needle prick, with resulting gush of blood correctly identifies the lesion. If any diagnostic uncertainty remains, a small punch biopsy will settle the issue.

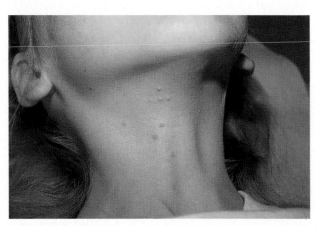

Figure C–85. Firm, waxy lesions of molluscum contagiosum on the neck of an 11-year-old girl. Close inspection reveals the diagnostic dell, or central umbilication.

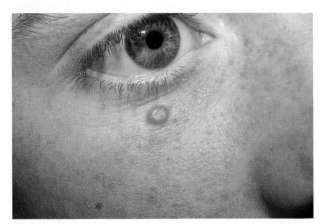

Figure C–86. Solitary molluscum contagiosum in a 19-year-old man. The flattened central indentation suggests the correct diagnosis.

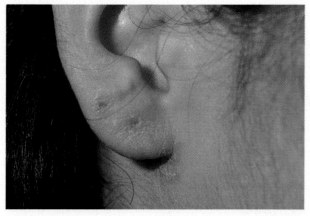

Figure C–87. Ear lobe dermatitis due to nickel allergy in a 23-year-old woman. Seborrheic dermatitis is another possible diagnosis.

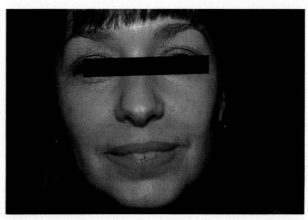

Figure C–90. Improvement following 1 month of tetracycline, 1 g daily, and stopping all corticosteroids. Three more months of tetracycline, in a gradually decreasing dose, were required to achieve complete clearing.

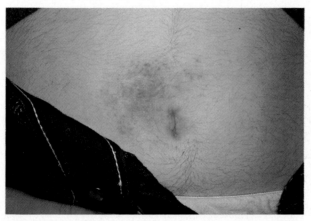

Figure C–88. Dermatitis on the same patient's abdomen corresponding to contact with the metal snaps of her jeans—a finding that strengthens the case for nickel allergy. A positive patch test later proved the diagnosis.

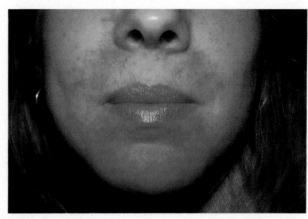

Figure C–91. Another example of the clinical appearance of perioral dermatitis.

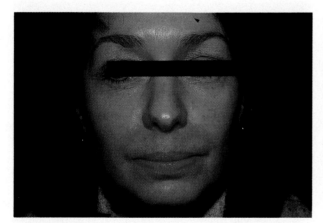

Figure C–89. Classic perioral dermatitis with papules and erythematous areas in a 42-year-old woman. The patient had been treated over 5 months with four different topical corticosteroids.

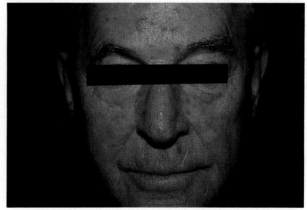

Figure C–92. Extensive rosacea in a 74-year-old man.

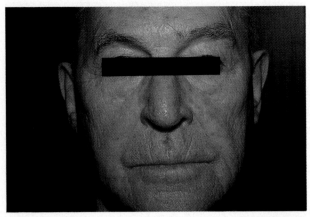

Figure C-93. Improvement is seen following 3 weeks of tetracycline, 1 g daily. The papulopustules of rosacea usually respond promptly to tetracycline. The erythema responds more slowly and not as completely.

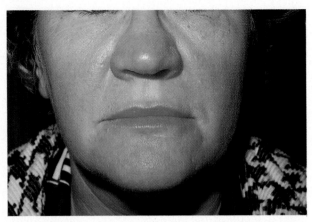

Figure C-96. The increased dose of tetracycline led to complete clearing 2 months later. It's possible that simply continuing 1 g of tetracycline a day for a longer time would have achieved the same result.

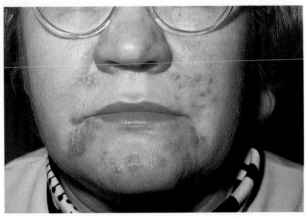

Figure C-94. Rosacea in a primarily perioral distribution in a 45-year-old woman.

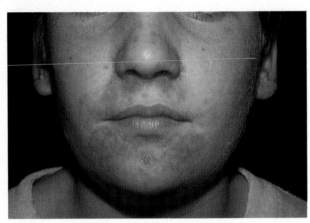

Figure C-97. Steroid rosacea resulting from more than 6 months of application of a potent corticosteroid to a minor facial rash in a 10-year-old boy.

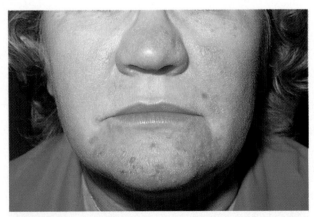

Figure C-95. Significant but unsatisfactory improvement after 24 days of tetracycline, 1 g daily. The tetracycline dose was increased to 1.5 g daily.

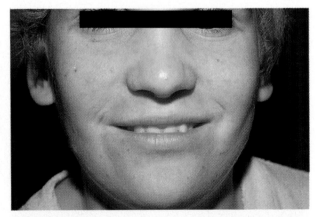

Figure C-98. Improvement following 25 days of treatment with erythromycin, 1 g daily. Because of the patient's age, erythromycin rather than tetracycline was employed. It took another 2 months of systemic erythromycin to completely heal the skin.

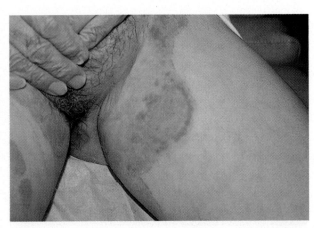

Figure C–99. Rosacea primarily affecting the nose, with swelling, pustules, and erythema. It has already led to rhinophyma. Tetracycline was prescribed and proved to be dramatically effective.

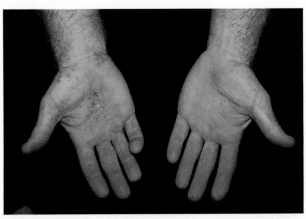

Figure C–102. Extensive tinea cruris in a 66-year-old man. Other skin sites are also involved. Note the patches of tinea corporis on the right thigh. Such widespread infections are best treated with systemic antifungal agents.

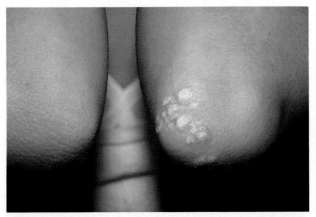

Figure C–100. Hyperkeratotic psoriasis of the left elbow in a 14-year-old girl.

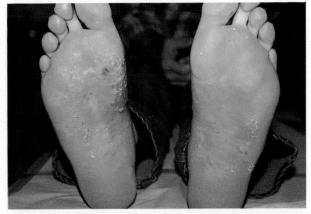

Figure C–103. Psoriasis of the palms in a 37-year-old man. Vesicles and pustules suggest an eczematous process, which has been called eczematous psoriasis.

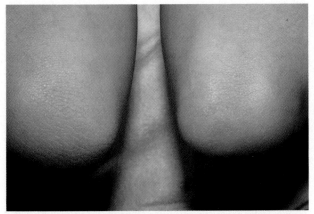

Figure C–101. Eighteen days after intralesional injection of a total of 0.7 ml of triamcinolone acetonide suspension, 10 mg/ml. Intralesional repository corticosteroids are an excellent treatment if the patient has only a few patches of psoriasis.

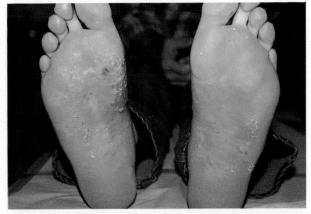

Figure C–104. The same patient's feet show a similar process. However, microscopic examination of KOH-cleared scrapings showed hyphae. The patient had both psoriasis and tinea pedis and required treatment directed at both disorders.

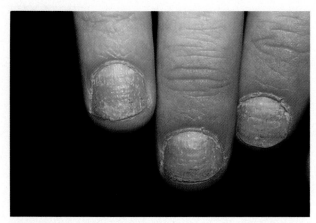

Figure C–105. A 17-year-old boy had pitting and ridging of all 10 fingernails. This is the classic picture of psoriatic nails; the patient denied other skin problems.

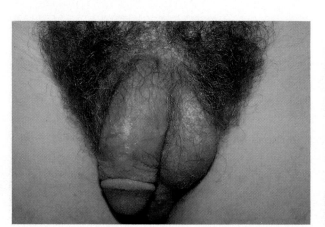

Figure C–106. Complete examination of the same patient's skin confirmed he had psoriasis of the skin restricted to the penis and scrotum.

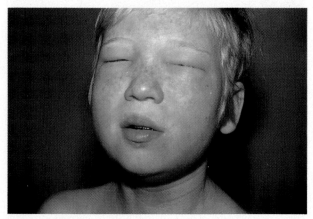

Figure C–107. The early edematous stage of severe poison oak contact dermatitis is rapidly reversible with high doses of systemic corticosteroids.

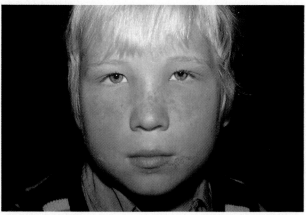

Figure C–108. The same patient 24 hours after administration of 100 mg of prednisone twice daily. This dose was rapidly tapered off over the next 9 days. While most patients with acute *Rhus* contact dermatitis will respond to initial doses of 60 to 80 mg of prednisone a day, severe cases require a few days of significantly higher doses.

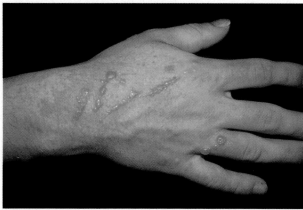

Figure C–109. Streaks and blisters typical of *Rhus* contact dermatitis.

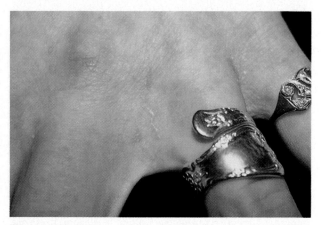

Figure C–110. Look at the finger webs and wrists for the diagnostic burrow of scabies. The rash of the trunk is a nonspecific hypersensitivity response.

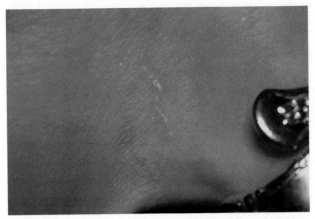

Figure C–111. Close-up view of a burrow. Note the uniformly slightly scaling surface. This uniformity and the wavy shape help to distinguish burrows from scratch marks.

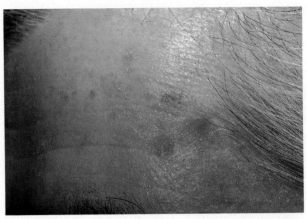

Figure C–114. Superficial curettage of the keratoses left these wounds, which were then packed with gelatin foam. Histology confirmed the clinical diagnosis.

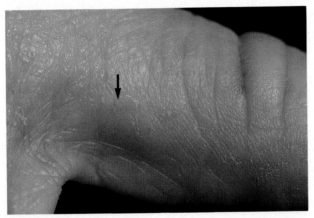

Figure C–112. Several burrows on the side of a patient's thumb. The brownish dot at the end of the unusually long burrow is the mite *(arrow).*

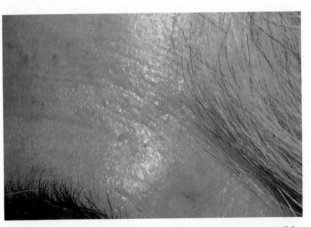

Figure C–115. Six weeks later, the treated sites are invisible. Superficial removal combined with nondestructive hemostasis produces far better cosmetic results than destructive hemostatic techniques such as Monsel's solution, aluminum chloride, or electrocautery.

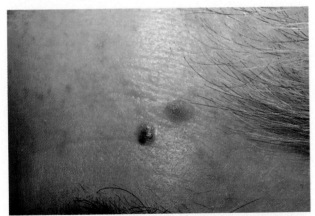

Figure C–113. Two seborrheic keratoses on the forehead of a 72-year-old woman. The lower, darker lesion could be a pigmented basal cell carcinoma or a melanoma.

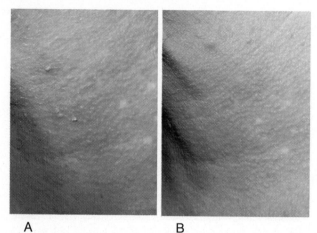

A   B

Figure C–116. *(A)* The scars on the neck of this 65-year-old woman from electrodesiccation of skin tags. Her current crop of five skin tags has just been frozen; hence, the redness surrounding them. These benign growths could be called either skin tags or pedunculated seborrheic keratoses. *(B)* Fifteen months later, the liquid nitrogen–treated growths have healed without a trace. Skin tags can be removed without detectable scarring by either freezing with liquid nitrogen or clipping them at the base with sharp scissors.

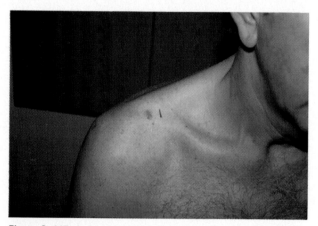

Figure C–117. A large, 17- by 11-mm basal cell carcinoma on the right shoulder of a 60-year-old man.

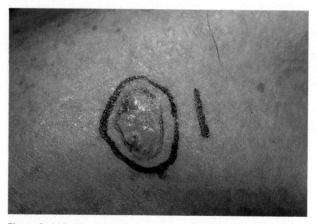

Figure C–118. The tumor is outlined in green ink. The margin of the intended disc excision is marked in black ink.

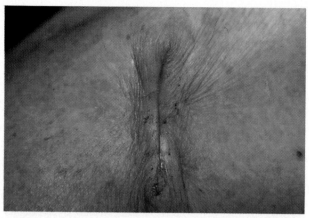

Figure C–119. Following excision, wide undermining and closure of the wound with four buried vertical mattress sutures of 2-0 polydioxanone. Significant dog-earing is evident at this point. Dog-ears were not excised.

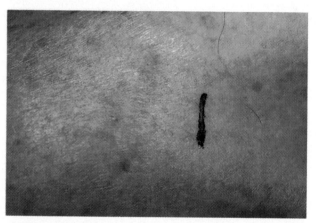

Figure C–120. Fifteen months later, the scar has shown the expected spreading but is flat, inconspicuous, and without crosshatch marks.

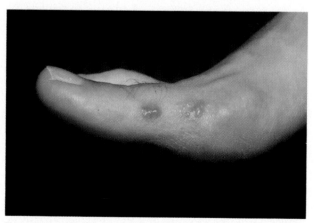

Figure C–121. Tinea pedis may cause blistering on the soles or sides of the feet, as in this middle-aged patient.

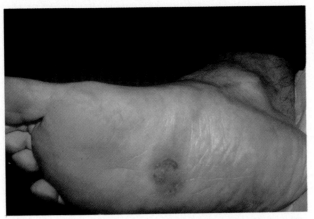

Figure C–122. Tinea pedis on the sole of a 47-year-old man. The pinkish streak of lymphadenitis extending medially is a sign of bacterial infection, which should be treated with antibiotics.

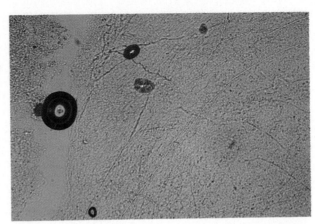

Figure C–125. High-power view of the same field shows typical hyphae with distinct walls. For KOH examination, the condenser must be racked down and the diaphragm partly closed to provide the oblique lighting required for maximum contrast.

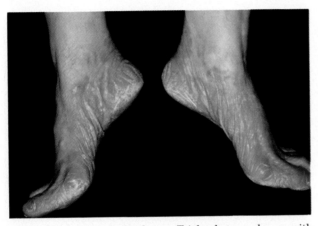

Figure C–123. Tinea pedis due to *Trichophyton rubrum,* with typical chronic, dry, hyperkeratotic skin and scaling patches. The extension onto the sides of this patient's feet makes it clear that the problem is not just dry skin. Psoriasis of the feet may mimic this presentation.

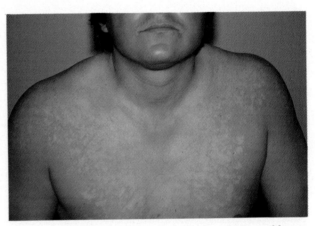

Figure C–126. Extensive tinea versicolor in a 34-year-old man. It sometimes is difficult to determine which is the patient's normal skin color; in this case, the hypopigmented areas are the ones affected by disease.

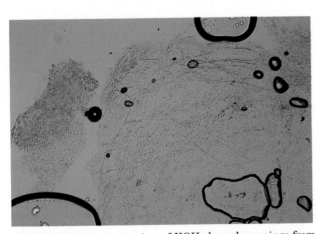

Figure C–124. Low-power view of KOH-cleared scrapings from the patient in Figure C–88 shows threadlike formations among debris, bubbles, and other artifacts.

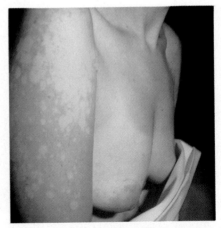

Figure C–127. This woman was diagnosed as having vitiligo by a physician who examined only her arms and didn't see the lesions on the untanned skin of her breast.

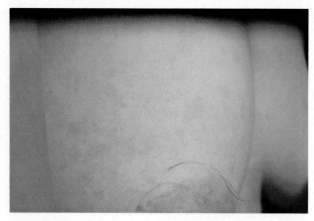

Figure C–128. Close-up view of the breast shows the scaly, light-tan patches of tinea versicolor that occur on skin shielded from the sun. Selenium sulfide cleared both arm and breast.

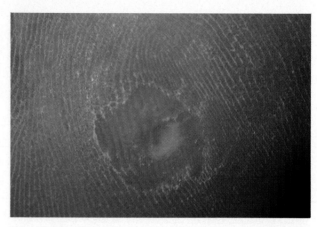

Figure C–131. Close-up view after the overlying keratosis was peeled away shows a corn over the scar produced by electro-desiccation. To prevent such permanent sequelae, I approach plantar warts gently, avoid surgery, and never electrodesiccate.

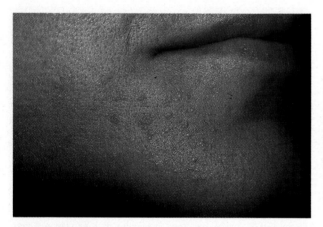

Figure C–129. Flat warts on the chin of an 18-year-old woman. These sometimes aren't recognized; this patient was told she had acne. Gentle peeling agents will avoid scarring and usually heal flat warts over a period of time.

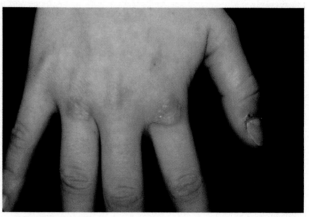

Figure C–132. Scars on a young woman's hand resulted from vigorous electrodesiccation of warts. Not only does the patient have unsightly scars, but warts remain at their peripheries.

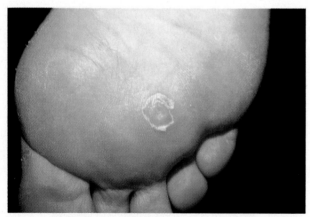

Figure C–130. Lesion on the plantar area was treated for longer than 20 years as a supposed plantar wart after it had been "destroyed with an electric needle."

Index

Note: Page numbers in *italics* refer to illustrations. Page numbers followed by t refer to tables.

Patient Instruction Sheets

P A R T

Patient Instruction Sheets

Contents

Acne

Acne is the term for the pimples and complexion problems that trouble many young people. Pimples occur mainly on the face, but often involve the neck, chest, back, and upper arms. Acne is only a skin problem and has nothing to do with your general health.

What Causes Acne?

Acne is caused by the oil glands of the skin breaking open. At puberty, the oil glands in the skin start producing an oily material called sebum. Sebum is discharged onto the skin's surface. Sometimes the wall of the oil gland breaks and spills the sebum within the skin. The sebum irritates the skin tissues and causes redness, swelling, and pus—in other words, a pimple.

Plugged oil glands may form blackheads and whiteheads. Blackheads are not caused by dirt. Removing blackheads will *not* prevent pimples. Try to ignore blackheads and whiteheads; they are small nuisances.

In mild acne, only a few oil glands break open; in severe acne, many do. How easily oil glands do this seems to be "built into" you. Acne runs in families. It's impossible to prevent acne, since there's no way of changing your oil glands.

Age and Acne

Acne usually begins in a mild form in the teens, gradually worsens, and then, after a time, improves. How long you will have acne is impossible to predict. Acne gets worse and improves by itself. There is usually no explanation for these ups and downs. Don't assume that because your acne gets worse you have done something wrong. And, if your acne gets better briefly, it may not have happened because of treatment. In women, acne frequently worsens about the time of their menstrual period.

Skin Hygiene

Dirt does *not* cause acne, despite what you may have been told. The oil on the skin's surface does no harm. Special soaps, astringents, abradants, and acne cleansers are a waste of money. Wash your face with ordinary soap and water only as much as you need to keep it clean. Too much washing and scrubbing can cause skin irritation. Cleanliness may be next to godliness, but it doesn't help acne.

Do not pick, squeeze, or otherwise manipulate your pimples, as it can leave scars.

Diet and Acne

Foods do *not* cause acne. Many persons try all sorts of diets and are frustrated because they don't help. In some people, certain foods do make acne worse. The most common foods are chocolate, nuts, cola drinks, and root beer. A few people who drink large quantities of milk (more than 1 quart per day) find that this worsens their acne.

Aggravation of acne by food varies from person to person. Many acne patients can eat chocolate without trouble, while others find that even a few pieces of chocolate cause new pimples. Find out for yourself if the foods previously mentioned aggravate your acne. Eliminate one food from your diet for 1 month and then test its effect by eating a large amount. If your skin improves when you stop eating a food and gets worse when you eat it, repeat the test. Acne has ups and downs of its own; make sure that the worsening is not just a coincidence. If certain foods worsen your acne, avoid them.

Nerves and Acne

Acne is not caused by nerves and worry, but may become worse under stress such as examinations or pressure at work. These are usually mild, temporary flare-ups. Some persons react to stress by picking, squeezing, or rubbing their pimples, and this can make their acne worse.

Treatment

Unfortunately, there is no medical cure for acne, *although it can be controlled until you outgrow it*. This often takes years; therefore, treatment may require many months or years.

Antibiotics are currently the best medicines for controlling acne. They may be taken by mouth or applied to the skin. If you have mild acne, antibiotics applied to the skin may control it. In persons with moderate or severe acne, antibiotics taken by mouth are usually needed. Antibiotics control acne only while they are being used and for a few weeks afterward. We do not know how antibiotics work in acne, or why they sometimes do not work.

Antibiotics do not remove blackheads and whiteheads. Retin-A (generic name: tretinoin; a prescription item) applied to the skin will gradually remove blackheads. Benzoyl peroxide, found in both prescription and over-the-counter acne remedies, also reduces the number of blackheads. Retin-A and benzoyl peroxide irritate the skin. They must be used carefully, and should *never* be used together. If you have only a few blackheads, you can safely ignore them. It is all right to hide blackheads with a little water-based makeup.

Accutane (generic name: isotretinoin) is a medicine taken by mouth that controls acne by reducing the activity of the oil glands of the skin. Accutane's effect usually lasts for 1 year or more after the medicine is stopped. Unfortunately, Accutane has many adverse effects and, if taken during pregnancy, causes severe birth defects. Patients taking Accutane must have periodic blood tests and checkups. We reserve Accutane for acne that has not responded to antibiotics.

Antibiotics Applied to the Skin

Antibiotics applied to acne skin are usually clear liquids, often in convenient "dab-on" applicator bottles. The liquid evaporates to leave an invisible film of antibiotic on the skin. It's important to leave this antibiotic film on for several hours; apply the medicine in the morning *after* washing or shaving and at bedtime. If you use makeup, apply the antibiotic first, then put the makeup over it. The antibiotic should be applied to the entire skin area involved with acne—don't just put it on a few pimples. Antibiotic solutions agree with most persons' skin, but some find them too drying. If this happens, we prescribe an antibiotic lotion or cream.

Antibiotics Taken By Mouth

Tetracycline, erythromycin, and minocycline are among the internal antibiotics used in treating acne. A combination of sulfa and trimethoprim, marketed as Bactrim or Septra, may be used if other antimicrobials fail to control acne. Sometimes it's necessary to try several different antibiotics, or a combination, before acne is controlled.

Sunshine

Sunlight benefits many acne patients, but also ages the skin. If sunlight improves your complexion, get moderate amounts of it. Don't allow yourself to sunburn or "bake" for hours. If the sun actually makes your acne worse, try to avoid heavy exposure. Do not bother with sun lamps, since they can't duplicate natural sunlight.

Camouflage

A water-based makeup or foundation lotion, or a flesh-tinted acne lotion, can be safely used to hide blemishes.

Actinic Keratoses

What Causes Actinic Keratoses?

Repeated, prolonged sun exposure causes skin damage, especially in fair-skinned persons. Sun-damaged skin becomes dry and wrinkled and may form rough, scaly spots called actinic keratoses. These rough spots remain on the skin even though the crust or scale is picked off. Treatment of an actinic keratosis requires removal of the defective skin cells. New skin then forms from the deeper skin cells, which have escaped sun damage.

Why Treat Actinic Keratoses?

Actinic keratoses are *not* skin cancers. Because they sometimes may turn cancerous, it is usually a good idea to remove them. In persons with many actinic keratoses, only those that show change, bleed, or are enlarging need to be removed.

Treatment

Actinic keratoses can be removed surgically with scissors or a scraping instrument called a curette. Another way of destroying actinic keratoses is to freeze them with liquid nitrogen. Freezing causes blistering and shedding of the sun-damaged skin. Sometimes, we are not sure whether the growth is harmless. When there's doubt, I prefer to cut the growth off and send it for microscopic analysis (biopsy). Healing after removal usually takes 2 to 4 weeks, depending on the size and location of the keratosis. Hands and legs heal more slowly than the face. The skin's final appearance is usually excellent.

When there are many keratoses, a useful treatment is the application of 5-fluorouracil (5-FU). The medication is rubbed on the keratoses for 15 to 25 days. 5-FU destroys sun-damaged skin cells. After 3 to 5 days, the treated area starts to get raw. The applications are continued until your physician determines that you have obtained the needed results. Healing starts when the 5-FU is stopped. 5-FU is effective in removing actinic keratoses from the face, but it often fails when used on the hands, forearms, or back.

Prevention

Sun damage is permanent. Once sun damage has progressed to the point where actinic keratoses develop, new keratoses may appear even without further sun exposure. You should avoid *excessive* sun exposure—but don't go overboard and deprive yourself of the pleasure of being outdoors. *Reasonable* sun protection should be your aim. It's described in a separate patient information sheet Sunlight and Your Skin.

Alopecia Areata

What Causes Alopecia Areata?

In alopecia areata, round patches of hair loss appear suddenly. The hair loss is often discovered by a barber or hairdresser. The hair-growing tissue stops making hair, and the hair then falls out from the roots. Why this happens is a mystery. Alopecia areata is not contagious, is not caused by foods, and is not the result of nervousness. It sometimes runs in families.

Alopecia areata has three stages. First, there is sudden hair loss. Then the patches of hair loss may enlarge. Finally, new hair grows back. This process takes months—sometimes more than 1 year.

Treatment

Hair usually grows back by itself, but slowly. Sometimes the new hair is temporarily gray or white, but after a while the original color usually returns. Cortisone injections often stimulate hair regrowth.

In the cortisone-injection treatment, a long-acting cortisone compound is injected into the hair-loss area. It remains in place for 2 to 3 months, signaling the hair roots to resume making hair. It generally takes 1 to 2 months after the injection before hair growth is visible. The cortisone acts only in the areas that have been injected; it does not prevent new areas of hair loss. However, if new areas of hair loss appear, regrowth may be helped by injecting the cortisone there.

Applications of minoxidil (Rogaine) to the scalp sometimes stimulate hair growth in male-pattern hair loss. Unfortunately, it doesn't grow hair in alopecia areata.

Skin Cancer (Basal Cell Carcinoma)

What Causes Skin Cancer?

The skin cancer (basal cell carcinoma) for which you are being treated is common and *always curable*. Basal cell cancers are the result of sun damage to the skin. Sunlight damages the skin cells, causing their growth to be disturbed. A basal cell cancer begins as a small spot that grows slowly and relentlessly until it is treated. Basal cell cancers enlarge steadily, but they *never* spread to distant parts of the body and *never* invade internal tissues. Microscopic examination is necessary to determine whether a growth is cancerous. The tissue is examined by a pathologist in a medical laboratory.

Skin cancers are most common on the face. They are practically never found in areas such as the buttocks, which are protected from the sun by clothing. Skin cancers occur more often in people living in sunny areas like Texas, Arizona, and California than in areas receiving less sunshine, such as New England. Fair-skinned individuals are more prone to skin cancer than darker-skinned persons, since skin pigment protects the skin. Persons of African ancestry with very dark skin practically never get skin cancer.

Treatment

Basal cell cancers are best treated early, when they are small, because it is simpler to remove a small growth than a large one. Surgical removal of basal cell cancers is almost 100 percent curative.

Very rarely, a cancer will grow back. In order to detect this rare event, the treated area should be checked periodically for 5 years. If you become concerned about the treated area or if other skin growths appear, please return to this office promptly.

Prevention

The skin-damaging effects of sunlight are permanent and build up slowly over time. Ordinary sun exposure and sunbathing produce gradual skin damage *even if sunburn is avoided*. As many as 10 years or more can pass between the time of sun exposure and the time the skin shows signs of sun damage. Thus, teenaged sun worshippers often pay for their deep tans when they reach their 40s or 50s. There is no way of undoing sun damage. You can prevent further skin injury by using the sun-protective measures outlined in a separate information sheet, Sunlight and Your Skin. Be *reasonable* about sun protection. Don't go overboard and try to avoid the sun completely. The damage has already been done; a *little* more sun won't make things worse. With the passage of time, skin cancer patients are likely to develop additional skin cancers. If you notice a new growth or a sore that doesn't heal or keeps coming back, be sure to have it examined. This summary is intended to answer common questions about skin cancer. If you have additional questions, be sure to discuss them at your next visit.

Boils (Furuncles)

What Causes Boils?

Boils are painful swellings of the skin caused by deep infection with staphylococcus bacteria. The bacteria enter the skin from the outside, usually through a hair opening. Boils begin as red, tender swellings. Later, the infection produces pus, which may ooze out through the skin. The source of the staph bacteria is usually not known. Most boils appear "out of the blue." Sometimes, boils develop after exposure to a person who has boils or another skin infection.

A few people have recurring boils. When this occurs, it's customary to test the urine and blood to check for any underlying disease, such as diabetes.

Treatment

Penicillin or other antibiotics taken by mouth usually speed healing in the early stages of a boil. If pus has formed, minor surgery to open the boil and drain the pus may be needed. Gentle heat provided by a heating pad, hot water bottle, or lamp held close to the skin for 20 minutes three or four times per day speeds healing. Movement worsens a skin infection. You can help a boil heal by moving it as little as possible.

Putting medicine directly on a boil won't help it heal, because the medicine doesn't penetrate into the infected area. If pus is oozing from the boil, a thin coat of antibiotic ointment (_____) and a Band-Aid over the boil will help keep the germs from spreading.

If your boil doesn't improve after treatment, please return. A different antibiotic or minor surgery may be needed.

Canker Sores (Aphthae)

What Causes Canker Sores?

Canker sores are common. They develop suddenly on the tongue, sides of the mouth, or gums and result from destruction of the protective lining of the mouth. You can recognize a canker sore; it is raw and open with a whitish yellow base. Contact with acidic, spicy, or salty foods usually is painful.

It isn't known why people get canker sores. Heredity may play a part, since canker sores often run in families. Occasionally, certain foods, such as peanuts, may trigger an attack of canker sores. Most canker sores appear without known reason. Canker sores are usually a small, occasional nuisance. However, some persons tend to get large, painful sores, which may occur frequently.

Contagion

Canker sores are *not* contagious and are *not* caused by bacteria or viruses ("germs").

Treatment

Unfortunately, we do not have a cure for canker sores. Small sores often clear in 1 week or less and can be ignored. For a sore that does not heal, your doctor may prescribe a strong cortisone ointment. Applying it to the sore six or seven times a day may speed healing and lessen pain. The cortisone ointment must be started early to prevent enlargement of the canker sore and should be used only for 2 or 3 days. Applying the cortisone ointment for more than 2 or 3 days will interfere with healing.

If your sore is very large and painful, your physician may inject cortisone into the base of the sore to provide immediate relief from pain and speed healing. When several painful canker sores occur at one time, your doctor may prescribe prednisone by mouth to be taken for 2 or 3 days. This treatment is safe, and the dosage of prednisone does not have to be tapered. Tetracycline mouthwash prescribed by a doctor is also effective against canker sores. At the first sign of a sore, swish 1 teaspoon of tetracycline suspension around your mouth for 4 to 5 minutes, and then spit it out. Do this four times per day for 5 days. Tetracycline treatment may need to be continued for 1 month or more. There is no harm if you accidentally swallow the tetracycline mouthwash—it is a safe, widely used antibiotic.

Summary

Most persons get prompt relief from canker sores by applying medicines directly to the sores. For the occasional person who suffers from frequent attacks of large, painful canker sores, both medicines taken by mouth and local treatment are usually needed to provide relief.

Cortisone Ointments

What is a Cortisone Ointment?

Cortisone skin preparations in the form of ointments and salves contain hydrocortisone or a similar chemical. Hydrocortisone is a natural chemical made by the body, but chemists have learned to manufacture stronger synthetic cortisones. Many skin medications contain these powerful synthetic cortisones.

Safety

Although cortisone taken by mouth can cause side effects, cortisone skin preparations are remarkably safe. Hydrocortisone ointment is even available without prescription in a 1 percent strength. Internal side effects from cortisone applied externally are rare, but you should check regularly with your doctor if any of the following conditions apply:

1. You are using strong cortisones over most of your body for many months.
2. Strong cortisones plus plastic covering, which increases penetration, are applied to much of the body surface.
3. Strong cortisones are used on *large* areas of a child or infant.
4. You are using an ultra-high-potency cortisone such as Diprolene, Temovate, Psorcon, or Ultravate.

Local Side Effects

Strong cortisone medications may damage the skin to which they are applied, especially on skin-fold areas, fingertips, and the face. Skin thinning (atrophy) is the most troublesome side effect. The stronger the cortisone, the greater the risk of atrophy; the risk of atrophy is increased when plastic covering also is used. Atrophy makes skin-fold sites, such as the groin, rectal area, and armpits, tender and raw. Cortisone atrophy of fingertip skin causes painful cracks. Cortisone atrophy of the face results in a flushed appearance with small blood vessels becoming noticeable.

Not every skin disorder responds magically to cortisones. They can worsen some diseases, such as athlete's foot, ringworm, and acne. Strong cortisones applied to the face may cause a red, pimply rash.

How to Use Cortisone Ointments

Use a *small* amount of the cortisone preparation and massage it gently into your skin. Ointment or salve left on the surface of the skin is wasted. Keep the medication away from your eyes. If your eyelids are to be treated, use a clean fingertip and apply only a tiny amount of the preparation carefully, avoiding your eyes.

Cortisone ointments and salves are some of our safest and most effective skin medicines. Internal side effects are rare, but the skin—especially on the face and at skin-fold areas—can be damaged by strong cortisone preparations. Use them only under your doctor's supervision.

Cortisone Taken Internally

When is Cortisone Taken Internally?

Cortisone is a chemical (hormone) made by the human body and essential for life. Cortisone and compounds related to it (called corticosteroids) are widely used in medicine. They control allergies, inflammation, and many disease processes. Cortisone compounds can be applied to the skin in the form of ointments or taken internally. We are describing the use of *cortisones taken internally,* either by mouth or by injection. Usually, cortisones are prescribed by mouth when an internal effect is required; when injections are used, we have a choice of fast- or slow-acting cortisones.

Safety

Cortisone has effects on the entire body; those that are not desired are called side effects. Side effects of cortisone include salt and water retention, increased stomach acid, increased appetite, mood and energy changes, facial flushing, and muscle soreness or weakness.

Cortisones are remarkably safe for most people when used for brief periods of several weeks or less. Some people taking cortisones for short periods have no unpleasant side effects. Disturbances of sleep patterns and increased appetite are common. Others will notice weight gain resulting from fluid retention, or changes in mood—usually, nervousness, trouble sleeping, and restlessness. Sometimes, cortisones cause indigestion. These side effects are usually minor and disappear after the cortisone is stopped. If you're having troublesome side effects, please contact me.

CAUTION. *Internal cortisones increase blood sugar and blood pressure.* These drugs may worsen diabetes and hypertension. If you are being treated for diabetes or hypertension, please inform me. Internal cortisones may also worsen or activate peptic ulcers; please tell me if you have ever had a stomach or duodenal ulcer.

Unfortunately, when cortisones are used for *many months or years,* serious side effects are common. Consequently, we use long-term cortisone treatment only when a disease threatens or seriously disturbs a patient's life.

Treatment

The most common internal cortisone treatment is prednisone taken by mouth. This medicine acts rapidly and is inexpensive. Most patients are told to take the entire day's dose of prednisone in the morning, because this coincides with the body's own rhythm of cortisone production. If you're being treated for a severe allergic reaction, you may be told to divide the day's prednisone ration into two or more doses.

The amount of prednisone prescribed for you depends on the severity of your skin problem. The starting dose is an estimate. It may have to be increased or decreased, depending on your response to it. Prompt improvement is important not just to clear your skin but also to hold down the severity of side effects. As your skin improves, the dose of prednisone will be gradually decreased. When your skin has cleared—or nearly so—the prednisone tablets will be stopped. If you have been taking prednisone for only 1 or 2 weeks, it's safe to stop taking it all at once.

If your skin does not improve promptly or if you are having trouble with side effects, please call me.

Cysts

What Causes a Cyst?

A cyst is a harmless, sac-like growth in the deeper layers of the skin. The cyst sac is filled with a soft, whitish brown material that sometimes oozes out onto the skin's surface. We don't know why cysts appear, nor do we know why some persons get many of them.

Cysts are a nuisance, but they *never* become cancerous or malignant. Occasionally, germs get into the cyst and cause an infection that resembles a boil. When this happens, antibiotics taken by mouth and minor surgery performed in the office may be needed to relieve the pressure and discomfort.

Treatment

Small cysts—those ¼ inch in diameter or less—ordinarily do not need treatment unless they mar your appearance. Larger cysts are usually removed because of their size and the danger of infection.

Cysts are treated by making a small surgical opening into the skin and removing the sac. This small operation is done in the office. A local anesthetic is used to numb the skin. Stitches are often used to close the skin opening and are usually removed 3 to 8 days later. Surgery usually cures cysts, but sometimes, a cyst comes back and requires a second treatment.

Dermatitis

What Causes Dermatitis?

Dermatitis is a harmless but annoying rash. It results from a combination of causes and is not contagious. Think of dermatitis as skin "misbehaving."

Treatment

Dermatitis is treated by applying a cortisone-type medicine. Your skin should start to improve within 1 week; sometimes treatment takes longer. As long as you follow directions, cortisone medicines are safe to use on the skin until your rash clears.

Skin suffering from dermatitis is easily irritated. Treat it gently. Because soap is irritating, keep it away from areas of dermatitis. Home remedies, over-the-counter medicines, and your neighbor's treatment suggestions rarely help and often make matters worse. Don't use them!

Please follow these directions:

1. Apply small amounts of cortisone to your skin as often as directed. Massage it in gently but thoroughly.
2. Do not apply anything to your rash except (1) water, (2) the medicine prescribed for your dermatitis, and (3) white petrolatum (plain Vaseline). If your skin is dry, you may apply white petrolatum as often as needed. Petrolatum is best used *after* you've applied the medicine. It may be most convenient to apply petrolatum sparingly at bedtime, when its greasiness is least objectionable.
3. Keep soap away from dermatitis. If you shower, it's all right to use a little soap on *normal* skin. Be sure to rinse it off well. If the dermatitis is widespread, you should shower or bathe with plain water and not use any soap.
4. Keep your skin well lubricated, using the cortisone and white petrolatum. When there is widespread dermatitis, lubrication with mineral oil is simple, effective, and inexpensive. Apply the mineral oil sparingly with your hands to your entire wet skin after a bath or shower. Put a few drops of mineral oil on your hands, spread it thinly over your skin, and repeat until your body is covered. The patient information sheet Dry Skin (Asteatosis, Xerosis) gives details on skin lubrication.
5. Wool and other rough clothing may aggravate dermatitis. Wear something smooth and soft next to your skin.
6. If your dermatitis doesn't improve with these measures, please call and make an appointment.
7. Keep your medicines and this sheet even after your dermatitis has cleared, because dermatitis tends to come back. If it does, resume the original treatment.

CAUTION. *Cortisone medicines are to be used only on dermatitis.* They may actually worsen other rashes such as athlete's foot or impetigo. Strong cortisone ointments may cause rashes when used on the face and may result in thinning of your skin when applied to skin-fold areas. Use your cortisone only for treating dermatitis and only for the areas prescribed.

Atopic Dermatitis (Atopic Eczema)

Atopic dermatitis, also called atopic eczema or just eczema, is a stubborn, itchy rash that occurs in certain persons with sensitive or irritable skin. Eczema is common in infants and young children and may disappear before adulthood. Eczema may clear for years, only to reappear later—often on the hands.

What Causes Atopic Dermatitis?

The cause of atopic dermatitis is not known. It's the result of a built-in defect of the skin that tends to run in families. Eczema is not contagious and is not related to your general health. Atopic dermatitis is also called "constitutional eczema"; this name emphasizes the built-in aspect of the condition. Persons with eczema have skin that is dry and easily irritated by soap, detergents, and rough woolen clothing. Very hot or very cold weather often aggravates eczema. Although certain allergies may worsen eczema, they do not cause it. Skin tests do *not* help, because eczema is *not* due to an allergy.

Treatment

Because eczema patients have a constitutional skin defect, no permanent cure is possible. Fortunately, we have effective ways of controlling eczema; most persons are able to live comfortably with their skin handicap.

Cortisone compounds applied to the skin are the best medicine for controlling eczema. Most cortisone salves can be used safely for years. When large areas of the body are treated with strong cortisone salves, periodic medical checkups are necessary. Certain cortisones should not be applied to the face, armpits, groin, or rectal area. In patients with severe eczema, it's sometimes necessary to take cortisone by mouth; however, this is done only for short periods and under the close supervision of a doctor.

Cortisone is applied to the skin in the form of lotions, creams, or greasy ointments. When the skin is very dry, ointments are often best. Whatever preparation you use, be sure to use only a little and massage it in well. If you wish to have more vigorous treatment, apply the medicine more often. Always remember to use just a little.

Other medicines are sometimes used. For stubborn eczema, salves containing coal tar can be helpful. Coal tar smells and stains clothes. You can minimize these nuisances by using it at bedtime.

In controlling your eczema, remember the following points:

1. Keep your skin well lubricated. If your skin is too dry, use a greasy cortisone salve or apply a little white petrolatum (Vaseline) after you rub in your cortisone cream or lotion. Using a bath oil in the tub or applying mineral oil

right after bathing will help keep your skin moist. The patient information sheet Dry Skin (Asteatosis, Xerosis) gives details on skin lubrication.

2. Keep soap away from your eczema. Soap irritates and dries the skin. Persons with eczema should avoid it. When bathing or showering, use plain water; limit soap to your face, armpits, genital area, and feet. If you must wash your hands frequently with soap, rinse them carefully and afterward apply a little cortisone cream or ointment.

3. Avoid overheating. Most persons with eczema find that hot weather and heavy sweating worsen their eczema. In hot weather, wear cool, loose clothing, and try to stay in air-conditioned buildings.

4. Avoid direct skin contact with wool or similar rough clothing.

5. Avoid anything that definitely aggravates your eczema. If certain creams, makeups, perfumes and so on cause itching or irritation, don't use them.

6. It is usually possible to find a treatment routine that lets you control your eczema. Most treatments involve cortisone ointments or creams. When properly applied, these medications can be used safely for years.

7. If your eczema worsens and you can't control it, please return so we can give you a different treatment.

Hand Protection for Hand Dermatitis

Hand dermatitis (hand eczema is another name for the same thing) is common. Hand rashes usually result from a combination of (1) sensitive skin and (2) irritation or allergy from materials touched. Everyone's hands routinely touch irritating soaps and detergents several times a day. Add the raw foods, solvents, paints, oils, greases, acids, glues, and so on that most of us touch at work or in the home, and you can see that the skin of your hands takes a beating.

Not everyone gets hand dermatitis. Many lucky persons have "tough" skin, but, unfortunately, some persons have skin that's easily damaged. The result is dermatitis. Persons with hand dermatitis often have dermatitis elsewhere, and frequently blood relatives have hand dermatitis. We can't toughen your skin, but we have effective treatment to heal your dermatitis.

Skin protection is an important part of treatment. This instruction sheet gives you detailed directions on how to protect your hands. Please read it carefully every day for a week to fix these instructions in your mind.

1. Protect your hands from direct contact with soaps, detergents, scouring powders, and similar irritating chemicals by wearing waterproof, heavy-duty vinyl gloves. Heavy-duty vinyl gloves such as Allerderm brand are better than rubber gloves, because you may become allergic to rubber. Heavy-duty vinyl gloves are usually available at paint and hardware stores. Buy four or five pairs so they can be conveniently located in kitchen, bathroom, and laundry areas. If a glove develops a hole, *discard it immediately*. Wearing a glove with a hole is worse than wearing no gloves at all.
2. The waterproof, heavy-duty vinyl gloves may be lined or unlined. You should have enough waterproof gloves so that the insides of the gloves can dry between wearings.
3. Wear waterproof gloves while peeling and squeezing lemons, oranges, or grapefruit, while peeling potatoes, and while handling tomatoes.
4. Wear leather or heavy-duty fabric gloves when doing dry work and gardening. Dirty your gloves, not your hands. If you keep house for your family, scatter a dozen pairs of cheap cotton gloves about your home and use them while doing dry housework. When they get dirty, put them in the washing machine. Wash your gloves, not your hands.
5. If you have an automatic dishwasher, use it as much as possible. If you don't, let a member of your family do the dishes. Do your laundry by machine, not by hand.
6. Avoid direct contact with turpentine, paint thinner, paints, and floor, furniture, metal, and shoe polishes. They contain irritating solvents. When using them, wear heavy-duty vinyl gloves.
7. If your hands are frequently exposed to solvents and other irritating chem-

icals, especially at work, ask an industrial hygienist about protective gloves.

8. When washing your hands, use lukewarm water and very little mild soap. Rinse the soap off carefully and dry gently. Although all soaps are irritating, some are less irritating than others.

9. Rings often worsen dermatitis by trapping irritating materials beneath them. Remove your rings when doing housework and before washing your hands.

10. When you are outdoors in cold or windy weather, wear leather gloves to protect your hands from drying and chapping.

11. Use only the prescribed medicines and lubricants. Do not use other lotions, creams, or medications—they may irritate your skin.

12. Protect your hands for at least 4 months *after* your dermatitis has healed. It takes a long time for skin to recover; unless you are careful, the dermatitis may recur.

There is no fast, "magic" treatment for hand dermatitis. Your skin must be given a rest from irritation. Follow these instructions carefully.

Overnight Plastic Occlusion for Hand Dermatitis

Covering skin overnight with plastic increases the penetration and effectiveness of cortisone medicines. For hand dermatitis, you should wear plastic gloves overnight after applying a cortisone to your rash. You will receive a special cortisone to be used *only at bedtime*. Please follow these directions carefully.

1. At bedtime, apply _____ (a cortisone) thinly to the rash areas only. Do *not* apply it to normal skin. Then put on the plastic gloves; take them off in the morning. The plastic gloves recommended are disposable vinyl examining gloves; they can be re-used for a few nights or until they develop holes. They are made in four sizes; your proper size is: Small   Medium   Large   Extra-large.   If your drugstore does not stock them, our receptionist can tell you where to buy them.

IMPORTANT. Use only vinyl (plastic) gloves. Do *not* use latex (rubber) gloves.

2. At first, wearing the plastic gloves may be a bit uncomfortable. It may take a few days to get used to them.
3. The cortisone ointment–plastic glove treatment can make your skin become thin. You should use it exactly as directed on this sheet. It's important to apply the cortisone medicine *only to the rash* when using plastic gloves. Do *not* apply the cortisone medicine to normal skin. If your fingertips are normal, cut the fingertips off your gloves, because the plastic covering softens skin. If your rash is on only one or two fingers, cut the proper number of fingers from a plastic glove and hold them in place with a nonirritating paper tape.
4. During the day, follow the patient instruction sheets Hand Dermatitis Treatment and Hand Protection for Hand Dermatitis. Apply the daytime lubricant thinly and often to the entire skin of both hands.
5. Keep your follow-up appointment. You will need an appointment 7 to 10 days after starting the cortisone–plastic covering treatment.
6. CAUTION. *Strong cortisones covered with plastic may cause your skin to thin and crack easily.* To prevent this, be sure to use the cortisone–plastic glove treatment less often as soon as directed.
7. Follow these instructions exactly until your next appointment. The cortisone–plastic covering treatment should be used only under medical supervision.

Hand Dermatitis Treatment

1. The most important part of your treatment is to apply a lubricating, mild cortisone cream to your hands many times a day. You should apply this medicated hand lubricant after each handwashing, and as often as possible at other times—at least 15 times each day. Apply the medicated hand lubricant very thinly to your whole hand like a hand cream, and massage it in well.

2. Do *not* apply any cream, lotion, or ointment to your hands except the one prescribed for you. There is one exception: If your skin is still too dry, you may apply plain white petrolatum (Vaseline) thinly *after* rubbing in your medicine.

3. When washing your hands, use lukewarm water and a very small amount of mild soap. Rinse the soap off well and dry gently. Then apply a little medicine and massage it in well.

4. Pamper your hands by following the instructions in the patient information sheet Hand Protection for Hand Dermatitis.

5. When your rash is *much* better, you may use the medicine less often. However, you should apply the medicine at least four times a day until your skin has healed completely.

6. Continue applying the medicine until your skin is completely normal. Pamper your hands for at least 4 months after healing. It takes a long time for skin to recover from prolonged inflammation.

7. Hand dermatitis is stubborn. If your hand rash improves at first and then worsens, it usually means that you need to use your medicine more often.

8. Hand dermatitis often recurs. If your hand rash comes back, you need to apply the medicine often and pamper your hands.

9. If you have dry, chapped hands and your dermatitis tends to recur, make it a permanent routine to apply the medicated hand lubricant several times a day. It's safe to do so indefinitely.

10. Cortisones keep for years at room temperature. As long as the prescriptions are refillable, take the *original container* to your pharmacist for a refill when you need more medicine. If you have used up all the authorized refills, please make an appointment for a checkup.

11. If your rash does not clear, please return to this office so we can re-evaluate your treatment.

Seborrheic Dermatitis

Seborrheic dermatitis is a common, harmless, scaling rash that sometimes itches. Dandruff is seborrheic dermatitis of the scalp. Seborrheic dermatitis may also occur on the eyebrows, eyelid edges, ears, the skin near the nose, and skin-fold areas such as the armpits and groin. Sometimes, seborrheic dermatitis produces round, scaling patches on the middle of the chest or scales on the back.

What Causes Seborrheic Dermatitis?

Seborrheic dermatitis results from skin not growing properly. The cause is not known. Seborrheic dermatitis is *not* related to diet and is *not* contagious. Nervous stress and any physical illness tend to worsen seborrheic dermatitis, but do not cause it.

Seborrheic dermatitis may appear at any age, either gradually or suddenly. It tends to run in families. Seborrheic dermatitis may last for many years and may disappear by itself. Often it gets better or worse without any apparent reason.

Treatment

There is no cure for seborrheic dermatitis; however, we can keep this nuisance under control. The treatment of seborrheic dermatitis depends on what part of the body is involved. Dandruff (seborrheic dermatitis of the scalp) can usually be controlled by washing your hair often with medicated shampoos. Sometimes it's also necessary to use lotions or gels containing tar, ketoconazole, cortisone, or other medicines. Remember that dandruff is a harmless nuisance. It does *not* cause hair loss.

In areas of smooth skin such as the face and ears, ketoconazole cream and cortisone-containing creams, lotions, or ointments are effective. Cortisones applied to limited areas of skin do not affect your general health.

When your seborrheic dermatitis is under control, gradually use your medicines less often. It may be possible to stop the medicines completely, but occasional treatment is usually needed. Seborrheic dermatitis often returns. If it does, resume the original treatment. If your seborrheic dermatitis isn't controlled by the treatment prescribed, please return for further evaluation.

Dermatofibromas

What Causes a Dermatofibroma?

A dermatofibroma is a round, brownish-to-purple growth commonly found on the legs and arms. Dermatofibromas contain scar tissue and feel like hard lumps in the skin. We don't know why people grow dermatofibromas. Some may be caused by insect bites. They are harmless and never turn cancerous.

Treatment

Dermatofibromas are best ignored. Sometimes, if the diagnosis is not certain, a piece may be removed for tissue analysis (biopsy). Dermatofibromas can be removed surgically, but because they are deep, this usually leaves an unsightly scar. When a dermatofibroma becomes bothersome—for instance, if it gets in the way of leg shaving or is irritated by clothing—it can be flattened by freezing with liquid nitrogen.

Taking a small punch biopsy can be combined with liquid nitrogen treatment as a simple, one-step procedure. If a tiny punch is used, the biopsy scar is barely visible, and the liquid nitrogen treatment flattens the growth to make it less noticeable. Liquid nitrogen freezing destroys only the upper part of the growth. Therefore, the dermatofibroma, after several years, may again become noticeable. Usually, any regrowth is slight and can be handled by another freezing. If there is any unusual change or marked regrowth of a dermatofibroma, please return.

Dry Skin (Asteatosis, Xerosis)

What Causes Dry Skin?

Dry skin is a problem for many people, especially in cool weather when the air is dry. Dry air causes the skin to lose moisture and then chap and crack. These chapped, cracked areas may become irritated and itchy. The dry skin rash sometimes forms round patches that resemble ringworm.

Treatment: Skin Lubrication

Skin is lubricated by moisture. Water will briefly moisturize your skin, but the moisture is soon lost by evaporation. Oils, ointments, creams, and lotions provide a coating that prevents water loss and keeps moisture in your skin.

The simplest way to prevent loss of skin moisture is to oil your skin with mineral oil immediately after a shower or bath *while your skin is still wet*. Oil your skin by pouring a few drops onto your palms, spreading it thinly over a wide area of skin, and repeating until you have covered your entire body. By having your skin wet when you apply the oil, it is possible to apply a very thin coating. Let the water evaporate rather than toweling yourself dry. If your skin feels greasy, too much oil was applied. Wipe off the excess with a tissue, and next time, use less oil.

Why mineral oil? It's a pure oil, without additives, perfumes, or irritants. Mineral oil is inexpensive and available without prescription at all drugstores. White petrolatum (Vaseline) is an excellent lubricant, but it is difficult to spread thinly. Other, less desirable lubricants are bath oils, baby oil, and lotions. Bath oil contains a substance that lets the oil mix with water. Baby oil consists of mineral oil and a perfume. Lotions contain additives that may irritate your skin. Bubble baths are *not* lubricants. Do not use bubble baths, because these irritate and dry the skin. If you are fond of baths, bath oil is a convenient way to lubricate the skin. A tablespoon of bath oil is enough for an entire tub. Soak for 15 to 20 minutes, and *do not use soap*. The bath oil–water combination will get you clean. Afterward, pat yourself dry with a towel; enough oil will remain on your skin to prevent moisture loss. If you add oil to your bath, be sure to use a commercial bath oil. Mineral oil or baby oil should not be added to the bath, because it does not mix with water.

CAUTION. Bath oils make the tub extremely slippery. Be very careful when you enter and leave the tub.

Treating Dry Skin Rash

When dry skin has developed into a rash that itches, a cortisone cream or ointment usually provides quick relief. The cortisone is applied thinly to the rash once a day and massaged in well; bedtime may be convenient. As the rash improves, the cortisone is used less often. Occasionally, rashes are severe enough to require a few days of oral medication.

Soap

Soap is bad for dry skin. It removes skin oils needed to hold in moisture. Soap should *not* be used on dry skin. Most of us use far too much soap; actually, plain water is often enough for a shower or bath. If you can't live without soap, it's all right to use a *little* soap (rinsed off well) for your face, feet, armpits, and groin, and to use shampoo or soap on your scalp.

Bathing

Persons with dry skin may bathe or shower once daily—not more often. Remember two things: (1) use no soap on dry skin areas; (2) lubricate your skin using one of the methods described on this sheet.

Long-Term Control

Dry skin is usually a long-term problem that recurs often, especially in winter. When you notice your skin getting dry, resume your lubricating routine, and carefully avoid the use of soap. If the itchy dry-skin rash returns, use both the lubricating routine and the prescription cortisone cream or ointment.

5-Fluorouracil Treatment

5-Fluorouracil (abbreviated 5-FU) has the ability to destroy sun-damaged skin cells. Applying 5-FU to the skin removes the rough spots resulting from sun damage (actinic keratoses). The skin is then smoother and more youthful-looking.

Apply 5-FU twice a day to the areas of the skin that need treatment. You may feel stinging or burning when you put 5-FU on your skin. This is normal. Three to eight days after you start using 5-FU, your sun-damaged skin will become red and irritated. As you continue treatment, sores and crusts will appear. These raw areas result from the destruction of defective skin cells. They are a necessary part of 5-FU treatment.

You should be seen 12 to 14 days after starting treatment to check on your progress and determine how long to continue using 5-FU. Usually 4 weeks of treatment are needed. When treatment is stopped, your skin will heal rapidly; in 2 or 3 weeks, healthy new skin will have replaced the sun-damaged skin destroyed by the 5-FU. After healing, the treated areas will be redder than normal; this redness will fade in several months.

Directions for Use

1. Treat the following areas with 5-FU: _____ _____ .
2. Two times daily, apply the medicine very thinly to the treatment area with your fingertip and massage it in well. Morning and evening applications are best; don't apply 5-FU at bedtime, because contact with pillows and bedding may cause undesirable spreading of the medicine.
3. After applying the 5-FU, rinse your finger thoroughly with water.
4. Do *not* get 5-FU into your eyes, and do *not* use it on your eyelids.
5. Keep 5-FU *off* your lips.
6. Use 5-FU with care in the area between the nose and cheeks, because the medicine may irritate the folds around your nostrils.
7. Do *not* sunbathe while using 5-FU.
8. If you wish, you may wash the area that is to be treated with plain water *before* applying 5-FU.
9. You may use makeup; be sure to apply the 5-FU before putting on makeup.
10. If you notice any unusual or severe reaction, stop the medicine and contact this office.
11. After 5-FU has caused the keratoses to become irritated and raw, applying petrolatum (Vaseline) thinly at bedtime will lessen the discomfort. Continue these bedtime petrolatum applications until the skin has healed.
12. CAUTION. *5-FU is a powerful, destructive medication and must be used exactly as directed.* Keep it away from your eyes and mouth. Keep your 5-FU locked up so other people can't mistakenly use it to treat a rash.

Fragile Skin Bleeding

What Causes Fragile Skin Bleeding?

Easy bruising and bleeding into the skin of the tops of the hands and forearms occurs in many middle-aged and older people, especially if their skin is fair. This easy bleeding, which can occur without apparent injury, is a result of the skin being made thin and fragile by years of sunlight exposure. It is *not* the result of a blood disorder or internal disease. The fact that bleeding occurs only on the sundamaged areas of the hands and forearms, and never on the covered parts of the body, clearly shows that it results from local skin damage.

Sun exposure over the years, even without sunburning, has thinned your skin and damaged its supporting fibers. These sun-damaged fibers can no longer adequately support your skin and its blood vessels. Even slight movement may cause an unsupported blood vessel to break. This releases blood into the skin and leaves unsightly purplish marks. Cortisones taken by mouth may cause skin thinning and worsen fragile skin bleeding. Anticoagulants (blood thinners), such as coumadin, may also cause you to bleed more easily.

Treatment

Fragile skin bleeding is a harmless nuisance. The skin damage produced by sunlight is permanent, and for that reason we have no treatment for your problem. You can prevent further sun damage by using the sun-protective measures described in the patient instruction sheet Sunlight and Your Skin.

Hair Loss in Women (Female-Pattern Alopecia)

Adult men tend to lose their scalp hair with age. The rate of this hair loss varies and depends on inherited (genetic) factors. Although balding and dramatic hair loss are a male characteristic, women also undergo gradual scalp hair loss. All women in their 70s have less hair than they did when they were 20. Such scalp hair loss may start in your 20s or 30s. Fortunately, women do *not* become completely bald from this type of hair loss.

What Causes Hair Loss in Women?

Scalp hair loss in women, as in men, is a biological (natural) event. It is also called female-pattern alopecia. In female-pattern alopecia, the hair roots gradually shrink, and the affected hairs become thinner and thinner until they disappear. The hair roots are controlled by inherited (genetic) factors, which cannot be changed. The inherited factor is obvious when there are female blood relatives with the same problem. However, we are not carbon copies of our blood relatives, and some women may have sparse hair, whereas close relatives will have large amounts of scalp hair.

Female-pattern alopecia has several important features:

1. The hair loss may follow a pattern and take place mainly on the temples and crown of the scalp, or it may occur evenly throughout the scalp.
2. The hair loss is limited to the scalp; the hair of the eyebrows, armpits, and genital area remains unchanged.
3. The hair loss often tends to occur in waves, with periods of heavy hair loss that may last for a few months.
4. Diet, general health, dandruff, and other factors do *not* cause female-pattern alopecia. Many women will notice episodes of *temporary* loss after a high fever, the birth of a baby, surgery, or other physical stress. Such "stress" hair loss is temporary, although it may last for many months.
5. Shampooing, hair care, dyeing of hair, and permanents do not cause or worsen female-pattern alopecia.

Female-pattern alopecia occurs when the hair roots deep within the skin stop making hair. It is virtually impossible to affect the growth of hair by any external method. For example, the growth of unwanted facial hair can be stopped only by electrolysis, in which the hair root is destroyed with an electric current. You can safely shampoo your hair as often as you like, dye it, and use the hair-care preparations you prefer. The hair lost during a shampoo would fall out a few days later anyway. The occasional stories you hear about women losing their hair after too much hair straightening or an incorrectly applied permanent refer to hair damage and *breakage,* not hair loss from the roots.

Treatment

There is no cure for female-pattern hair loss. Although claims are made that massage, vitamins, hair treatments, and scalp applications will grow hair, except for minoxidil (trade name: Rogaine), these treatments are completely worthless. The many over-the-counter scalp preparations and treatments aimed at revitalizing hair growth are frauds.

Minoxidil applied to the scalp stimulates hair regrowth in both men and women. In men with male-pattern alopecia, significant hair growth recurs in about one out of 10 patients treated with Rogaine applications. Unfortunately, in women with female-pattern hair loss, *cosmetically significant* hair regrowth appears to be even more infrequent and has not been documented in scientific studies. It requires 4 to 6 months of treatment before hair growth—if it is to occur—becomes noticeable. If minoxidil is stopped, any new hair that may have grown falls out; therefore, minoxidil applications need to be continued indefinitely. A few reports have described minoxidil treatments to the scalp causing an increased growth of facial hair. Minoxidil appears to be safe; occasionally it causes scalp irritation. Whether minoxidil applications will prevent worsening of female-pattern alopecia is not known. Minoxidil is expensive, costing about $2 per day.

Most women are content to live with this cosmetically annoying but quite harmless natural process once they understand that (1) they will not go bald; (2) it is perfectly all right to wear a wiglet or wig; and (3) they can use their usual hair-care routines.

Herpes Simplex

What Causes Herpes Simplex?

Herpes simplex, commonly called cold sores or fever blisters, may occur once or recur again and again. It's caused by the herpes hominis virus. There are two kinds of herpes virus: Type 1 and type 2. Type 1 virus causes the cold sores common on the lips and face. Herpes of the genital area is usually caused by type 2 virus.

Herpes simplex begins as a group of small red bumps that blister. You may have noticed itching or discomfort before the rash appeared. The blisters begin to dry up after a few days and form yellow crusts. The crusts gradually fall off and leave slowly fading red areas. The whole process takes about 10 to 14 days. No scars form.

These mild symptoms are typical of *recurring* herpes simplex. The very first infection with type 1 herpes simplex virus usually happens in childhood. It may go unrecognized, but often it causes fever, general illness, and much local soreness. Once you have had a herpes simplex infection, the virus becomes permanently established in your nerve tissue. Recurring herpes results from activation of this virus. Between attacks, it lives quietly in nerve tissue.

Fever and sun exposure are the most common triggering factors for type 1 herpes simplex virus. That's when cold sores or fever blisters break out. Often, the virus becomes activated without any apparent reason.

Contagion

Like most other viruses, herpes simplex virus is contagious to people who have never had the infection before. Anyone who's had a fever blister or cold sore on the face is resistant to type 1 virus. Herpes simplex type 1 virus is not very contagious. Close contact such as kissing is necessary to transmit the infection.

Genital herpes (type 2) is usually spread through sexual intercourse and is essentially a disease of adults. It's highly contagious when in the active stages. Unfortunately, herpes simplex also may be contagious between attacks, when the skin is normal. Recurring herpes is not a reinfection but an activation of virus present in a quiet form in nerve tissue.

Treatment

Acyclovir, the first medicine effective against herpes simplex, became available in early 1985. To be effective, acyclovir (trade name: Zovirax) must be taken by mouth. Acyclovir ointment (Zovirax ointment) does *not* work.

Acyclovir interferes with the growth of the virus, and it is important to start treatment early. If you can recognize the early signs of herpes (itching, burning, and redness) *before* blisters develop—that is the best time to start taking acyclovir.

The purpose of acyclovir is to stop the spread of the virus. It does not speed the healing of blisters and scabs already there. For *recurring* herpes simplex, acyclovir is usually given for 3 or 4 days. For the *first* attack of herpes simplex (primary herpes), acyclovir is continued for 7 or 8 days. Side effects from acyclovir are rare. If you are pregnant, acyclovir (like other medicines) should be taken only if approved by the physician responsible for your prenatal care.

Acyclovir is *not* a miracle drug that banishes herpes simplex. If you begin treatment early, it will shorten the course of your disease. Once blisters and crusts have formed, time is required for their healing. Two simple remedies will make you more comfortable while you are getting over herpes:

1. If there is oozing and crusting, apply cool tap water with a clean cloth for 10 to 15 minutes two or three times a day.
2. Later, when the blisters become yellow and crusted, you can relieve any cracking and dryness with small amounts of plain white petrolatum (Vaseline).

Recurring herpes is usually only an uncomfortable nuisance. One exception is herpes of the eye. Because it may lead to eye damage, you should see an eye doctor (ophthalmologist) immediately. Fortunately, eye involvement is rare with herpes simplex. Herpes simplex *around* the eye is *not* dangerous unless it involves the eye.

Prevention

At present, there are only two ways to prevent recurring herpes simplex: (1) Continuous daily intake of acyclovir; and (2) protection from sunlight, if sun is a triggering factor. Taking acyclovir on a daily basis over many months *may* be of benefit if you are plagued with frequent and disabling attacks of herpes.

If sunlight activates your herpes simplex, use a sunscreen on and around your lips when you go outdoors. You can use a heavily pigmented lipstick or a colorless sunscreening lip pomade on your lips, and a sun block cream or lotion on the skin around your lips. Both the lip pomade and the sun block should have an SPF (sun protection factor) of at least 15 and preferably over 25.

Summary

Fever blisters or cold sores are a harmless infection caused by the herpes hominis virus. Acyclovir, a medication taken by mouth, will stop the spread of herpes and make attacks less severe *if started early in each attack*. Fortunately, herpes heals without leaving scars. Sometimes, repeated attacks can be prevented if a triggering factor, such as sunlight, can be found and avoided. Herpes simplex is moderately contagious to people who have never had the infection.

Herpes Zoster (Shingles)

What Causes Shingles?

Shingles (herpes zoster) is a nerve infection caused by the chicken-pox virus. Shingles results from activation of chicken-pox virus that has remained in your body since you had chicken pox—perhaps many years ago. The virus activation is limited to a nerve root. That accounts for the pattern of the rash, which always stops at the body's midline. The nerve involvement explains the stinging, burning, or pain common in shingles. Some patients have discomfort before the rash appears.

The rash of shingles begins as red patches that soon develop blisters. The blisters may remain small or can become large. They heal in 2 to 4 weeks. They may leave some scars.

Many patients mistakenly believe that nervousness causes shingles. This is incorrect; shingles is a viral infection of a nerve and has nothing to do with being nervous.

Contagion

You don't have to quarantine yourself. Until your rash has healed, however, you should keep away from persons who have never had chicken pox, are ill, or are unable to fight infection because of a disease or a medication. Small children or infants can catch chicken pox from someone with shingles. Persons whose resistance to infection is lowered by illness or certain medications, such as cortisone, can also catch shingles. Contact with healthy adults appears to be safe.

Treatment

The antiviral drug acyclovir helps to control the skin eruption. Acyclovir is *not* a cure, but it helps to heal the rash, provided treatment is started early. Acyclovir is taken by mouth.

Even taking acyclovir may not eliminate discomfort, burning sensations, or pain. If the discomfort is mild, take aspirin or a similar mild painkiller. If you have much pain, we can order a prescription painkiller to take until the pain subsides. The pain is caused by neuritis (inflammation of a nerve). The blistering rash usually clears in a few weeks. The discomfort may persist longer.

Treat your rash gently. Don't open your blisters. As long as there is blistering or crusting, water compresses will make you more comfortable. Compress the blisters by applying lukewarm tap water on a clean cloth for 10 minutes twice daily. It is all right to bathe, but do not use soap, because it irritates the blisters. Stop the compresses when the blisters have dried up. Later, when the crusts and scabs are separating, your skin may become dry, tense, and cracked. If this happens, rub on a small amount of plain white petrolatum (Vaseline) three or four times a day.

Hives (Urticaria)

Hives are itching red welts or small bumps that last from 15 minutes to several hours. They usually appear suddenly and leave no trace when they disappear. Crops of hives may appear several times a day. They may come and go for days or weeks, sometimes longer. Hives are harmless except when they cause throat swelling; this is rare but requires immediate treatment.

What Causes Hives?

Hives may be caused by something taken internally, most often a medicine such as penicillin or aspirin. Sometimes foods cause hives; shellfish and strawberries are well-known examples. Hives are sometimes caused by infections such as infectious mononucleosis or are the result of an internal disease. Occasionally, physical agents such as pressure or cold can cause hives. Often, the cause cannot be found. Fortunately, we can usually treat hives successfully—even though their cause may remain a mystery.

Treatment

In treating your hives, we try to find their cause. Medicine is prescribed to control the rash and itching.

Because medicines are the commonest cause of hives, please list all the medicines you've been taking, including headache tablets, allergy pills, medicines for stomach discomfort, laxatives, tranquilizers, cough medicines, and painkillers. Think of what your medicine cabinet contains. List any unusual foods you ate in the 2 days before the hives first appeared. Have you had any recent illnesses? Answers to these questions may help find the cause of your hives. Meanwhile, you'll be given medicines to control them.

Hives are usually controlled with antihistamines. Often, one type of antihistamine is prescribed for daytime use, and a different antihistamine for bedtime.

CAUTION. *Antihistamines sometimes cause drowsiness; if you feel sleepy, do not drive.* Do not drink alcoholic beverages when taking antihistamines.

Injections of epinephrine (Adrenalin) may be used for treatment of severe hives. Sometimes, epinephrinelike medicines taken by mouth are used in combination with antihistamines. If these drugs don't stop hives, it's likely that cortisone will.

Hives usually improve with these medicines in 24 hours or less. If you are not better within 24 hours, call this office.

Medicines applied to your skin (for example, lotions, creams, and sprays) won't help your hives. However, cooling the skin often relieves severe itching. A cold shower is the simplest method of cooling the skin; if your hives are confined to a small area, an ice pack is useful. Because warmth worsens itching, avoid overheating and hot baths.

When your hives have cleared, keep taking the prescribed medicines in the same way for 2 more days. Once you have been free of hives for 2 days, *gradually* take less of your medicines over the next 5 to 7 days while your body eliminates the cause of your hives. If hives recur while you're tapering off the medicines, resume the original amount until the hives disappear.

Although hives usually clear quickly with treatment, they can be stubborn, and we may have to try different medicines. Sometimes, the amount of medicine needs to be increased. If your hives don't go away in a few days, or if they last more than 3 weeks, call this office.

Treatment Schedule

A. Take 1 _____ tablet _____ times a day. Do *not* take more than _____ tablets each day.

B. Take _____ tablets _____ times a day. If the medicine causes drowsiness, decrease to _____ tablets _____ times a day. If your hives are not controlled, you may increase the dose to _____ tablets _____ times a day.

C. At the end of supper, take _____, and before bedtime take _____. If groggy or "hung over" the next day, eliminate the supper dose. If the hives are only partly controlled, you may increase the bedtime dose to _____ or _____ tablets.

_____ is over-the-counter

_____ is over-the-counter

_____ requires a prescription

_____ requires a prescription

Hyperhidrosis

What is Hyperhidrosis?

Hyperhidrosis is the medical term for excessive sweating. The problem may be limited to the armpits, but often the palms and soles also sweat excessively. Excessive sweating becomes noticeable after puberty. Stressful situations such as examinations, job interviews, or an important date often aggravate excessive sweating. Unfortunately, most over-the-counter antiperspirants do not control hyperhidrosis.

Treatment

Treatment aims to control excessive sweating; it is not a permanent cure. The best control method is aluminum chloride hexahydrate in absolute alcohol. In the United States, a 20 percent aluminum chloride hexahydrate alcoholic solution is available by prescription under the name of Drysol. An over-the-counter preparation containing 13 percent aluminum chloride hexahydrate is sold over the counter under the name of Certain-Dri. Here is how to use your medicine:

1. Armpits: Apply the medicine at bedtime to your dry armpits. To prevent irritation, wash the medicine off in the morning with plain water. Do not use your regular daytime deodorant. Repeat the treatment nightly until the sweating is under control; then treat every other night, then every third night, to find the treatment frequency that prevents excessive sweating.

   Most people can control excessive armpit sweating by overnight applications of aluminum chloride hexahydrate. Sometimes, it is necessary to increase the medicine's penetration by covering the area with plastic film overnight. After applying the aluminum chloride medicine to your dry armpits at bedtime, cover them with a pliable plastic film such as Saran Wrap. Keep the plastic film in place with a T-shirt or similar light garment. In the morning, remove the plastic film and gently wash your armpits with plain water.

   Aluminum chloride may irritate your skin; if your armpits become sore or itchy, contact this office for advice. Until your excessive armpit sweating is controlled, apply only the aluminum chloride medicine and water to your armpits. Later, when the sweating is under control, you may try adding your daytime deodorant.

2. Palms and soles: The thick skin of the palms and soles is more resistant to aluminum chloride's effect. At first, apply the medicine at bedtime to your dry palms or soles, and in the morning, wash the medicine off with plain water. If in 10 to 14 days you do not see a decrease in sweating, cover your hands and feet overnight with plastic film. For your hands, use thin, pliable, plastic disposable gloves available at most drugstores. After applying the medicine, allow it to dry, and then put on the plastic gloves. Remove the gloves in the morning and wash your hands with plain water. For the feet, use plastic bags held in place with socks. Cut the plastic bags to size so that

they cover only your feet and not your legs. In the morning, remove the plastic bags and wash your feet with plain water. Repeat the aluminum chloride applications and plastic covering nightly for 1 to 2 weeks until you get the desired effect, then treat less often.

Usually, local applications of aluminum chloride hexahydrate provide satisfactory sweat control; when they fail, we can try internal medicines or electrophoresis. For almost everyone troubled by excessive perspiration, there is a treatment to control the problem.

Impetigo

What Causes Impetigo?

Impetigo is a skin infection caused by germs. It is most common in children and is contagious. Impetigo forms round, crusted, oozing spots that grow larger day by day. The hands and face are the favorite locations for impetigo, but it often appears on other parts of the body.

How does one get impetigo? While the germs causing impetigo may have been caught from someone else with impetigo or boils, impetigo usually begins out of the blue, without any apparent source of infection.

Treatment

When there are only a few spots, impetigo is best treated by applying mupirocin (trade name: Bactroban) ointment four times a day to every spot of impetigo. If you have thick crusts (scabs), it helps to remove them before applying the mupirocin. To loosen the crusts, apply a cloth wet with lukewarm water for 5 to 10 minutes, and then gently wipe off the crusts with a tissue. Next, apply a thin layer of mupirocin ointment to every spot of impetigo. Continue to apply the ointment until the skin has healed. You must use mupirocin ointment, because other antibiotic ointments are not effective.

When impetigo is widespread, it is best treated with antibiotics taken by mouth. It's important that you take the antibiotic until the prescribed supply is completely used up. If there is a lot of crusting, remove the crusts with water as described previously. If the crusts dry out and crack, apply _____ ointment; it can be purchased without a prescription.

Contagion

Impetigo is contagious when there is crusting or oozing. While it's contagious, take the following precautions:

1. Patients should avoid close contact with other people.
2. Children should be kept home from school for 1 or 2 days after beginning treatment.
3. Use separate towels for the patient. Towels, pillowcases, and sheets should be changed after the first day of treatment. The patient's clothing should be changed and laundered daily for the first 2 days.

These measures are necessary only during the contagious (crusting or oozing) stage of impetigo. Usually, the contagious period ends within 2 days after treatment starts. Then children can return to school, and special laundering and other precautions can be stopped. If the impetigo does not heal in 1 week, please return to this office for evaluation.

Isotretinoin (Accutane)

What is Isotretinoin?

Isotretinoin (trade name: Accutane) is a powerful drug used in the treatment of acne. Acne medicines aim to control acne until nature cures it; often, this takes years. Isotretinoin is unique in that it controls acne for months or years after the end of treatment. Four to five months of isotretinoin treatment usually lead to clearing of acne for 1 year or more *after medicine is stopped*. All other acne-controlling medicines are antibacterial agents, which are effective only while they are used.

Side Effects

Why shouldn't all acne patients take isotretinoin? Isotretinoin has significant side effects:

Side Effect	Frequency (%)
Chapped lips	100
Dry skin and itching	90
Dryness of nose, mild nosebleed	80
Irritation of eyelids and eyes	40
Joint and muscle pains	40
Temporary hair thinning	10
Rash	15
Intestinal symptoms	5
Urinary symptoms	5
Headache	5
Increased sensitivity to sunburn	5
Mood changes	1–2

Isotretinoin may increase the level of blood fats, sometimes to risky levels. Occasionally, it may affect the liver. This is why regular blood tests are necessary when you are taking isotretinoin; these tests must be done after you have fasted for 12 hours (no breakfast), so that the blood fat determinations are reliable. Baseline blood chemistry levels are established before patients start isotretinoin.

The most damaging side effect of isotretinoin is serious birth defects if taken during pregnancy. It is critically important for women not to take isotretinoin while pregnant and not to become pregnant while taking this drug. Women who are, or expect to be, sexually active while taking isotretinoin must use two effective methods of birth control. A woman who does get pregnant while taking isotretinoin must be prepared to have an abortion and must state this in writing before I will prescribe isotretinoin for her.

Isotretinoin may cause birth defects as long as 2 months after it is stopped. After that time, it is safe to become pregnant. Because the birth defects caused by isotretinoin are so serious, it is important not to share the pills with others.

We don't know whether isotretinoin taken by men can cause birth defects. It is best to not father a child while taking isotretinoin. If your partner is not using birth control, you should use a condom.

How Does Isotretinoin Work?

Isotretinoin decreases the amount of oil produced by the skin's sebaceous (oil) glands. It may be as long as 2 months before you see improvement in your skin. There's no medicine we can add to speed isotretinoin's action. In fact, sometimes acne gets worse during the first month or so of treatment. *Side effects, such as lip dryness, begin before the acne starts to clear.*

Treatment

Isotretinoin works best when taken with food, so remember to take it at mealtime. Taking the entire daily dose with supper is convenient and effective. Do not take vitamin A while being treated with isotretinoin; serious side effects may occur. Isotretinoin and vitamin A are closely related chemically. You should also stop any other acne treatment by mouth, because antibiotics may interact with isotretinoin. You may continue to apply medicine to your acne if you wish, but do not use Retin-A (tretinoin) while being treated with isotretinoin.

While you are taking isotretinoin, you will be checked monthly for your general condition and any side effects. Samples of your blood will be drawn for laboratory tests. If you tolerate any side effects and your blood tests are normal, isotretinoin will be continued for 4 to 5 months. After that time, acne usually is controlled. In most patients, improvement continues for 1 year or more after isotretinoin is stopped.

Serious problems from isotretinoin are rare, but everyone gets mild side effects such as chapped lips. You will be given a patient information sheet, Managing Side Effects of Isotretinoin (Accutane), dealing with these annoying but harmless side effects. If you feel you are having a serious reaction to isotretinoin, stop the medicine and call this office.

Long-Term Results

Isotretinoin is not a permanent cure for acne, although it often clears acne until nature clears your skin. Your skin may stay clear for months, even years, after isotretinoin is stopped. As long as it does, there's no need to return to this office.

In about one person in 10, acne comes back after 1 year. About one person in four has acne again after 2 years. If your acne returns, antibiotics may work, or you may be treated with isotretinoin again.

Keloids

What is a Keloid?

A keloid is greatly enlarged scar that projects above the skin surface. Skin heals by formation of scar tissue, which at first is often red and somewhat prominent. As time passes, a scar usually becomes flat. Unfortunately, sometimes scars enlarge to form firm, smooth, hard growths called keloids.

What Causes Keloids?

No one knows why keloids form. Although most persons never form keloids, others develop them after minor injuries or even insect bites or pimples. Keloids may form on any part of the body, although the upper chest and upper back are especially prone to keloid formation. Dark-skinned persons form keloids more easily than Caucasians. Keloids are a cosmetic nuisance and never become malignant.

Treatment

There is no satisfactory treatment for keloids. Surgical removal of a keloid usually results in a second keloid that is worse than the first. The best treatment is to inject a long-acting cortisone into the keloid itself. The cortisone acts slowly, and the keloid should be checked in 6 to 8 weeks. At this time, most keloids are flatter, and the injection is repeated, sometimes with a stronger cortisone. Although occasionally a single injection results in satisfactory flattening of a keloid, usually several injection treatments are needed.

Tretinoin (trade name: Retin-A) cream applied twice daily for at least 3 months often helps to flatten keloids. Because tretinoin cream irritates the skin, start by using it only once every other day. As the skin adjusts, apply it once daily. After another 2 to 3 weeks, use it two times a day. Continue the twice-daily applications for at least 3 months.

Covering a keloid with silicone gel sheeting is often effective in flattening a keloid. How this happens is not known. The sheeting must be kept in place 12 to 24 hours a day; it is customary to remove it once a day for cleaning and reapplying. Generally, it takes 2 to 3 months for the keloid to flatten.

Liquid Nitrogen Treatment

Liquid nitrogen is a cold, liquefied gas with a temperature of 196° below zero Celsius (−321° Fahrenheit). It is used to freeze and destroy superficial skin growths such as warts and keratoses. Liquid nitrogen causes stinging and pain while the growth is being frozen and then thaws. This discomfort usually lasts less than 15 minutes.

After liquid nitrogen treatment, your skin will become swollen and red; later, it may blister. Then a scab (crust) will form. It will fall off by itself. The skin growth will come off with the scab, leaving healthy new skin. Growths treated on the face heal fairly quickly, usually in about 2 weeks. The chest, back, and arms take longer to heal, often 4 to 5 weeks, whereas the lower legs may take 6 or more weeks to heal. Smaller lesions heal faster than larger ones.

If your growth required deep freezing, there may be considerable blistering and swelling, especially if your hands, scalp, or eyelids were treated. Sometimes, a blood blister may appear. The blisters and swelling are part of the treatment and will gradually heal by themselves. If a blister is annoyingly large, you may puncture it with a sterile needle and absorb the fluid with a tissue. Afterward, cover with a Band-Aid for 4 to 10 hours.

No special care is needed after liquid nitrogen treatment. Just ignore it. You can wash your skin as usual and use makeup or other cosmetics. If clothing irritates the area, cover it with a Band-Aid.

Sometimes, liquid nitrogen treatment fails. If the growth is not cured by liquid nitrogen, please make a return appointment.

Hair Loss in Men (Male-Pattern Alopecia)

What Causes Male-Pattern Hair Loss?

Men lose hair as they age. This is called "male-pattern hair loss" or "male-pattern alopecia," alopecia being the medical name for hair loss. Another name for the condition is androgenetic alopecia, referring to the two factors causing the hair loss: male sex hormones (androgens) and heredity (genes). Unfortunately, neither can be changed.

In male-pattern alopecia, the hair roots gradually shrink, and the hair becomes thinner and thinner until it disappears. This occurs in the deep layers of the skin and is not influenced by shampoos, hair applications, how long your hair is, or whether you dye your hair. You *cannot* make male-pattern hair loss *worse*.

Treatment

"Not good" summarizes the available forms of treatment for male-pattern alopecia. Until recently, only surgical hair transplants were of value in treating male-pattern alopecia. A few years ago, minoxidil (Rogaine) was introduced as a medicine that causes hair growth. Unfortunately, it has been disappointing.

When minoxidil was given internally as tablets for control of high blood pressure, patients grew unwanted hair on their faces, arms, and elsewhere. Naturally someone had the bright idea: "Will it grow hair if we apply it to the skin?" The answer is "Sometimes, but not very well." Minoxidil produces significant hair regrowth in about one out of five men when applied to the crown of the scalp, *if* they're young and have *early* hair loss. It is less effective in front of the scalp above the forehead. Four to six months of treatment with minoxidil are needed before hair growth becomes noticeable. If minoxidil is stopped, any new hair falls out; therefore, the applications need to be continued indefinitely. Although minoxidil is expensive, (about $2 a day), it appears to be safe; occasionally, it causes scalp irritation.

Will minoxidil prevent additional hair loss in men with early alopecia? Although minoxidil will cause significant hair regrowth in fewer than one out of five men, it's the *only* application that stimulates any hair growth at all. There are hundreds of tonics, lotions, stimulants, and hormone agents for which hair growth claims are made; none of them work.

Surgical hair transplants are the other treatment for male-pattern alopecia. Plugs of hair-bearing skin are taken from the back of the scalp—an area that resists male-pattern hair loss—and transplanted to the area of hair loss. This surgical approach grew out of an experiment performed by Dr. Norman Orentreich in New York in the 1950s to settle the question of whether poor circulation caused male hair loss. In men with early hair loss, he transplanted hair-bearing skin from the nape of the neck to just behind the forehead scalp line. The skin he took from the front of the scalp was transferred to the donor site on the back of the head. With time, as the hairline receded, the skin grafted onto the front of the scalp continued to grow hair. However, the skin transplanted from front to back lost its hair as the hairline receded.

This experiment proved the genetic difference between the hair roots of the front and back of the scalp. It also proved that blood supply is not a factor in causing hair loss, because only the hair roots, and not the blood supply, were transplanted. Dr. Orentreich realized that this was a way of treating hair loss, and hair transplantation has become an established technique for treating men with hair loss. Hair transplants require special expertise, are expensive, and are practical only in men with a plentiful supply of hair on their back scalp.

Wigs, hair weaving, and other techniques for augmenting scalp hair are popular. They do *not* influence male-pattern hair loss.

The most practical approach to male-pattern hair loss is to ignore this cosmetic nuisance. It has nothing to do with your general health. Vitamins, tonics, or massage will not grow hair. On the other hand, you cannot make it worse. Remember to wear a hat or use a sunscreen to prevent sunburn and sun damage to your scalp.

Managing Side Effects of Isotretinoin (Accutane)

Everyone who takes isotretinoin gets mild side effects. These are nuisances, and usually respond to the measures outlined on this sheet. Severe side effects are rare and are an indication for you to contact this office or your personal physician. Occasionally, it is difficult to determine whether a sore throat, fever, or other illness is a side effect of isotretinoin or the result of another illness, such as a viral infection. If this occurs, contact this office. Sometimes we stop the isotretinoin for a week to sort things out. It does no harm to interrupt the isotretinoin treatment temporarily.

Side Effect	What to Do
Chapped lips	Apply Vaseline (petrolatum, petroleum jelly) or a lip pomade such as Chapstick
Dry skin	Avoid soap. Apply mineral oil, Vaseline, or a lubricating lotion to your wet skin after bath or shower
Nosebleed	Gently apply Vaseline sparingly four to six times a day to the insides of the nostrils with a fingertip or Q-tip. Do *not* pick at scabs or crusts
Dry eyes	May cause problems for wearers of contact lenses; if so, wear glasses. If severe, consult your eye physician (ophthalmologist). Very rarely, patients on isotretinoin have reported significant visual problems. Should you experience any difficulty with night or daytime vision, stop the isotretinoin and consult an ophthalmologist.
Headache	If minor, take Tylenol or aspirin; if severe or persistent, stop isotretinoin and call my office
Joint or muscle pain	If mild, avoid strenuous exercise and take Tylenol or aspirin. If severe, call my office
Sun sensitivity	Use a sunscreen, preferably with an SPF (sun protection factor) of 25 or more
Mood changes	Depression can occur, but is rarely severe. If you experience a significant change in mood, stop isotretinoin and call my office

Cautions to Keep in Mind

1. Sexually active women must use two methods of contraception.
2. Do not take vitamin A or vitamin supplements containing vitamin A.
3. Avoid tetracycline and tetracycline-type antibiotics while taking isotretinoin.
4. Be sure to inform any physician whom you are seeing for any medical problem that you are taking isotretinoin.

Melanoma (Malignant Melanoma)

What is a Melanoma?

Melanoma, also called malignant melanoma, is a serious skin cancer. Melanoma develops from the pigment-producing cells of the skin, called melanocytes. Moles are groups of melanocytes. A melanoma may start from a cluster of melanocytes in a mole or from one of the melanocytes scattered throughout ordinary skin.

Melanoma is dangerous because it *can* spread to a distant part of the body (metastasize). Most other skin cancers, such as the common basal cell carcinoma, do not metastasize. If melanoma is treated before it metastasizes, it is curable; this is why we urge early diagnosis and treatment.

Melanoma has become much more common in the past 10 years. It is estimated that one of 100 Caucasians will develop it. Because dark skin color affords protection from melanoma, melanoma is much more common in Caucasians than in blacks or other darkly complected races.

What Causes Melanoma?

Melanoma is related to sun exposure, but not in the same way that most skin cancers are. The usual skin cancer—a basal cell carcinoma—appears on the exposed skin of persons who work outdoors, such as farmers, gardeners, sailors, and construction workers. However, melanoma is most common in fair-skinned, indoor workers who occasionally get sunburned. A history of repeated *severe* sunburns in childhood relates to melanoma. Although ordinary skin cancers are usually found on the most heavily sun-exposed areas such as the face and nose, melanomas often occur on the back and legs.

Recognizing a Melanoma

Melanomas are almost always colored and resemble a mole. How do you tell a mole from a melanoma? The only certain way is to have the growth surgically removed and examined microscopically. Because this cannot be done for every colored spot on your body, there are guidelines for which growths must be seen by a physician. Melanomas grow, and often do so irregularly. Their borders are usually notched or angular, and their color varies in different parts of the growth. Melanomas tend to be *asymmetrical,* have an irregular *border,* have variations in *color,* and have a *diameter* of more than 6 mm (¼ inch). These characteristics have been referred to as the ABCDs of melanoma and are best understood by comparing photographs of melanomas with benign moles. The Skin Cancer Foundation produces an excellent illustrated brochure on melanoma.

Most babies are born without moles. It's normal for children to grow new moles and have moles that change color, especially before and during puberty. Parents should not be alarmed by this normal process. Melanoma is *very* rare in children under the age of 16.

CAUTION. In an adult, a change in the color, shape, or size of a mole or the appearance of a new pigmented lesion is a reason to consult a physician.

Risk Factors for Melanomas

Your risk of developing a melanoma is increased in the following situations:

1. You have had a previous melanoma.
2. A close blood relative has had a melanoma.
3. You are fair-skinned, especially if you are a redhead who never tans and always burns.
4. You have atypical moles. Also called dysplastic moles, these are large, irregularly colored moles.
5. You have large numbers of moles.
6. You have had numerous severe sunburns.
7. You have a congenital nevus or birthmark mole—that is, a mole that was present at birth. Congenital nevi may have an increased risk of developing melanoma. Many physicians recommend that such birthmark moles be surgically removed in the mid-teens to prevent the possibility of their becoming a melanoma.

Treatment

Melanomas are treated by surgical removal. When a growth or mole is suspected of being a melanoma, it is customary to remove it for microscopic analysis. This procedure is called a biopsy. If the microscopic examination reveals it to be harmless, or benign, nothing more is needed. However, if the growth proves to be a melanoma, additional surgery is required, and a border of normal skin is removed to ensure that all skin cancer cells have been removed.

The success of surgery depends on whether the melanoma has been removed before it has had a chance to spread to a distant site (metastasize). Early, thin melanomas usually have not yet metastasized. If the melanoma is less than 0.76 mm thick (about 1/30 inch), we can be 98 percent certain that surgical removal will be curative. The older and thicker the melanoma, the greater the danger of metastasis. Fortunately, the majority of people with melanomas now see their doctor early and are cured of the disease.

What Should You Do?

Avoid excessive sun exposure, especially sunburns. It's especially important to protect children from sunburn with clothing or regular applications of an effective sunscreen. Adults should consult a doctor if any of the following occur:

1. There is change in size of a mole or obvious growth of a new mole.
2. A new or old mole has an irregular shape or notched border.
3. A mole develops various colors, especially shades of black or reddish violet.
4. A mole oozes, crusts, itches, or bleeds.

Moles

What Causes Moles?

Moles are harmless skin growths that may be flat or protruding. They vary in color from pink flesh tones to dark brown or black. Everyone has moles; some of us have many, others have only a few. The number depends on our genes and sun exposure. Moles sometimes appear in "crops," especially during the early teens. Sunlight causes moles to enlarge and new moles to grow. This is an additional reason to avoid the sun and never deliberately tan.

Moles begin to grow in infancy. New moles can develop at any age. When a mole develops, it usually stays for many years without becoming a problem. Some moles disappear by themselves; the elderly have fewer moles than do middle-aged adults. A growing or changing mole *in a youngster* is almost always harmless. On the other hand, if an adult's mole markedly changes in color or size or bleeds, it should be checked by a physician.

Sometimes, the skin around a mole loses its color so the mole appears to be surrounded by a white ring. This is called a "halo nevus" and is harmless. We leave it alone. In time the white ring often disappears.

Malignant melanoma, a rare cancerous growth that may resemble a mole, is dangerous and should be removed surgically. It seldom appears before the age of 16 years. Persons with a family history of melanoma have an increased risk of developing one.

Treatment

Most moles are harmless and safe to ignore. Moles may be treated under the following conditions:

1. A mole that has bled, has an unusual shape, is growing rapidly, or has changed color noticeably is giving warning signs of *possible* malignancy.
2. A mole that is irritated by your clothing, comb, or razor is only a nuisance, but your doctor can remove it to prevent ongoing irritation.
3. A mole that is unsightly can be removed for cosmetic reasons.

Treating a protruding mole is a simple procedure. After numbing the skin, the doctor removes the projecting part of the mole with scissors or a scalpel. The removed portion is sent to a laboratory for microscopic examination. The wound heals to leave a flat mole, but the color generally remains the same. As a rule, dark moles leave dark spots.

Complete destruction of a mole requires removing the full thickness of skin. The resulting scar may be more noticeable than the mole was. For that reason, I avoid complete removal of facial moles and urge you to forget about treatment. Instead, think of moles as beauty spots.

Moles sometimes grow annoyingly coarse hair, which may be safely removed by shaving or plucking. Permanent removal of the hair, which has roots deep within the skin, requires electrolysis or complete surgical excision of the mole.

The great majority of moles are harmless and best ignored. Protuberant moles that annoy you can easily be converted into flat moles by simple office surgery. Bleeding, rapid growth, unusual appearance, and sudden change in a mole are urgent reasons to consult your physician.

Molluscum Contagiosum

What is Molluscum Contagiosum?

Molluscum contagiosum consists of small, harmless skin growths caused by a virus. They resemble pimples at first. Later, when they enlarge, they often have a waxy, pinkish look and a small central pit.

Molluscum contagiosum can be spread from person to person by direct skin contact. It is harmless and never turns cancerous.

Treatment

There is no single perfect treatment of molluscum contagiosum, because we are unable to kill the virus. Individual lesions can be destroyed by a blistering agent, by liquid nitrogen, or by superficial surgical removal.

Sometimes, new lesions will form while existing ones are being destroyed. New growths should be treated when they become large enough to be seen.

Molluscum lesions may become red and sore when the body tries to reject the virus. Sometimes, a rash appears around the growths. These symptoms are harmless and can be safely ignored.

Nickel Allergy

What Causes Nickel Allergy?

Nickel allergy, like other allergies, may develop at any age. We don't know why some persons become allergic to nickel while others never do. Once you've become allergic to nickel, you are likely to have the allergy for many years.

Nickel allergy is especially common in women. It often prevents them from wearing jewelry. Persons allergic to nickel may break out from contact with nickel-containing or nickel-plated objects such as bracelets, earrings, zippers, bra hooks, and metal eyeglass frames. Although many coins contain nickel, they don't usually cause rashes.

Some persons are highly allergic to nickel and get a rash from even brief contact with nickel-containing metals, whereas others break out only after a long period of skin contact with nickel. All jewelry contains nickel; there is less nickel in 14- or 18-karat gold jewelry than in inexpensive costume jewelry. As a result, many are able to wear high-quality gold jewelry but break out when they wear cheaper costume jewelry.

Persons allergic to nickel can touch stainless steel without trouble, unless it's nickel-plated. Therefore, you don't have to worry about contact with stainless-steel instruments, tools, sinks, cutlery, or cooking utensils.

Treatment

Nickel-allergy rashes usually clear up when contact with nickel-containing metal is stopped and a cortisone medicine is applied to the rash. *Preventing* nickel-contact rashes requires avoiding skin contact with nickel-containing metals. This may be awkward, especially as far as wearing jewelry is concerned. When you want to wear your wedding ring or other "essential" jewelry, please try this compromise approach: Wear the jewelry only for short periods of time when you're away from home, and apply a cortisone cream to your skin before putting your jewelry on.

If your ears are pierced, you can obtain hypoallergenic earrings from companies such as H&A Enterprises, Inc., 143-19 25th Avenue, Whitestone, N.Y. 11357. Write and ask for a catalog.

Desensitization

There is no way to desensitize a person with nickel allergy with shots, pills, or any other method. Nickel allergy remains for years, although sometimes it gradually becomes less severe.

Perioral Dermatitis (Rosaceaform Dermatitis)

What is Perioral Dermatitis?

Perioral dermatitis is a rash of the skin around the mouth. It is seen mainly in women aged 20 to 50 years. Perioral dermatitis produces small, pimplelike bumps along with redness and scaling on the upper lip, chin, and cheeks. At times, it may itch or burn. This rash tends to come and go. Although it's cosmetically annoying, perioral dermatitis is harmless and does not scar.

Sometimes, the rash spreads to the upper cheeks, eyelids, and forehead. Then it's called rosaceaform dermatitis.

What Causes Perioral Dermatitis?

We don't know why women get perioral dermatitis or why it's rare among men. Perioral dermatitis is *not* caused by diet, cosmetics, germs, or viruses, and it is *not* contagious. We do know strong cortisone ointments applied to the skin can cause or aggravate perioral dermatitis, even though the rash seems to fade at first. But the improvement is only temporary; when the strong cortisone is stopped, the rash gets worse. Applying the strong cortisone again will set up a vicious cycle of ever-worsening redness, bumps, scales, and itching.

Treatment

Tetracycline taken by mouth usually produces improvement in 2 to 3 weeks. If you can't take tetracycline, other antibiotics by mouth are effective. Why tetracycline is effective in treating this condition remains a mystery, because perioral dermatitis is *not* an infectious disease. If you wish to avoid internal treatment, antibiotics applied to the skin are of benefit but are less effective than antibiotics taken by mouth.

If you have been applying a strong cortisone to your face, you must stop. You must not resume it, even though your rash gets worse. This flare-up is temporary. It usually goes away after 2 to 4 weeks of antibiotic treatment. If the flare-up is very severe, you may need to take cortisone by mouth for a short time.

Perioral dermatitis is unpredictable. In many patients, it disappears after 4 to 8 weeks of internal antibiotics. However, some patients need to take their antibiotic much longer. Perioral dermatitis may recur after months to years. If perioral dermatitis recurs, resume the treatment that worked previously. Remember, any strong cortisone ointment will make your perioral dermatitis worse. Don't use it on your face.

Pityriasis Rosea

What Causes Pityriasis Rosea?

Pityriasis rosea is a common, harmless skin disease. The cause is unknown, but we do know that:

- Pityriasis rosea is *not* contagious.
- Pityriasis rosea usually clears in about 3 to 6 weeks, sometimes a little longer. When clear, the skin returns to its normal appearance. There will be no scars.
- Pityriasis rosea is not related to foods, medicines, or nervous upsets.
- Pityriasis rosea always disappears by itself.
- A single, scaling spot often appears 1 to 20 days before the general rash. The rash covers mainly the trunk but may spread to the thighs, upper arms, and neck. Pityriasis rosea usually avoids the face, although sometimes a few spots spread to the cheeks.
- Second attacks of pityriasis rosea are rare.

Treatment

Nature always cures this disorder, but sometimes slowly. Treatment does not speed the cure. The rash of pityriasis rosea is irritated by soap; bathe or shower with plain water. This rash makes the skin dry; it helps to put a thin coating of mineral oil on wet skin after a shower or bath.

If the rash itches, treatment with a cortisone ointment usually brings prompt relief. Occasionally, when there is severe itching, 1 to 2 weeks of cortisone by mouth may be needed to bring the itching under control. The cortisone does not cure pityriasis rosea; it will only make you more comfortable while getting over the rash.

Poison Ivy and Poison Oak Allergy (Rhus Allergy)

What Causes Poison Ivy Rash?

Poison ivy and poison oak rashes are caused by allergy to the juices of these plants—called *Rhus* plants. You don't have to come in direct contact with the leaves, roots, or branches of *Rhus* plants to get the rash. The plant juice can reach your skin indirectly when you touch clothing or a pet that carries the plant juice.

Like other allergies, *Rhus* allergy is acquired; you're not born with it. Although some lucky people never become allergic to *Rhus* plants, most persons become sensitized at some time and remain allergic. Unfortunately, there's no way to desensitize persons allergic to *Rhus* plants. The many drops, tablets, and injections that supposedly produce immunity are of little value. Some have caused unpleasant side effects. I don't recommend them.

Contagion

Poison ivy or poison oak rash is not contagious. The fluid in the blisters does not spread the rash. *Rhus* rash doesn't appear immediately after exposure to the plant juice, but only after a time called the latent period. This latent period between exposure to the plant and appearance of the rash may be as short as 4 hours or as long as 10 days, depending on individual sensitivity and the amount of plant contact. Sometimes, more rash appears after treatment has begun. These new patches are areas that had a longer latent period.

Treatment

Rhus rashes are self-limited: eventually, they clear without treatment. Letting nature take its course is reasonable with mild *Rhus* rash, but severe rashes need treatment to ease the misery and disability they cause. Cortisones taken by mouth are dramatically effective in treating *Rhus* rash. It's safe to take these drugs for a short period (2 or 3 weeks). If you have a peptic ulcer, high blood pressure, or diabetes, you should take cortisone only under close medical supervision.

Medicines taken by mouth are usually needed during the early, severe stages of *Rhus* rash, because remedies applied to your skin may not penetrate deeply enough. For crusted or oozing areas, apply cool water compresses for 15 minutes two to four times daily. Ice packs or cold showers or baths will temporarily relieve itching. Some persons find they get more relief by putting very hot water on the itchy areas. After 12 to 24 hours, cortisone will control your rash and itch.

Improvement in your rash should be prompt and steady. Improvement depends on getting enough cortisone. If you don't improve steadily, please telephone this office so I can modify your treatment. Treatment changes can usually be managed by telephone; you probably won't have to make a return visit.

When the swelling has gone down, a regular-strength cortisone cream or ointment will help your rash heal. You will be given a prescription for a cortisone cream. Please don't use it until the swelling is gone and blistering has stopped; otherwise you will waste it. Don't put anything on your rash except the prescription cream and water. You may bathe or shower as usual; keep the water as cool as you can stand, and don't use soap on your rash, because it irritates.

Regular-strength cortisone ointments are not effective when there is swelling and blistering. However, an ultra-high-strength (class 1) cortisone ointment may help during the early stages of *Rhus* dermatitis. If the rash is mild or confined to a small area, the ointment alone may be able to control it.

Prevention

The only way to prevent *Rhus* rash is to avoid contact with the plant juice. It is traditional advice to wash with strong soap after poison ivy or poison oak exposure. This does no harm, but in order to prevent a rash, you must wash within 15 minutes of exposure. If you can do so, simple washing with water and mild soap will effectively remove any plant juice from clothing, pets, or tools. Strong soaps are unnecessary. *Rhus* plants may cause rashes throughout the year. Roots and stems of *Rhus* plants can cause a rash as easily as the leaves. If you can't recognize poison ivy or poison oak plants, have friends or neighbors point them out so you can avoid them.

Pruritis Ani (Rectal Itch)

What Causes Pruritus Ani?

Itching of the skin about the anus (opening of the rectum) is a common complaint. The skin is exposed to irritating digestive products in the stool; this may lead to an itchy rash, especially when stools are frequent. Often, the rash is worsened by vigorous use of toilet tissue or scrubbing with soap and water.

Anal itching is usually an isolated skin complaint in otherwise healthy persons, but in some people, it is part of a disorder involving other areas of the skin. Whether pruritus ani is an isolated problem or part of another skin disorder, irritation from stools and from cleansing after bowel movements keeps the rash going. You may find that coffee and spicy foods make it worse. These foods irritate the digestive tract and increase the number of stools or amount of mucus (liquid) secreted from the rectum.

Treatment

Treatment is intended to reduce irritation of the anal skin. Unfortunately, it is impossible to eliminate all irritation, because it is impossible to avoid contact of stool with the inflamed skin. Careful, thorough, gentle cleansing after bowel movements is *very* important. Moisten toilet paper with lukewarm water; dry toilet paper does not cleanse as well and also irritates your skin. Never use soap on the anal area. Cleansing with plain water, in either the shower or bathtub, will do the job.

You will be given a soothing preparation, which you should apply thinly with your fingertips after each bowel movement, at bedtime, and at other times during the day as directed. *Do not apply any other remedy, suppository, or medicine to your rash.* Only the prescription medicine, water, moist toilet paper, and clean underwear should ever touch inflamed anal skin.

Pruritus ani is frequently stubborn and requires months of local medication and gentle skin care. Pruritus ani often recurs. Therefore, don't throw your medicines away when you are free from itching, but keep them on hand in case your trouble returns. Some persons need to continue using the medication once or twice daily indefinitely, because the itching returns whenever they stop. Anyone who has had pruritus ani should, for at least 1 year, keep soap off the anal skin and use only wet toilet paper for cleansing after bowel movements. If the medicine no longer controls your rash, please return.

Psoriasis

What Causes Psoriasis?

Psoriasis is a common skin disorder affecting about 1 in 40 persons. In the United States, more than 4 million people have psoriasis. The cause of psoriasis is not known. Many persons with psoriasis have blood relatives with this disorder, which indicates that heredity plays a role.

In psoriasis, areas of the skin grow much faster than normal and form red, scaling patches. The scalp, elbows, and knees are the most common sites, but almost any part of the skin may become involved. Fortunately, psoriasis is only a skin condition and does not affect your general health. In rare cases it may be associated with arthritis. Psoriasis is a problem only because it itches and is unsightly. It is *not* contagious.

Psoriasis usually begins in young adulthood, although it can start in childhood or first appear in old age. In most cases, psoriasis is mild and is limited to a few areas of the body. In a small percentage of cases, large areas of the body may become involved. Psoriasis is unpredictable; patches may clear by themselves and even disappear for months or years.

Treatment

You will be given detailed, individualized instructions for treatment of your psoriasis. Treatment is temporarily effective, and may need to be continued for quite a while. You will find it reassuring to know the following: (1) diet does *not* affect psoriasis; (2) psoriasis does *not* cause baldness; and (3) psoriasis is *not* caused by nerves. A nervous upset sometimes worsens psoriasis, just as nervous upsets may worsen any illness.

It is important to keep your skin lubricated, because psoriasis tends to begin in dry, scaly skin. Go easy on soap and follow a skin-lubrication routine.

If you have psoriasis of the scalp, it helps to wash your hair often. A medicated shampoo is not necessary. Some other treatments used in psoriasis include the following:

1. Moderate sunlight exposure is often helpful. Don't get sunburned, because psoriasis may settle in areas of injured skin.
2. Ultraviolet light by itself often helps psoriasis. Ultraviolet light is even more effective when used with tar or anthralin.
3. PUVA treatment combines Psoralen (an internal medicine) with ultraviolet light A (i.e., PUVA = *P*soralen + *U*ltra *V*iolet *A*). This therapy is available only at certain centers, because it requires specialized light equipment. Although PUVA is an effective treatment for extensive psoriasis, like all other treatments, it is only of temporary benefit.
4. Etretinate (Tegison), given by mouth, is justified only in very severe psoriasis because it has many adverse effects.
5. Cytotoxic drugs such as methotrexate, given by mouth or injection, are used only for very severe psoriasis. *Cytotoxic* means *poisonous to cells,* and these drugs are used only with special precautions. Although psoriasis is an unsightly nuisance, it should not prevent you from leading a full, active life.

Anthralin Treatment of Psoriasis

What is Anthralin?

Anthralin is a medicine applied to the skin of people with psoriasis. It controls the extra-rapid growth of skin cells. It is not a cortisone, but a strong medicine that can cause the skin to become sore and irritated. Use it carefully, and only where directed.

Anthralin often produces lasting improvement in psoriasis. This is an advantage over cortisone ointments, which usually provide only temporary improvement. Anthralin stains clothing permanently and may temporarily discolor your skin.

Treatment

Anthralin is available both as a cream (Drithocreme) and as a greasy ointment (Anthra-Derm ointment) in concentrations of 0.1, 0.25, 0.5, and 1 percent. Sometimes, stronger concentrations of anthralin are needed; these must be prepared by a pharmacist.

In short-contact therapy, anthralin is applied for period of 5 to 30 minutes and then washed off. After washing off the anthralin, apply _____ to prevent skin irritation and staining. As your skin improves, gradually increase the time of application of anthralin. The longer anthralin stays on the skin, the stronger its action will be. When you get up to 30 minutes of anthralin contact, it's time to increase the strength of the anthralin medicine.

In using anthralin, please follow these directions:

1. Use only a very small amount of anthralin; apply it exactly to your psoriasis, and gently rub it in. If you apply too much anthralin, remove the excess with tissue. Start with _____ percent anthralin.
2. Do not apply anthralin to skin-fold areas. The armpits, groin, genital and rectal regions are "off limits" for anthralin because severe soreness may result.
3. After about _____ minutes, take a shower, and gently wash off the anthralin with a little soap. Dry yourself with an old towel, because anthralin may stain the towel.
4. Right after drying, apply _____ to all patches of psoriasis. It will minimize skin irritation and discoloration.
5. After a few days, gradually increase the time anthralin is left on your skin. The longer it is left on, the greater its effect. When you reach 30 minutes of anthralin contact, it is time to switch to a stronger concentration.
6. Repeat the treatment daily. However, if the anthralin causes annoying redness and tenderness, use it only *every other day* until your skin gets used to it. If there is severe irritation, please contact this office.
7. Please keep your follow-up appointment. Successful anthralin treatment requires close cooperation between you and your physician.

Retin-A for Acne

Retin-A (chemical name: tretinoin) is a relative of vitamin A that is applied to the skin to treat the blackheads and whiteheads of acne. Tretinoin gradually opens the plugged oil glands that cause blackheads and whiteheads. However, it has little effect on red, inflamed pimples. For these, other treatments are needed.

Tretinoin must be used carefully. It can irritate the skin and cause redness, dryness, and scaling. It's available in different strengths as a cream, gel, or liquid. For acne, we usually start with the 0.025 percent cream applied thinly at bedtime. For the first 2 weeks, use tretinoin only every other night so your skin adjusts to its drying effect. If you find every-other-night use too irritating, use it every third night. Apply only water, mild soap, and what your doctor has prescribed to your face. Do not apply astringents, drying agents, abrasive scrubs, or harsh soaps to your face while using tretinoin. Tretinoin may make you more sensitive to sunlight. Apply a sunblock to your face before spending time in the sun.

After using tretinoin every other night for 2 weeks, try using it every night. If nightly use causes too much drying and scaling, go back to using tretinoin every other night. You do not need to irritate the skin for tretinoin to work. If you develop anything more than mild redness and scaling, use tretinoin less often.

When using tretinoin, apply nothing to your face except (1) other medicines prescribed by me; (2) water; (3) a little soap once or twice daily; and (4) water-based makeup applied thinly during the day and washed off at night.

Tretinoin works slowly; it usually takes 2 months before your skin is better. Two to three months after starting treatment, please return for an evaluation of the result and possible adjustment of the medicine's strength. If you have pimples, you will need additional treatment with an antibiotic, either applied to the skin or taken by mouth.

Rosacea

What is Rosacea?

Rosacea is a fairly common annoying face rash of adults. The rash of rosacea has red areas and pimples. It is especially noticeable on the nose, mid-forehead, and chin. Rosacea pimples resemble the acne pimples of teenagers, and years ago rosacea used to be called acne rosacea. Rosacea is only a skin condition and is not related to your general health. Sometimes, eye irritation occurs in rosacea. Although in some persons rosacea causes mild itching or burning, its unsightly appearance is the usual reason for treating it.

What Causes It?

The cause of rosacea is unknown. Rosacea is stubborn and often lasts for years. Foods or beverages that cause facial flushing, such as alcohol, spicy foods, and hot soups and drinks, may make rosacea more noticeable. Strong cortisone ointments, when applied to the face, will worsen rosacea. If you have rosacea, avoid applying any cortisone medicines to your face.

Treatment

Antibacterial medicines are usually effective in controlling rosacea. Why antibacterial medicines work is not known; rosacea is not an infectious disease. Most persons improve with a locally applied antimicrobial called metronidazole. This comes in a gel form (trade name: MetroGel). It should be applied thinly in the morning and at bedtime. You may apply makeup over it.

MetroGel usually improves rosacea in 3 to 4 weeks. If your rosacea is not satisfactorily controlled after 2 months of MetroGel treatment, please return.

When rosacea is severe, or when there is eye irritation, we prescribe an antibiotic to be taken by mouth in addition to the MetroGel. Also, if your rosacea doesn't clear with MetroGel, you may be given an antibiotic to be taken by mouth instead. I usually use tetracycline, a widely employed antibiotic with a 30-year safety record. When tetracycline is prescribed, we ask that you return in 3 weeks to determine the response and future dose required.

Rosacea is usually a long-term problem that is only *controlled* by treatment. Most persons with this condition need to continue their treatment for months and even years.

Scabies

What Causes Scabies?

Scabies—also known as "the itch"—is an intensely itchy rash caused by a tiny mite or bug that lives in the skin. Because it is only 1/60 inch long, the scabies mite is almost impossible to see without magnification. The mite causing scabies usually lives on the hands, wrists, ankles, groin, and armpits. The *rash* of scabies is caused by allergy to the mite and may affect the entire skin except for the face. You may have only six or seven scabies mites but be covered with hundreds of itchy spots. The itching areas are an allergic reaction, and no mite can be found in them.

Scabies often resembles other rashes. The only way to find out whether you have scabies is for a doctor to scrape off a piece of skin and examine it under a microscope. Sometimes we treat scabies because we suspect it, even though we cannot find the mite.

Contagion

Scabies is spread by skin-to-skin contact. All members of your family and any sexual partners you may have *must* be treated at the same time you are being treated. The early stages of scabies may not itch; be sure all close personal contacts are treated, even if they are not itching. All contacts must be treated at the same time to prevent back-and-forth spread of the mites.

Scabies is *not* spread by clothes, towels, bedding, or eating utensils. There is no need to sterilize sheets, towels, blankets, or clothing.

Treatment

Treatment consists of applying a mite-killing medication to the entire skin of the body except the face and scalp. It is *very* important to apply the medicine to every bit of your skin below the face, including the genital area, feet, and hands. The medicine should remain on the skin for 24 hours. Please follow these directions exactly:

1. At bedtime, apply the medicine thinly to the entire skin from the neck downward. Rub it on every bit of skin, including the genital area, and be sure to apply it well to the hands, wrists, feet, and ankles.
2. If you wash your hands in the next 8 hours, put more of the medicine on your hands and wrists afterward.
3. The next day, reapply the medicine to your hands and wrists after breakfast and again after lunch. Try not to wash your hands for 1 hour after putting the medicine on your hands.
4. Shower 24 hours after applying the medicine to thoroughly remove it. You have finished your treatment. Do *not* use the medicine more often than directed by your doctor.

After the treatment, avoid soap, because scabies causes sensitive skin. If your skin is dry, apply a lotion or Vaseline at bedtime. The itching and rash may continue even though all the mites have been killed. This results from allergy to the mites and is called postscabetic dermatitis. Postscabetic dermatitis is not scabies, and it requires special treatment. Don't try to treat it with the mite-killing medicine. We advise a return visit 10 to 14 days after treatment to be sure that you are cured and comfortable.

Seborrheic Keratoses

What Causes Seborrheic Keratoses?

Seborrheic keratoses are harmless, common skin growths that first appear during adult life. As time goes by, more growths appear. Some persons have a very large number of them. Seborrheic keratoses appear on both covered and uncovered parts of the body; they are not caused by sunlight. The tendency to develop seborrheic keratoses is inherited.

Seborrheic keratoses are harmless and never become malignant. They begin as slightly raised, light brown spots. Gradually, they thicken and take on a rough, wartlike surface. They slowly darken and may turn black. These color changes are harmless. Seborrheic keratoses are superficial and look as if they were stuck on the skin. Persons who have had several seborrheic keratoses can usually recognize this type of benign growth. However, if you are concerned or unsure about any growth, consult a dermatologist.

Treatment

Seborrheic keratoses can easily be removed in the office. The only reason for removing a seborrheic keratosis is your wish to get rid of it—if it's unsightly, itches, or annoys you by rubbing against your clothes.

Skin Aging and Treatments

To have a pleasing appearance is a basic human desire. Everyone is bombarded with advertising for products that claim to help skin stay healthy and young-looking. What is true and what is fiction? Here are some facts that may help you develop your own skin-care routines.

Common Concerns

1. Skin aging. Everyone develops wrinkles with age. Remember that much of wrinkling results from sun damage, not age. Fair-skinned persons who have spent much time in the sun usually have skin that is much more wrinkled and weatherbeaten than people with dark skin. Fortunately, effective sunscreens are available so people can continue an active outdoor life while partially protecting themselves from the wrinkling and aging effects of the sun. Details are provided in the patient information sheet Sunlight and Your Skin. If you value your youthful looks, never deliberately sunbathe. Stop using tanning parlors. The ultraviolet rays they use damage the skin, although the operators will tell you otherwise.

2. Except for tretinoin (trade name: Retin-A), there is no antiwrinkle cream. Scientists have spent much effort and money in the search for a substance that will stop wrinkling and reverse skin aging. So far, they have only come up with tretinoin (Retin-A), which sometimes is mildly beneficial. This fact has not kept the market from being flooded with cosmetics, creams, and lotions that claim to make your skin more youthful and attractive. Usually, there is a "magic" ingredient, which may be called a vitamin, a hormone, royal jelly, placenta extract, collagen, aloe vera, or some other product of the promoter's imagination. These products are all worthless. If someone really had developed an antiwrinkle cream or preparation that preserved the youthfulness of skin, he wouldn't have to advertise. His only problem would be how to make enough to keep up with the demand.

3. Tretinoin has not lived up to its advertising as an antiwrinkle cream. Prolonged, regular applications sometimes produce modest improvement in fine wrinkling. In my experience, not more than one out of three feel it's worthwhile. Tretinoin may be more beneficial in evening out irregular, spotty tan discoloration.

    Tretinoin iritates the skin. Many people have had to stop using it because they couldn't tolerate the redness, dryness, and stinging it causes. Even when tolerated, tretinoin makes the skin sensitive. Persons using it must limit their sun exposure and should not undergo wax removal of facial hair. It appears that any improvement achieved by tretinoin requires continued tretinoin applications for maintenance.

4. Do moisturizers work? Yes and no. For most people, these products produce *temporary* lubrication and smoothing of the skin. After a few hours, the skin will be the same as before. Moisturizers do not prevent wrinkles or skin aging. Which moisturizer or lubricant to use? The one that feels best to you. If you have dry skin, find an inexpensive moisturizer or lubricant and use it

wherever you have dry skin—eyelids, neck, face, hands—and whenever you like. There is no point in having special moisturizers for certain areas or in having separate day and night creams. Do *not* use price as a guide. With expensive brands, you often pay mainly for packaging and advertising.

5. What's the best way to cleanse your skin? Use water and a *little* mild soap. If you have very dry, sensitive skin and cannot tolerate soap, water will get you clean enough. If you wear heavy makeup, use a cold cream to remove it and then use water to remove the cold cream. For most people, the kind of soap used makes little difference. Find one that your skin tolerates and you like. Then stick with it. Don't be sold on the idea that "deep cleansing" is necessary to rid your skin of dirt and "impurities." This is advertising hype. The same applies to abrasives, skin peelers, and beauty masks to "restore," "desquamate," or "renew" your skin. All these agents do is peel off dead, outer layers of skin, which, if left alone, would peel off spontaneously in a few days.

6. Can makeup cause pimples? Sometimes. Heavy, greasy makeup (such as stage makeup) can cause blackheads and pimples or aggravate acne in people who already have it. Most, but not all, water-based makeup is safe and does not worsen acne. If this matter concerns you, please discuss it with your dermatologist. No matter what makeup you use, thoroughly remove it at night, using a lot of water and a little soap.

7. Do facial exercises prevent wrinkles? No, they do *not*. The opposite is true. Facial movements cause wrinkles. Wrinkles actually flatten out and sometimes disappear in persons whose face muscles are paralyzed because of a stroke or nerve disease.

8. What can you do about wrinkles? By yourself, nothing. Tretinoin (Retin-A) provides modest improvement in fine wrinkling in a minority of users. Some physicians use face lifts, dermabrasion, deep chemical peels, or collagen injections to smooth out wrinkles. Face lifts, dermabrasion, and deep chemical peels are significant surgical procedures. They are expensive, painful, and require several weeks for recovery. Although sometimes these produce a great deal of improvement, this is not always the case. There may be a poor result or scarring.

9. Injecting wrinkles with material to puff them out has become popular. The three materials currently used are collagen, Fibrel, and the patient's own fat. Collagen is a protein derived from cattle, and there are concerns about injecting a foreign protein into a human. Negative skin tests are required; even then, there is a rare, unpleasant local reaction to collagen. When skillfully done, collagen injections can provide impressive short-term smoothing of wrinkles. Unfortunately, the improvement is temporary. After 6 to 12 months, the collagen is absorbed and the skin becomes as wrinkled as it was before the treatment. Fibrel is the trade name for a mixture of gelatin, the patient's plasma, and a chemical. Its results are less predictable than collagen's, and it is not widely used. Injecting your own fat cells would seem ideal. So far, this technique has not proven itself as the injected fat cells are usually absorbed in a matter of months.

If you value youthful looks and wish to avoid wrinkling, protect yourself from the sun. This is especially important if you are fair-skinned. Aside from that, there is nothing that prevents wrinkling or delays skin aging.

Cosmetics are a safe way to temporarily lubricate your skin and conceal blemishes and imperfections. Keep your cosmetic routine simple, and stick to a few products that agree with your skin. Don't get involved in elaborate routines with products such as cleansers, astringents, "deep cleansing," night creams, day creams, antiwrinkle creams, or skin tighteners. Keep in mind that cosmetics only conceal, they don't heal.

Skin Tags

What Causes Skin Tags?

Skin tags are little growths some persons develop about the neck, armpits, or groin. Their name perfectly describes them, for they look like little bits of skin. The medical name for a skin tag is acrochordon. The tendency to develop skin tags is inherited. Skin tags sometimes turn tan or brown. They are harmless and *never* become cancerous or malignant. At times, a skin tag may become sore from rubbing against clothing or jewelry. Although annoying, this is *not* dangerous.

Treatment

Skin tags are harmless and are treated only if *you* find them unsightly or a nuisance. Removal of skin tags is a simple office procedure. They may be frozen with liquid nitrogen or snipped off with surgical scissors. Healing is usually complete in 1 or 2 weeks.

New skin tags may form even if *all* existing tags are removed. There's no way of preventing them.

Sunlight and Your Skin

Why Avoid the Sun?

Sunlight permanently damages skin. Ordinary sun exposure during tanning and outdoor sports causes permanent skin changes. These changes build up over the years, so that even moderate repeated sun exposure causes visible skin damage. Most of the wrinkling, roughening, and freckling that appear on the face, hands, and arms of Caucasian adults come from sun damage, not age. You can see this if you compare less sun-exposed areas, such as the undersides of your arms, with sun-exposed areas such as your face, neck, or upper surfaces of your arms. The natural coloration of your skin (pigment) protects you from the damaging effects of sunlight. Persons with fair skin, who have little pigmentation, are more prone to sun damage than dark-skinned individuals.

The Skin-Damaging Effects of Sunlight

The skin-damaging effects of sunlight gradually lead to roughening, freckling, and wrinkling. Many people in their 30s and 40s are unhappy because their wrinkled, roughened, sun-damaged skin makes them appear 10 or 15 years older. Unfortunately, there's no way to undo these changes. Young people should realize that they'll ultimately pay a very steep price for the temporary glamour of a deep suntan.

A more serious effect of sun damage is skin cancer. Sun damage is the chief cause of skin cancer. Again, fair-skinned individuals are much more susceptible to skin cancer. Skin cancer rarely occurs in blacks. As you might expect, skin cancer tends to occur on sun-exposed areas such as the face, neck, shoulders, and arms. Although skin cancers can usually be removed by minor surgery in a doctor's office, it's better to prevent them.

Ultraviolet Rays—The Invisible Enemy

Sunlight contains both ordinary, harmless, visible light and shorter, invisible light rays called ultraviolet light. Tanning, burning, and skin damage from sunlight are caused by ultraviolet rays. Because ultraviolet rays produce both tanning and skin damage, it's impossible to tan "safely" and avoid permanent skin damage. Discussions on sunbathing that describe "safe" tanning refer to the avoidance of sunburn. With proper timing, most persons can get a deep tan without a sunburn. However, no one can get a tan without some skin damage. The ultraviolet light used by tanning parlors, spas, and gymnasiums causes skin damage despite claims of safety. Avoid tanning parlors.

Instant Tanning Lotions

Instant tanning lotions are a safe way to "tan" without the sun. There are many different brands. All of them require repeated application to maintain a darkened skin color. This artificial "tan," although safe, does *not* protect against sunburn.

Sun-Protective Measures

There are two basic ways of protecting your skin from the damaging effects of ultraviolet rays: (1) by blocking out all light with opaque material such as clothing and (2) by using a chemical sunscreen that selectively absorbs ultraviolet rays. Blocking out all light with clothing is most effective. Clothing varies in its ability to stop the sun's rays. Thin T-shirts provide poor protection. Several manufacturers now make lightweight sports clothing designed to block the sun's rays. Certain sun protectives depend on the same principle. They coat the skin with a paintlike pigment that mechanically blocks light. These "chemical-free" products work well, but they're messy and rather unsightly.

There are many clear sunscreens that absorb ultraviolet light; the better ones are often called sunblocks. These "clean" sunscreens usually contain several ultraviolet-absorbing chemicals. Some persons are allergic to certain sunscreens, so test any new sunscreen on a small skin area before spreading it all over your body.

Many sunscreens irritate sensitive skin, especially about the eyes. If you find that one product irritates your skin, try another brand. Eye irritation can be a problem when heavy sweating causes sunscreen to run from the forehead into the eyes. One way to prevent this is to apply a barrier strip of a greasy, pomade-type sunscreen just above the eyebrows.

Sun protectives are labeled with a number called a sun-protection factor (SPF). The higher the SPF number, the better the protection. The best sunscreens have an SPF of 25 or more, and these products are what you should use. Women can use makeup along with a sun-protective. The sun protective should be applied first, and the makeup can be applied over it. The makeup itself, especially if heavily colored, provides some sun protection.

Water removes many sunscreens. Fortunately for swimmers, surfers, and sailors, sun blocks with significant water resistance are available. These products are usually labeled "waterproof" or "amphibious formula." Waterproof sun protectives should be applied 20 to 40 minutes before water exposure so they can bind to the skin.

Remember to put on another coat of sunscreen after swimming or bathing. If you're sweating heavily, use some more sunscreen every 1 or 2 hours. If you're in very bright sunlight, it's wise to protect your skin as much as possible with clothing (e.g., long sleeves, gloves, wide-brimmed hats) and use one of the "clean" chemical sunscreens on the parts of your skin exposed to the sun.

Protect your lips from sun damage. The darker lipstick shades are effective for women. Men and women who don't wear lipstick should use an ultraviolet-absorbing lip pomade. These greasy, stick-type, pomade sun protectives are also useful for applying about the eyes, because they don't run into the eyes. Choose a pomade with an SPF over 15.

You should aim to minimize sun exposure, not avoid it. Being outdoors is fun and healthful; *do not* let fear of sun damage keep you inside during sunny weather. *Do* use sun protectives when enjoying sports or a walk in the sun.

The Skin Cancer Foundation has prepared a set of guidelines for sun protection; the following rules have been adapted from their list. Think of them as the "Twelve Commandments" for preserving your skin.

1. Minimize sun exposure between 10 A.M. and 3 P.M. (11 A.M. to 4 P.M. daylight saving time), when the sun is strongest.
2. Wear a hat, long sleeves, and long pants when in the sun. Choose tightly woven materials for greater protection from the sun's rays.
3. Apply a sunscreen before every exposure to the sun, and reapply it liberally every 2 hours as long as you stay in the sun. The sunscreen should be reapplied after swimming or perspiring heavily. Use a sunscreen with a sun-protective factor (SPF) of 25 or more.
4. Use a sunscreen during high-altitude activities such as mountain climbing

and skiing. At high altitudes, there is less atmosphere to absorb the sun's rays, and your risk of burning is greater. The sun also is stronger near the equator.

5. Don't forget to use sunscreens on overcast days, because the damaging ultraviolet rays penetrate clouds.

6. Individuals at high risk for skin cancer (e.g., outdoor workers, fair-skinned individuals, persons who have already had skin cancer) should routinely apply sunscreens in the morning as basic sun protection. Reapply the sun protective every 2 hours while exposed to the sun.

7. Photosensitivity (an increased sensitivity to sun exposure) is a possible side effect of certain medications, drugs, cosmetics, and birth control pills. If this occurs, you may need to be extra careful to avoid sun exposure.

8. If you develop an allergic reaction to your sunscreen, change sunscreens. One of the many products on the market today should agree with your skin.

9. Beware of reflective surfaces. Sand, snow, concrete, and water can reflect more than half the sun's rays onto your skin, even when you're sitting in the shade.

10. Avoid tanning parlors. The ultraviolet light in tanning booths causes premature aging and increases your risk of developing skin cancer.

11. Keep young infants out of the sun. Begin using sunscreens on children at 6 months of age, and allow sun exposure only in moderation.

12. Teach children sun protection early. Sun damage occurs with each unprotected sun exposure and accumulates over a lifetime.

Surgery Done in the Office

Your skin growth will be excised (removed surgically) in the office and will be sent for microscopic examination to be certain it has been completely removed. Unless otherwise instructed, please eat normally and take all regularly prescribed medications. After surgery, most patients may resume their usual activities; sometimes, there are temporary restrictions on sports, dancing, or other physical activity. You will be able to drive.

Cosmetics

Do not apply *any* cosmetics or creams to the area of surgery and the surrounding skin. If you are scheduled for surgery on the face, do not apply any cosmetics to your face, eyelids, or eyebrows. Do not use any blusher, foundation, moisturizer, mascara, eyeliner, eyebrow pencil, or any other cosmetic.

Anesthesia

We use Xylocaine for local anesthesia; it stings briefly when injected, but there is *no* pain during surgery. The anesthetic numbs only the area of surgery. You will be conscious during surgery, and afterward, you will be able to drive home.

Cautions

Please tell us if:

1. You are taking blood thinners.
2. You have ever had a reaction to a local anesthetic such as Novocain or Xylocaine.
3. You have heart trouble.
4. You have a pacemaker.
5. You are taking aspirin.
6. You are taking anti-inflammatory or anti-arthritis medicines.
7. You are taking propranolol (Inderal) or another beta-blocker.
8. You are allergic to antibiotics.
9. You are allergic to tape.
10. You have been advised to take antibiotics before surgery.

A caution about aspirin: Aspirin makes people bleed more easily, and we prefer that patients not take it for 7 days before surgery and for 2 days after surgery. If you are taking aspirin or an aspirin-containing medicine *on your own,* please stop it for 7 days before surgery. However, if you are taking aspirin on a doctor's order, ask your doctor if you can temporarily stop it and *inform us* of the decision *before* the surgery date.

Stitches

Stitches (sutures) are used to close the wound after surgery. The type of stitch we use depends on the surgery and your skin. Stitches that need removal are usually taken out 4 to 14 days after surgery. Stitch removal tickles, and takes only a few minutes. Sometimes we use stitches that dissolve by themselves.

Postoperative Care

Your wound will be bandaged, and you will be given written instructions telling you exactly how to take care of it.

Discomfort

Postoperative discomfort is usually mild, and lasts only 12 to 24 hours after surgery. If it lasts longer, or if you have severe pain, please call this office. If a painkiller is needed, take Tylenol. Remember, *no* aspirin for 48 hours after surgery.

Scarring

When cut skin heals, it does so by forming a scar. Every effort will be made to minimize the scar produced by your surgery. Often, a scar may be barely visible, especially if the skin is wrinkled. However, on the chest, shoulders, back, arms, and legs, scars may spread, often become thickened, and may be noticeable.

Questions

If you have any questions or concerns, please ask. If you'd like to bring someone with you, please do. You may also have them present during surgery.

Care After Superficial Surgery

The scab (crust) that covers your skin surgery site is nature's bandage, and healing takes place beneath the scab. The scab will fall off by itself when healing is nearly complete. Please follow these directions:

1. Apply _____ (once) (twice) daily to the scab with a cotton-tipped applicator.
2. Leave the scab uncovered overnight.
3. During the day, either leave the scab uncovered or cover it with a Band-Aid, whichever you prefer.
4. You may apply makeup or powder over the scab.
5. It's best to keep the scab dry. You may get it wet temporarily, provided you dry the scab gently afterward. When swimming, protect the scab with a Band-Aid. Be sure to remove the wet Band-Aid when you come out of the water.
6. If the scab cracks or oozes, buy a tube of _____ ointment (no prescription needed) and apply it thinly five times a day.
7. If the skin around the wound becomes red, swollen, and painful, you may have an infected wound. Call this office promptly.

Wound Care

Following these directions will speed up the healing process:

1. While the wound is raw or oozing, cover it with a Band-Aid to which you have applied a little Polysporin or bacitracin ointment.
2. Polysporin and bacitracin ointments are two antibiotic ointments available without prescription. Antibiotic ointments prevent wound infection and keep the bandage from sticking to the wound surface.
3. When washing your skin, avoid the wound area. There's no harm in getting the bandage temporarily wet; if you do, apply a fresh bandage with a little antibiotic ointment.
4. Wipe off any pus on the wound surface with a clean tissue when you change your bandage.
5. Wounds may bleed. Bleeding will usually stop if you apply pressure over the bandage for 10 minutes by the clock.
6. When the wound has healed or is covered by a dry crust, remove the bandage and leave the wound exposed. Any sticky tape remnants around the wound can be removed with a cotton-tipped applicator moistened with nail-polish remover.
7. If the skin around the wound becomes red, swollen, and painful, you may have an infected wound. Call this office promptly.

Care of the Sutured (Stitched) Wound

Keep your wound dry and covered with a bandage for the first 2 days after surgery. If you change the bandage, use sterile gauze or a Band-Aid to which you've applied a small amount of Polysporin or bacitracin (antibiotic) ointment. No prescription is needed. After 2 days, you may get the bandage wet. If you do, remove the wet bandage promptly and replace it with a dry bandage spread with antibiotic ointment.

Removal of the stitches is painless and, depending on the type of surgery, is done 2 to 14 days later. The wound will then be left open, or tape may be used to protect it and keep it closed. You may get the tape wet. Leave it on until it becomes loose (in 4 to 10 days).

Discomfort and swelling are usual between 6 and 20 hours after surgery. If they're annoying, take acetaminophen (Tylenol) or a similar mild, *non-aspirin* pain-killer. Avoid aspirin and medicines containing aspirin for 2 days after surgery, because they may cause easy bleeding. If the pain continues or if severe discomfort or swelling develops, please call this office promptly.

Bleeding sometimes occurs after surgery. You can ignore a little bleeding, but you should control heavier bleeding by putting firm pressure on the wound with a tissue or a clean cloth. Do this, without stopping, for 10 minutes by the clock. Should the amount of bleeding concern you, or if it is not controlled after continuous pressure for 10 minutes, please call this office.

Care of Wounds Closed with Dissolving Stitches

Your wound has been closed with stitches that dissolve by themselves. They will fall out as the wound heals. They do not need to be removed by a physician.

The wound is covered with two different dressings. Next to the skin is a tape support that *must be left in place*. On top of the tape support is a gauze bandage.

1. Keep the wound dry for 2 days. After that, you may get it wet.
2. Remove the gauze bandage on _____.
   Underneath the gauze dressing is a tape support. *Do not remove the tape support.*
3. Leave the tape support, which helps the wound to heal, in place until _____ or longer, if possible. After that, if the tape loosens, you may gently remove it.
4. When the tape is off, remove any remaining tape adhesive with nail-polish remover or acetone.
5. From 6 to 20 hours after surgery, you may expect some discomfort and swelling. You may take a mild painkiller such as acetaminophen (Tylenol). If the pain continues or if severe discomfort or swelling develops, please call this office promptly. Do not take aspirin.
6. Bleeding sometimes occurs after surgery. You can ignore a little bleeding, but you should control heavy bleeding by putting firm pressure on the wound with a clean tissue or cloth *for 10 minutes by the clock*. If the amount of bleeding concerns you, or if it's not controlled after continuous pressure for 10 minutes, please call this office.

Tetracycline Treatment of Skin Disorders

Tetracycline is an antibiotic taken internally for the treatment of acne and other skin conditions such as rosacea, perioral dermatitis, and rosaceaform dermatitis. Because tetracycline does not cure but only suppresses these skin disorders, the antibiotic needs to be continued until the disease runs its course. It may be necessary to continue taking tetracycline for months or years. Long-term treatment with tetracycline is remarkably safe; we have had over 30 years of experience with it.

Dosage

Patients differ in the amount of tetracycline they need. The amount necessary to control your skin disorder may be as little as one pill a day or as much as 12 pills a day. Whatever the total amount of pills, take them twice daily with a full glass of water on an empty stomach. Take half the total daily amount on arising, and the other half in the midafternoon or early evening, both with a full glass of water. A good system is to count out the entire daily amount first thing in the morning when you are in the bathroom. Take half of that dose immediately, and put the other half in a small glass or dish near your toothbrush as your *memory device*. If the "memory device" glass isn't empty when you brush your teeth at bedtime, it means that you forgot to take the pills earlier and it is time to take them now with a full glass of water. It's best to take the tetracycline in the afternoon or evening, but if you forget, take it at bedtime.

Tetracycline should be taken on an empty stomach, because food—especially dairy products—interferes with the absorption of tetracycline into the blood. Dairy products form an insoluble calcium-tetracycline complex, preventing the medicine from getting into your blood. You may take tetracycline 1 hour before or 1.5 hours after meals. The morning is an exception: If you take your tetracycline on arising with a full glass of water, you may have breakfast in 30 minutes. If you forget to take your tetracycline on an empty stomach, don't skip the dose; take it on a full stomach.

Cautions

Tetracycline is a remarkably safe medicine. Many people have taken it for more than 10 years without problems. However, no medicine is without side effects, so please read the following precautions:

1. Tetracycline may interact with birth control pills, and *may possibly* cause birth control pills to fail. Birth control pills are not 100 percent effective; there have been rare pregnancies even when they were taken faithfully. We don't know whether tetracycline or other antibiotics used in treating acne significantly increase this failure rate. For many years, women have suc-

cessfully combined birth control pills with tetracycline in treating their acne. Most dermatologists continue to prescribe tetracycline for women taking birth control pills.

2. Tetracycline may make you sunburn more easily. The sun sensitivity depends on the amount of tetracycline you are taking. On one or two pills a day, there is little increase in sun sensitivity. On four pills a day, it's wise to be cautious at the beach, when skiing, or at other times of intense sun exposure. If you are taking more than four pills daily, use a sunscreen if you are going to be exposed to strong sunlight or if you will be outside in spring or summer, even on an overcast day. Ultraviolet light, which causes sunburn, passes through clouds.

3. Tetracycline causes a vaginal yeast infection in one of eight women; it may result in genital itching and a vaginal discharge. This side effect is annoying, but harmless. It responds promptly to treatment with antiyeast suppositories or cream while you continue your tetracycline. If you develop yeast vaginitis, please call this office for advice.

4. Stomach and intestinal side effects may occur. A little nausea or mild cramps may disappear as you get used to the medicine. However, if vomiting, severe cramps, or diarrhea occur, you should stop the medicine and call this office or your personal physician.

5. Tetracycline interacts in the digestive tract with calcium, iron, and antacids to form insoluble compounds. As a result, you do not absorb the tetracycline, and you do not benefit from the iron, calcium, or antacids. If you are taking iron, calcium, or antacids, be sure you allow at least 2 hours between taking tetracycline and any of these medicines.

Reasons for Not Taking Tetracycline

1. Pregnancy.
2. Nursing an infant.
3. Age under 8 years, because tetracycline may cause permanent discoloration of the teeth.
4. Taking barbiturates or phenytoin (Dilantin), because tetracycline interacts with them.
5. Lithium, because tetracycline interacts with it.

Tinea Cruris ("Jock Itch")

What Causes Tinea Cruris?

"Jock itch" refers to any itching groin rash of men and is not a medical term. There are many causes for "jock itch"; when caused by a fungus, the rash is known as tinea cruris. The fungus causing tinea cruris is a microscopic plant that grows in the outer skin and prefers moisture. When this fungus infects the feet, it is called athlete's foot (tinea pedis).

Contagion

Fortunately, tinea cruris is not contagious. Direct person-to-person spreading is not a problem. The patient's own case of athlete's foot is the usual source of infection and reinfection of the groin.

Treatment

Tinea cruris is treated by applying the antifungal medicine _____ thinly twice a day with your fingertips. Spread the medicine on sparingly, and massage it in gently until it disappears. To prevent recurrences, continue to apply the antifungal medicine for 2 weeks after the rash has cleared.

Apply nothing else to your groin except water. Cleanse your groin with plain water, because soap aggravates groin rashes.

Tinea cruris usually clears promptly with antifungal medicines applied to the skin. If it doesn't, you may need 10 to 14 days of treatment with an antifungal antibiotic taken by mouth. Tinea cruris is only *one* cause of groin itching. If your rash does not improve, please return for further evaluation.

Prevention

Tinea cruris often recurs. Warmth and moisture encourage the fungus to grow. You can help prevent recurrences by drying thoroughly after bathing, wearing loose cotton underwear, and dusting a bland powder on your groin once or twice daily. After swimming, put on dry clothes right away; do not wear a wet swimsuit for long.

Tinea Pedis ("Athlete's Foot")

What Causes Tinea Pedis?

Athlete's foot is a skin infection caused by a type of mold called a fungus. The fungus that causes athlete's foot prefers moist, warm skin; this is why athlete's foot rash favors the folds between toes and is often worse in hot weather. Not all foot rashes are athlete's foot—only those caused by fungus growing in the skin.

Athlete's foot fungus may stay in the skin indefinitely. Even if the rash seems to have been cured, microscopic examination may reveal the fungus to be present. Although medicines will clear the rash, the fungus may merely be "lying low" and may cause the same rash again.

Spread

Athlete's foot rash rarely spreads to other parts of the body. Sometimes the same fungus that causes athlete's foot will cause a groin rash in men (jock itch). However, a fungus rash of the groin is a different problem and is not related to the treatment or activity of athlete's foot.

Contagion

Can you give athlete's foot to other people? It's possible. However, special precautions at home are pointless, because there is no way your family can avoid exposure to the fungus *outside* the home. In our society, everyone is exposed to the fungus causing athlete's foot; why only some people get it is not known.

Treatment

Athlete's foot is usually well controlled by application of antifungal liquids, creams, or ointments. For control of your athlete's foot, apply _____ *very* thinly once daily with the fingertips and massage in well. Continue until the skin looks normal.

Severe cases of athlete's foot may require an antifungal medication taken by mouth. Sometimes, infection with bacteria complicates athlete's foot, and antibiotics are needed to kill the germs.

Athlete's foot may come back, especially in hot weather or when you wear poorly ventilated shoes. To prevent this, keep your feet dry. Dry well after bathing, change socks frequently, and wear well-ventilated shoes, especially in summer. An antifungal powder such as _____ (available without a prescription) applied to the feet in the morning also helps prevent reactivation of athlete's foot.

Should your athlete's foot rash return, resume daily use of the antifungal medicine originally prescribed. If the rash does *not* improve rapidly, return to this office for further medical care and evaluation.

P–117

Tinea Versicolor

What Causes Tinea Versicolor?

Tinea versicolor is a harmless skin disorder caused by a germ living on normal skin. Usually this germ—which all of us have on our skin—grows sparsely and is not visible. In some individuals, it grows more actively. This causes the slightly scaling patches on the trunk, neck, or arms known as tinea versicolor. On untanned skin, tinea versicolor rash is pink to coppery tan. On tanned skin, the tinea versicolor patches are lighter, because tanning doesn't occur in the rash areas. The failure to tan is temporary; the skin tans normally after the rash has cleared.

Tinea versicolor is *not* contagious. Tinea versicolor is more common in hot, humid climates and often comes back in the summertime.

Treatment

Although many treatments will temporarily clear tinea versicolor, we do not have a permanent cure. Tinea versicolor—being caused by a normal skin inhabitant— tends to recur. When tinea versicolor recurs, repeat the treatment you've found to succeed. We'll describe a number of different treatments, since more than one approach may be necessary. Any of the following treatments will clear more than 90 percent of cases of tinea versicolor.

1. Selenium sulfide suspension, 2.5 percent, applied to the affected area before showering. Massage in well and allow to remain on the skin for 10 minutes before rinsing off. Repeat once daily for 7 days. Selenium sulfide may also be used as a *single* treatment; apply it at bedtime, leave it on overnight, and shower it off the next day. Repeat once a month until clear.
2. Shampoos containing zinc pyrithione, applied to the skin 10 minutes before showering. Continue this treatment daily for 2 weeks. Rub the shampoo in thoroughly (a bath brush is recommended), and let it remain on the skin for 10 minutes. Shampoos containing 2 percent zinc pyrithione are available over the counter.
3. Propylene glycol, 50 percent in water, applied twice daily for 2 weeks. Propylene glycol is a clear liquid without stain or odor, and it is inexpensive. Apply it thinly and massage it in thoroughly.
4. Certain prescription antifungal creams, applied thinly once or twice daily, are an effective but expensive treatment.
5. Ketoconazole, taken by mouth for 2 days. Take two ketoconazole tablets in the morning with orange juice, grapefruit juice, lemonade, or similar citrus juice 2 days in a row. This course of a total of four tablets is the simplest and best treatment when tinea versicolor involves large areas of your skin. However, because any internal medicine may cause undesirable side effects, ketoconazole treatment is reserved for extensive or stubborn cases of tinea versicolor. Usually, the tinea versicolor clears 3 to 4 weeks after taking the ketoconazole. If the tinea versicolor recurs, you may take another 2-day course of ketoconazole, provided you have waited at least 3 months before repeating the dose.

Warts

What Causes Warts?

Warts are harmless skin growths caused by a virus. They have a rough surface on which tiny dark specks may be seen. They may grow on any part of the body. Their appearance depends on their location. On the face and tops of the hands warts protrude, while on such pressure areas as the palms of the hands and soles of the feet, they're pushed inward. Warts on the bottoms of the feet (called plantar warts) grow inward from the pressure of standing and walking and are often painful.

Warts are common. They may bleed if injured. However, they never turn cancerous.

Since warts are caused by a virus, they are slightly contagious. Warts may spread on the body, since a wart is the source of a virus that can seed other areas. We don't know why some persons get warts easily while others never get them. There's no way to prevent warts.

People have been trying to cure warts for thousands of years. The "success" of folk remedies for warts is due to the fact that warts often disappear by themselves, especially in young children. This spontaneous disappearance is less common in older children and adults.

Treatment

There is no single perfect treatment of warts, because we are unable to kill the virus. Treatment consists of destroying the wart. Warts can be destroyed with surgery, by freezing with liquid nitrogen, or with chemicals. The treatment to be used on your warts depends on their location and size, your type of skin, and the physician's professional medical judgment.

Sometimes, new warts will form while existing ones are being destroyed. All we can do is treat the new warts when they grow large enough to be seen.

Warts in the genital area require special consideration. Although genital warts are *not* cancerous, in women, they may cause cancerous changes in the cervix. Women with genital warts should have a Pap smear performed by their personal physician or gynecologist. In adults, genital warts are usually transmitted through sexual intercourse. To prevent further contagion, genital warts should be faithfully treated until they have cleared. Men with penile warts should use condoms to prevent transmission of warts to their sexual partners.

No matter what treatment is used, warts occasionally fail to disappear. They may also return weeks or months after an apparent cure. Don't become concerned if a wart recurs. Please make an appointment for a return visit. The treatment will be repeated, or a different method will be used to destroy the wart.

Plantar Warts

What Causes Plantar Warts?

Plantar warts are ordinary warts of the sole, or plantar surface, of the foot. Since plantar warts are on a pressure area, they grow inward and are often tender and painful. Like other warts, plantar warts are caused by a virus and are harmless.

Treatment

There are many ways of treating plantar warts. All involve destroying the warts. So far, we don't have a perfect treatment for plantar warts. I prefer to treat plantar warts by destroying them chemically. This treatment is painless and will let you engage in your usual activities. It usually succeeds if carried out according to instructions. It will take several weeks or months.

You will be given a prescription that is to be used as follows:

1. At bedtime, put a tiny amount of wart-destroying medicine exactly on your warts with _____. Put the medicine only on the warts; it may irritate normal skin.
2. If the wart-destroying medicine is a liquid, let it dry for 5 minutes so it won't spread to normal skin when covered with tape.
3. Cover your warts with waterproof adhesive tape. The tape keeps your skin moist. The moisture softens the surface of the warts so the medicine will penetrate them. It's all right to get the tape wet.
4. In the morning, remove the adhesive tape. If your skin tears when you do this, loosen the tape by painting nail-polish remover between your skin and the tape with a cotton-tipped applicator.
5. After a few days, the outside of the warts will start to turn gray. This means the chemical has begun to destroy them. Scrape this gray wart tissue off with the point of a metal nail file every second or third day. Do the scraping after a bath or shower has softened the wart's surface. Be sure to remove *every bit* of dead wart tissue; otherwise, it will keep the wart-destroying medicine from reaching the living tissue underneath. Sometimes, a small, curved scissors or a pumice stone helps in removing the dead wart tissue. Whatever you use for scraping your warts should not be used for anything else, because warts are somewhat contagious.
6. If the warts become sore, stop the treatment for a few days.
7. If you don't see much progress after 2 to 3 weeks, try leaving the tape on until noon, or even longer. Stubborn warts may need to be covered continuously with tape.
8. If your plantar warts hurt when you stand or walk, wear a pad cut out of Dr. Scholl's Foot and Shoe Padding (available without prescription). Cut a hole or holes corresponding to where the warts are. This will take the pressure off the warts.
9. Continue the treatment until you believe the warts are gone. If you can

see the lines of your skin crossing the treated area, the warts are probably gone. If it turns out that after you stop treatment the warts are still there—it happens—start treating them again until you feel more certain that the warts have gone away.

10. If necessary, continue the treatment for 4 months. If the warts have not been destroyed after 4 months of treatment, return; a different approach will be used.

11. If the warts become painful or infected, return at once.

Chemical Destruction of Warts

Chemical destruction of warts is a painless alternative to office surgery. Chemical destruction is also used when there are many warts and surgical removal is not practical.

You will put a medicine on your wart at bedtime, then cover it with tape. The tape covering holds the medicine in place and helps it penetrate the wart. The medicine gradually eats the wart away. Dead wart tissue builds up on the surface; you *must* scrape it off. Continue the treatment until all traces of the wart have been destroyed. This usually takes 1 to 3 months.

Follow these steps for treating your warts:

1. At bedtime, put a tiny amount of wart-destroying medicine exactly on your wart with _____. Put the medicine *only on the wart* as it will irritate normal skin.
2. If the wart-destroying medicine is a liquid, let it dry for 5 minutes so it will not spread to normal skin when covered with tape.
3. After applying the medicine, cover the wart with waterproof adhesive tape. The tape keeps your skin moist. The moisture softens the surface of the wart so the medicine will penetrate more deeply. It's all right to get the tape wet.
4. In the morning, take off the adhesive tape. If your skin starts to tear when you remove the tape, loosen the tape by painting nail-polish remover (use a cotton-tipped applicator) between your skin and the tape.
5. After a few days, the outside of the wart will start to turn gray. That means the chemical has begun to destroy the wart. Scrape this gray wart tissue off with the point of a metal nail file every second or third day. Do the scraping after a bath or shower has softened the wart's surface. Be sure to remove *every bit* of dead wart tissue; otherwise, it will keep the wart-destroying medicine from reaching the living tissue underneath. Sometimes, a small, curved scissors or a pumice stone helps in removing the dead tissue. Whatever you use for scraping your wart should not be used for anything else, because warts are somewhat contagious.
6. If the wart becomes sore, stop the treatment for a few days.
7. If you do not see much progress after 2 to 3 weeks, try leaving the tape on until noon, or even longer. Stubborn warts may need to be covered continuously with tape.
8. Continue the treatment until you believe the wart is gone. If it turns out that the wart is still there after you stop treatment, start treating it again until you feel more certain it has gone away.
9. If after 3 months, the wart hasn't been destroyed, please return for re-evaluation.

Long-Term Tetracycline Treatment

Long-term treatment with tetracycline is remarkably safe; we have had over 30 years experience with tetracycline. The aim of long-term treatment with tetracycline is to take the smallest number of pills that will control your skin problem. You will need to find that smallest amount by *gradually* decreasing your tetracycline dose. Remember to decrease your tetracycline gradually, since tetracycline has a lag time of 2 to 3 weeks between taking the medicine and its effect on the skin. Allow at least 4 to 6 weeks between each reduction in dose. Keep reducing your dosage until you start to break out—then continue taking the smallest dose that previously controlled your eruption.

Dosage Reduction Schedule

Please use the following schedule to determine the smallest dose of tetracycline you need to control your skin problem:

1. On _____, reduce your tetracycline pills to _____ pills on arising and _____ pills in the evening.
2. If your eruption is well controlled on __ pills a day, on _____, reduce to __ pills on arising and __ pills in the evening.
3. If __ pills a day keeps your eruption under good control, on _____ decrease your daily dose by one pill.
4. When you are down to one pill a day, try reducing your dosage to one pill every other day. Then, if one pill every other day is enough, try stopping tetracycline, as you may not need it anymore.

It is important to keep on reducing your dosage gradually until you start to break out—then continue taking the smallest dose that previously controlled your eruption.

What if your skin problem gets worse after many months of being controlled on low daily doses of tetracycline? This is not uncommon and means you should boost your tetracycline intake back to the full dose used initially. Usually, this will control your outbreak in 6 to 8 weeks, and then you may again gradually decrease your dose. The amount of tetracycline needed to control your skin may vary, and it is perfectly all right to adjust your dose, providing you (1) Do not exceed the original full dose, (2) decrease the tetracycline dose *gradually,* and (3) record the changes on your calendar.

If a flare-up of your skin problem does *not* respond after 6 to 8 weeks of full-dose tetracycline, please return to this office for re-evaluation and a change in your treatment.